PHARMACOLOGY - RESEARCH, SAFETY TESTING AND REGULATION

ACETAMINOPHEN

PROPERTIES, CLINICAL USES AND ADVERSE EFFECTS

PHARMACOLOGY - RESEARCH, SAFETY TESTING AND REGULATION

Additional books in this series can be found on Nova's website
under the Series tab.

Additional E-books in this series can be found on Nova's website
under the E-book tab.

PUBLIC HEALTH IN THE 21ST CENTURY

Additional books in this series can be found on Nova's website
under the Series tab.

Additional E-books in this series can be found on Nova's website
under the E-book tab.

PHARMACOLOGY - RESEARCH, SAFETY TESTING AND REGULATION

ACETAMINOPHEN

PROPERTIES, CLINICAL USES AND ADVERSE EFFECTS

ATASH JAVAHERIAN
AND
PASHA LATIFPOUR
EDITORS

Nova Science Publishers, Inc.
New York

For permission to use material from this book please contact us:
Telephone 631-231-7269; Fax 631-231-8175
Web Site: http://www.novapublishers.com

LIBRARY OF CONGRESS CATALOGING-IN-PUBLICATION DATA

ISBN: 978-1-61942-374-9

Published by Nova Science Publishers, Inc. † New York

CONTENTS

PREFACE

This book presents current research in the study of the properties, clinical uses and adverse effects of acetaminophen. Topics discussed include advanced methods for the removal of acetaminophen from the water supply; acetaminophen overdose, biomarkers and management; acetaminophen hepatotoxicity and potential interactions with dietary supplements; sesame oil and sesamol for treating acetaminophen-overdose-associated liver injuries and paracetamol use in the elderly.

Chapter 1 - Acetaminophen (paracetemol) is a non-opioid analgesic and antipyretic widely used for a large variety of mild to moderate pain conditions in a large variety of patient populations. In addition to over-the-counter oral and rectal formulations, there is a more-recently approved intravenous formulation. Some of the common uses of acetaminophen include the pain associated with headaches, muscle aches, menstrual periods, colds and sore throats, toothaches, backaches, osteoarthritis, and the reduction of fever. In addition to its use as a single agent, acetaminophen is also commonly used in fixed-ratio combinations with other analgesics in order to enhance pharmacokinetic or pharmacodynamic characteristics. In some cases the combination can result in a synergistic analgesic effect. The exact mechanism responsible for acetaminophen's analgesic effect is not known despite its long history of use, but it appears to involve actions on both the central and peripheral nervous systems. The safety profile of acetaminophen is considered to be very good and most side effects are mild and transient at recommended doses. However, severe hepatic toxicity has been associated with prolonged exposure, in combination with alcohol, or in cases of intentional or accidental overdose. Accidental overdose is a particular current concern because of the prevalence of acetaminophen in multiple over-the-counter products and the cumulative effect of inadvertent ingestion of an excess amount in aggregate. Overall, when used safely and properly, acetaminophen is a very good mild to moderate pain reliever for the general consumer and postoperative patient. It is particularly useful in situations where a nonopioid analgesic with good GI tolerability is desirable.

Chapter 2 - Acetaminophen (APAP) overdose frequently results in the development of severe liver injury in both humans and experimental animals. In humans, APAP-induced hepatotoxicity is currently the main cause of acute liver failure in the Western world. APAP-induced hepatotoxicity in the mouse is an extensively used experimental paradigm for dissecting the mechanisms of drug-induced liver injury. Even though a decrease of body temperature is a well-known effect of APAP, body temperature has rarely been measured in experimental studies of APAP-hepatotoxicity. Importantly, active maintenance of body temperature by external warming has been shown to decrease survival and to worsen the development of liver injury in the mouse with APAP-hepatotoxicity, suggesting that body temperature should be carefully monitored in order to adequately interpret results from this model. Induction of mild hypothermia is a potentially effective therapeutic approach for controlling episodes of intracranial hypertension in patients with APAP-induced acute liver failure.

Chapter 3 - Acetaminophen (N-Acetyl-4-aminophenol), also known as APAP or paracetamol, is one of the most widely used analgesics (pain reliever) and antipyretics (fever reducer). According to the U.S. Food and Drug Administration (FDA), currently there are 221 approved prescription and over-the-counter drug products containing acetaminophen as an active ingredient. When used as directed, acetaminophen is very safe and effective; however when taken in excess or ingested with alcohol hepatotoxicity and irreversible liver damage can arise. In addition to well-known clinical application as pain relief and fever reduction, recent laboratory and pre-clinical studies have demonstrated that acetaminophen may also have beneficial effects on blood glucose control, skeletal muscle function, and potential use as cardioprotective and neuroprotective agents. Extensive laboratory and pre-clinical studies have revealed that these off-label applications may be derived from the ability of acetaminophen to function as an antioxidant. Using our recent work as a reference point, herein, we will highlight these novel applications of acetaminophen, and attempt, where possible, to highlight how these findings may lead to new directions of inquiry and clinical relevance of other disorders.

Chapter 4 - During the last decades, the scientific community has become increasingly concerned about the potential public health impact of new environmental contaminants originating from industrial, agricultural and human activities. These compounds, known as emergent pollutants, include prescription and non-prescription human and veterinary pharmaceutical compounds, personal care products, household chemicals, pesticides, fertilizers and so forth. Among them, the occurrence of pharmaceuticals in water represents an outstanding environmental issue due to their therapeutic and/or biological activity, even at trace levels. The development of analytical techniques with low detection limits and high sensibility has enabled undertaking ambient monitoring studies to control the occurrence and fate of these emergent pollutants. Acetaminophen, a non-prescription analgesic widely consumed worldwide, is among the six pharmaceutical ingredients most often detected in drinking water. This is a direct consequence of the low efficiency of conventional water treatment processes for the removal/degradation of these compounds, along with their continuous discharge in the environment. To overcome the emergent environmental challenge associated with the occurrence and persistence of pharmaceuticals in water and wastewater, novel advanced water treatment techniques are currently being extensively investigated. In this chapter, a comprehensive review of recent advances on the development of new strategies to improve the water quality is made; special emphasis is paid to methods based on adsorption and degradation processes including adsorption, photo- and electro-assisted degradation techniques, etc.

Chapter 5 - Acetaminophen is manufactured in huge quantities worldwide. Approximately 3.2 thousand million tablets of acetaminophen are consumed by the public every year in the UK (mean of 55 tablets/person). Acetaminophen poisoning accounts for up to 48% of all poisons admissions to hospital. It is a weak inhibitor of COX-1 and COX-2 in peripheral tissues and possesses no significant anti-inflamatory effects. The oral dose of acetaminophen is 0.5-1g per 4-6 h to a maximum of 4 g in a day. Approximately 95% of acetaminophen is metabolised to glucuronide and sulphate conjugates which are excreted in the urine. About 5% of acetaminophen is metabolised through the cytochrome P-450 2E1 to produce a highly reactive toxic metabolite, N-acetyl-p-benzoquinonimine (NAPQI). At therapeutic doses, the small amounts of NAPQI produced by acetaminophen metabolism are detoxified by liver stores of hepatic glutathione and is excreted in bile or urine as mercapturic acid conjugate. In overdose, stores of glutathione become depleted. Without the glutathione substrate, NAPQI becomes available to bind to proteins and DNA of hepatocytes causing direct cellular injury. Generation of reactive oxygen species and nitric oxide, lipid peroxidation, mitochondrial dysfunction, disruption of calcium homeostasis and induction of apoptosis are all mechanisms have suggested that may be involved in acetaminophen-induced hepatotoxicity. Severe liver damage has been defined as an increase in plasma activities of aspartate aminotransferase (AST), alanine aminotransferase (ALT), sorbitol dehydrogenase (SDH), ornithine carbamyltransferase (OCT), lactic dehydrogenase (LDH), hydroxybutyrate dehydrogenase (HBDH), glutathione S-transferases, and F-protein. Increase in prothrombin time, plasma concentrations of creatinine, biliverdin, bilirubin, and phosphate, and reduction in blood pH, bicarbonate, and glucose have also been demonstrated as biomarkers of acetaminophen overdose. We recently showed an increase in plasma concentration of taurine as a probable biomarker of acetaminophen poisoning. Different antidotes such as: cimetidine, cysteamine, methionine, and glycyrrhizin have already used for the treatment of acetaminophen overdose. However, N-acetylcysteine (NAC) is a clinically approved drug which is used with three treatment regimens: a 20-hour continuous infusion of NAC, a 48-hour regimen of intermittent intravenous infusions and a 72-hour regimen of intermittent oral doses. NAC should be given if the plasma acetaminophen concentration is above a line joining 200mg/L (1.32mmol/L) at four hours after ingestion and 30mg/L (0.20mmol/L) at 15 hours on a semilogarithmic plot. Few adverse reactions have been reported in 5% of patients who receive NAC particularly in intravenous forms. The most of these reactions are anaphylactoid such as flushing, pruritus, urticaria, angioedema, cough, headache, shortness of breath, wheezing, hypotension, status epilepticus, and cortical blindness.

Chapter 6 - Acetaminophen (APAP) is the leading cause of drug-induced acute liver failure in the United States. At normal therapeutic doses, APAP is a safe drug when used by itself. Problems arise when multiple products containing APAP are used and the therapeutic dose is exceeded. A recent US FDA Advisory Committee concluded that other factors such as ethnicity, genetics, and nutrition may also play a role in a person's susceptibility to APAP-induced liver injury. One nutrition factor that is likely to play a role is dietary supplements. Dietary supplement use continues to rise and many consumers consider these products as inherently safe by themselves or in combination with other products, including drugs, since they are "natural". However, the safety of most dietary supplements by themselves has not been adequately tested and even less data are available on potential drug – dietary supplement interactions. APAP is metabolized by the liver to a reactive metabolite, NAPQI, that causes a wide array of cellular effects such as depletion of cytoprotective molecules, covalent binding to cellular macromolecules, oxidative stress, and impaired mitochondrial function. Dietary supplements that increase the metabolism of APAP are likely to increase the hepatotoxicity of APAP; whereas, those that decrease APAP metabolism are likely to provide protection. Dietary supplements that affect endpoints downstream of APAP metabolism could also either reduce or increase APAP hepatotoxicity depending on the magnitude and direction of the effect. This chapter reviews the key areas of potential interaction between APAP and dietary supplements and reviews the available data on specific dietary supplements.

Chapter 7 - Acetaminophen is an analgesic and antipyretic. It is safe when taken as directed but can cause extreme harm and even death in amounts above recommended doses. N-acetylcysteine is the standard clinical antidote for treating overdoses of acetaminophen. However, the optimal dose, route, and duration of N-acetylcysteine therapy remain unknown despite more than 30 years of experience with this antidote. The search for a novel and effective antidote for acetaminophen overdose continues. Sesame oil has been widely used in Chinese and Indian herbal medicine. Sesame oil and its lignan sesamol have been proved effective for treating various drug-induced and chemically induced liver injuries. Sesame oil and sesamol not only maintain glutathione levels but also reduce mitochondrial oxidative stress by inhibiting the generation of reactive oxygen species during acetaminophen intoxication. Sesame oil and sesamol's multi-beneficial actions may be useful for treating acetaminophen-overdose-associated liver injuries.

Chapter 8 - Paracetamol is an effective agent for pain relief and is generally regarded as a safe medication at therapeutic doses. It is widely used in elderly patients with recommendations that are common to those for adults. Recent reports have however questioned the safety of recommended doses and suggest that the elderly patient might be at an increased risk of developing adverse events when on paracetamol treatment. Glutathione depletion, polymedication including CYP450 inducing drugs and anticoagulant therapy, increased incidence of organ insufficiency with age, malnutrition, dehydration, fragility are factors that may favour the development of serious adverse events. While the benefit/risk ratio of paracetamol is evident in clinical practise, clinicians should be aware of the potential and preventable adverse side-effects of this centenarian pain treatment favourite analgesic.

In: Acetaminophen: Properties, Clinical Uses
Editors: Atash Javaherian and Pasha Latifpour
ISBN: 978-1-61942-374-9

Chapter 1

ACETAMINOPHEN (PARACETAMOL): PROPERTIES, CLINICAL USES, AND ADVERSE EFFECTS

***Robert Taylor Jr.*[1]*, Joseph V. Pergolizzi Jr.*[2] *and Robert B. Raffa*[3]**
[1]NEMA Research, Naples, FL, US
[2]Department of Medicine, Johns Hopkins University, Baltimore, MD, US;
Department of Anesthesiology, Georgetown University School of Medicine, Washington, DC, US,
and Department of Pharmacology, Temple University School of Medicine, Philadelphia, PA, US
[3]Department of Pharmaceutical Sciences,
Temple University School of Pharmacy, Philadelphia, PA, US

ABSTRACT

Acetaminophen (paracetemol) is a non-opioid analgesic and antipyretic widely used for a large variety of mild to moderate pain conditions in a large variety of patient populations. In addition to over-the-counter oral and rectal formulations, there is a more-recently approved intravenous formulation. Some of the common uses of acetaminophen include the pain associated with headaches, muscle aches, menstrual periods, colds and sore throats, toothaches, backaches, osteoarthritis, and the reduction of fever. In addition to its use as a single agent, acetaminophen is also commonly used in fixed-ratio combinations with other analgesics in order to enhance pharmacokinetic or pharmacodynamic characteristics. In some cases the combination can result in a synergistic analgesic effect. The exact mechanism responsible for acetaminophen's analgesic effect is not known despite its long history of use, but it appears to involve actions on both the central and peripheral nervous systems. The safety profile of acetaminophen is considered to be very good and most side effects are mild and transient at recommended doses. However, severe hepatic toxicity has been associated with prolonged exposure, in combination with alcohol, or in cases of intentional or accidental overdose. Accidental overdose is a particular current concern because of the prevalence of acetaminophen in multiple over-the-counter products and the cumulative effect of inadvertent ingestion of an excess amount in aggregate. Overall, when used safely and properly, acetaminophen is a very good mild to moderate pain reliever for the general consumer and postoperative patient. It is particularly useful in situations where a nonopioid analgesic with good GI tolerability is desirable.

Keywords: Acetaminophen, paracetamol, analgesia, non-opioid analgesic, overview

1. INTRODUCTION

The purpose of this chapter is to give a broad overview of the properties, clinical uses, and adverse effects of acetaminophen (*N*-(4-Hydroxyphenyl)ethanamide or *N*-(4-Hydroxyphenyl)acetamide), also called paracetamol (*para*-Acetylaminophenol) or APAP (*N*-Acetyl-*para*-aminophenol), and to direct the reader to the relevant primary literature.

Acetaminophen is a synthetic nonopioid analgesic and antipyretic. Because it is not significantly anti-inflammatory, it is not an NSAID (nonsteroidal anti-inflammatory drug), although in general its analgesic and antipyretic efficacy are equivalent to those of NSAIDs.

Acetaminophen has a relatively long history. Acetanilide (*N* –Phenylacetamide) was serendipitously discovered to have antipyretic properties in the latter half of the 1800s and it was marketed under the name Antifebrin. However, concerns over toxicity prompted a search for a safer alternative. An aniline derivative of acetanilide, phenacetin (*N*-(4-Ethoxyphenyl) acetamide), was selected and marketed, but it also had unacceptable toxicity. It was subsequently discovered that the toxicity of acetanilide and phenacetin were attributable to a metabolite and that analgesic and antipyretic actions were retained in a different, but common, metabolite – acetaminophen. Acetaminophen was reintroduced in 1955 under the brand name Tylenol™ and in 1956 as Panadol™. It is currently one of the most commonly- and widely-used nonopioid analgesics worldwide.

2. PROPERTIES

2.1. Chemistry

The chemical structure of acetaminophen is shown in Figure 1 where it is used to illustrate its various components as described at http://en.wikipedia.org/wiki/Paracetamol (1). Acetaminophen has a core aromatic (benzene) ring substituted in *para* orientation by two groups: a hydroxyl and an acetamide (ethanamide). Multiple portions of the molecule are conjugated, including the benzene ring, the hydroxyl oxygen, the amide nitrogen, and the carbonyl carbon and oxygen. As a result, the benzene ring is highly reactive toward electrophilic aromatic substitution (all positions being about equally activated), both oxygens and the nitrogen much less basic, and the hydroxyl acidic.

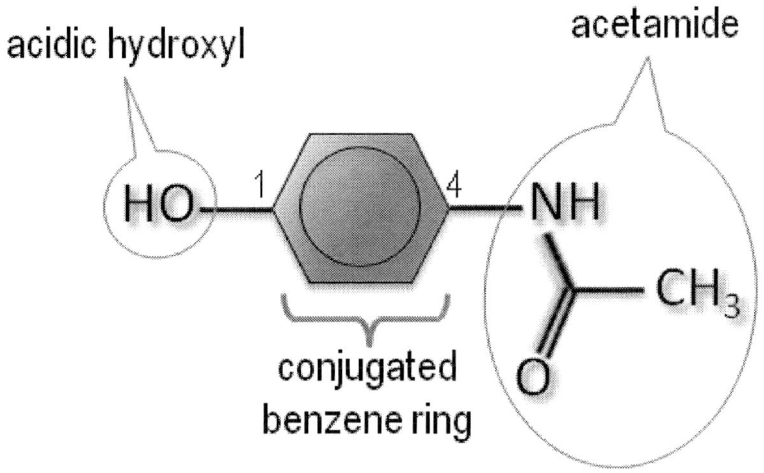

Figure 1. Chemical structure of acetaminophen (paracetamol)(N-(4-Hydroxyphenyl)ethanamide or N-(4-Hydroxyphenyl)acetamide or N-Acertyl-para-aminophenol), highlighting active components.

2.2. Pharmacokinetics

2.2.1. Absorption

2.2.1.1. Immediate Release

Rapid absorption of orally administered acetaminophen primarily occurs through the small intestine of the gastrointestinal tract, with minimal uptake by the stomach (2, 3). This absorption route allows acetaminophen to achieve a relative bioavailability of 85% to 98% (4). Studies have shown for individual adults administered a 1000 mg dose that maximum acetaminophen plasma concentrations of 7.7 to 17.6 μg/mL occur within the first hour and can reach a steady-state range from 7.9 to 27 μg/mL while administered 1000 mg every 6 hours (5).

2.2.1.2. Extended Release

Current extended-release caplet or gelcap formulations of acetaminophen consist of 650 mg total dose. The outer layer releases 325 mg of acetaminophen immediately upon entering the stomach, following which the absorption rate and bioavailability is similar to that of immediate-release formulations. The other 325 mg is released slowly from a specialized matrix located within the caplet or gelcap. Studies conducted on these formulations have shown release of up to 88% and 95% of acetaminophen within 3 and 5 hours (6). Maximum plasma concentrations in adults range from 6.9 to 14.1 μg/mL and occur within 0.5 to 3 hours.

2.2.1.3. Intravenous

Compared to oral acetaminophen, IV acetaminophen has a similar AUC (38 - 43 μg*h/mL), but a greater (~70%) Cmax value (IV mean 28 - 31 μg/mL). In general, the pharmacokinetic parameters (AUC, $t_{1/2}$) for IV administration are similar for adults, adolescents and children (> 2 years of age), but they are higher in infants and neonates (7).

2.2.2. Distribution

Plasma protein binding of acetaminophen is relatively low (10 - 25%) and distributes widely throughout the body with a volume of distribution of 0.7 - 1.0 L/kg in both adults and children (8-11). Acetaminophen metabolites do not bind to plasma proteins (12).

2.2.2.1. Spinal Fluid

Due to its low protein binding and low molecular weight, acetaminophen readily passes through the blood-brain barrier and achieves a maximum concentration in cerebrospinal fluid within 2 to 4 hours (13-15)

2.2.2.2. Placental Barrier

Acetaminophen has been shown to be safe when administered during pregnancy or labor when given at therapeutic doses. Passage into the fetal circulation through the placenta can occurs within 30 minutes of ingestion by the mother (16). Following delivery, serum concentrations in the mother and fetus are similar (5.925 +/- 2.15 mg/mL and 7.875 +/- 2.22 mg/mL, respectively)(16).

2.2.2.3. Breast Milk

Maternal ingestion of therapeutic doses of acetaminophen during periods of breast-feeding does not pose a risk for the nursing infant (17). Multiple studies have documented minimal concentrations of acetaminophen in breast milk, with a peak concentration representing less than 2% of the ingested dose by the mother (range 0.1% to 1.85%) (18-20).

2.2.3. Metabolism

Metabolism of acetaminophen can occur by three main pathways, all of which primarily take place in the liver. These pathways consist of conjugation with glucuronide; conjugation with sulfate; and oxidation via the cytochrome P450 (CYP450) enzyme pathway. In addition, acetaminophen can undergo hydroxylation to form 3-hydroxy-acetaminophen and methoxylation to form 3-methoxy-acetaminophen, which may be further conjugated to glucuronide or sulfate (21, 22).

The major CYP450 isoenzyme involved in the oxidation of acetaminophen is CYP2E1, with CYP1A2 and CYP3A4 having minimal contribution (23, 24). The main reactive metabolite of the oxidation process, *N*-acetyl-*p*-benzoquinone imine (NAPQI), is hepatoxic, but is normally rapidly converted to an inert cysteine and/or mercapturic acid metabolite by conjugation with glutathione (25). However, buildup of the toxic metabolite can occur if this pathway is saturated or glutathione stores are depleted for any reason. The consequence is serious hepatic toxicity, possibly resulting in liver failure.

2.2.4. Elimination

The elimination half-lives are similar with age (>2 years), but may vary slightly with different ethnic and medical backgrounds. The elimination $t_{1/2}$ for healthy adults (25, 26) is approximately 2 to 3 hours and about 1.5 to 3 hours in children. In neonates (4), cirrhotic patients (27-29), and in some ethnic groups (viz., Nigerians, Hong Kong, Chinese) (30, 31) the half life is roughly 4 hours. Acetaminophen is primarily excreted in the urine, with a majority eliminated in the glucuronide form (40 - 65%), sulfate form (25 - 35%), and as unchanged acetaminophen (3.5%) (32, 33)

2.2.5. Fetus, Neonates, Infants, and Children

Use of acetaminophen in this patient population is considered to be safe and efficacious when administered at recommended dosages. Just as in adolescents and adults, there is a risk of hepatoxicity and proper precautions need to be taken. Pharmacokinetic parameters for children more than 2 years of age and adults are similar, but vary with decreasing age from < 2 years to newborns.

Oxidation of acetaminophen to the reactive hepatoxic metabolite is approximately ten-times slower in the fetal liver than adult and increases with fetal age. Fetal livers primarily use sulfate conjugation to detoxify acetaminophen and not glucuronic acid (34). Though the fetus is able to detoxify acetaminophen, the generation of the hepatotoxic metabolite still is a risk if mothers are exposed to an excess amount (34).

2.2.6. Geriatric

Administration of acetaminophen does not require special dosage adjustment in the elderly. It is the preferred analgesic by the American Geriatrics Society as the first line treatment for mild to moderate musculoskeletal pain (35). Characterization of single or multiple doses of acetaminophen has been well documented in the elderly and studies have shown that the pharmacokinetics is similar to adults (36-42). Many of these studies have documented similar elimination half lives and clearance times for the glucuronide and glutathione metabolites. However, the formation clearance of the sulfate conjugates are reduced (36), and frail elderly might have a slight increase in elimination half live (38). Overall, acetaminophen is generally considered a safe and tolerable analgesic in the elderly, with the precautions indicated.

3. Clinical Uses

3.1. Antipyresis

Acetaminophen has been tested in multiple clinical trials in adults and children for its role in reducing body temperature. Many studies have documented acetaminophen to be superior to placebo and non-pharmacologic methods (sponging) in adults (43-46) and children (47-49). Its antipyretic efficacy is equivalent to aspirin or ibuprofen (50-57). In many of these studies, acetaminophen's therapeutic effect was evident within 30 - 60 minutes of initial administration and peaked at 2 - 3 hours.

The exact antipyretic mechanism of action of acetaminophen is still unclear, but it has been shown to block the formation and release of prostaglandins in the CNS in addition to inhibiting the endogenous pyrogens within the brain's thermoregulatory regions (58-60). A rise of prostaglandin E (PGE) in cerebrospinal fluid has been linked to an increased production of endogenous pyrogens by leukocytes (61). Excessive PGE impedes heat loss and increases heat gain, generating a fever.

3.2. Analgesia

Many pain models and clinical trials have documented acetaminophen's efficacy for conditions associated with mild to moderate pain. Clinical studies have documented successful pain reduction with acetaminophen use after dental, gynecologic, or orthopedic surgery (62-64), in addition to post-episiotomy pain (65, 66) and pain associated with tonsillectomy and sore throat (45, 67-71). Guidelines set forth by the European League Against Rheumatism (72-74), and the American Pain Society (75) recommend acetaminophen for Arthritis Pain (osteoarthritis of knee, hip, hand) based on multiple studies testing its safety and efficacy in this patient population (4, 76-82). Similar recommendations have been put forth by the National Headache Foundation (83) based on acetaminophen's effectiveness in relieving headache tension and pain (84-90). Other uses include relieving cyclic perimenstrual pain and discomfort (91), pain associated with fractures, acute musculoskeletal and soft-tissue injuries (4), and low back pain (4, 92).

Acetaminophen's mechanism of analgesic action is not known with certainty. It appears to act in the CNS (both the brain and spinal cord) and in the periphery. Multiple hypotheses have been proposed. Some of these have been discounted, others remain a possibility, but to date no hypothesis is backed by sufficient evidence to be considered definitive. In fact, no single mechanism has been able to describe all of acetaminophen's actions sufficiently and it seems reasonable to infer that acetaminophen likely interacts with a variety of physiological pathways and produces its analgesic effect by a combination of such actions. A recent comprehensive review details the major mechanisms that have been proposed to account for the analgesic action of acetaminophen (93). A partial list of proposed mechanisms can be summarized as follows: (94, 95).

- *Inhibition of cyclooxygenase (EC 1.14.99.1, COX).* Acetaminophen has periodically been proposed to inhibit one or more of the cyclooxygenase (prostaglandin synthase, PGHS) isozymes involved in the conversion of arachidonic acid to prostanoids and other chemical mediators of inflammation, fever, pain, platelet aggregation, and mucous production in the gastrointestinal tract. Acetaminophen's lack of the strong anti-inflammatory and antiplatelet effects displayed by conventional COX inhibitors such as the NSAIDs argues against this mechanism, but counter-explanations have been forwarded, for example that acetaminophen might be more potent as a COX inhibitor in the CNS than in the periphery. The antinociceptive (analgesic) activity of acetaminophen is attenuated in COX-1 knockout, but not in COX-2 knockout, mice, suggesting that acetaminophen requires COX-1 but not COX-2 to produce its full analgesic effect. A recent study reports that acetaminophen inhibits COX-2 to a comparable extent as NSAIDs and COX-2 inhibitors. However, the connection of COX-2 inhibition to acetaminophen's analgesic action has not been established. Because COX-3 is a variant of COX-1, most of the same evidence that supports a COX-1 mechanism of action for acetaminophen also supports a COX-3 mechanism. However, COX-3 does not mediate acetaminophen's antinociception in rats and it does not seem to be present in humans. For these and other reasons it seems unlikely that COX-3 has clinical relevance for acetaminophen's mechanism of analgesic action.

- *Peroxidase.* It has been proposed that acetaminophen might inhibit COX enzymes indirectly. Specifically, that acetaminophen might disrupt the tyrosyl radical step of the COX pathway. Another mechanism might be decreasing peroxide tone by scavenging or otherwise reducing free peroxides. This hypothesis is supported by evidence that suggests that acetaminophen may inhibit mild to moderate peroxide stimulation, but not higher amounts or all types of peroxides present in inflammatory responses.
- *Nitric Oxide Synthase.* Nitric oxide (NO) amplifies neuronal activity and facilitates nociception; inhibition of NO synthesis attenuates nociception. It has been suggested that acetaminophen might inhibit NO synthesis. Although acetaminophen has been reported to lack direct inhibitory effect on NO synthesis *in vitro* (96), perhaps the effect is indirect.
- *Cannabinoid.* Endogenous cannabinoid (marihuana-like) substances are involved in – and exogenous cannabinoid substances can modulate – various physiological processes, including pain, and the endocannabinoid system has been proposed to be involved in the mechanism of analgesic action of acetaminophen. Although acetaminophen does not have significant affinity for cannabinoid receptors (97), one of its metabolites displays cannabinoid-like activity, so acetaminophen might activate the endocannabinoid system by acting as a pro-drug. However, this proposal is still speculative in regards acetaminophen's clinical analgesic effect.
- *5-HT (5-hydroxytryptamine, serotonin).* There is evidence that acetaminophen's mechanism of analgesia involves descending serotonergic pathways that exert an inhibitory (analgesic) effect. Acetaminophen does not have affinity for 5-HT receptors or neuronal 5-HT reuptake sites (97), but it might work on 5-HT systems by an indirect mechanism. Two studies in human volunteers lend support to the idea that acetaminophen might produce its analgesia through a 5-HT-related mechanism. Both studies found that the analgesic effect of acetaminophen in a clinical setting was significantly reduced by 5-HT receptor antagonists.
- *Self-Synergism.* When acetaminophen is administered into the brain and spinal cord in close time proximity, synergistic antinociception is produced and this property of acetaminophen has been dubbed analgesic "self-synergy" (98). An opioid receptor antagonist administered by spinal injection attenuates this synergism, suggesting that perhaps the endogenous opioid system is somehow involved. Further study is needed to determine any clinical relevance of this finding.

4. Special Populations

4.1. Chronic Liver Disease

It has been theorized that the increased activity of CYP450 or reduction in glutathione stores that have been associated with some patients with chronic liver disease may increase the hepatoxic risk of acetaminophen. However, many patients with various types of chronic liver disease (e.g., acute viral hepatitis, cirrhosis, fatty liver) have normal to reduced CYP450 activity and increased levels of glutathione (99-103). Pharmacokinetic studies using single and multiple doses of acetaminophen have shown that the elimination half life is slower (1 to 2 hour increase) in patients with diseased livers (104-108), but the excretion percentage of various metabolites in urine is not affected (27-29). Overall, there has been minimal evidence to support an increased risk of hepatotoxicity in this patient population when acetaminophen is taken as recommended and due to its less effect on platelets, the gastrointestinal tract, or the kidney, acetaminophen is recommended over NSAIDs in this patient population (109)

4.2. Renal Disease

Clinical research suggets no significant concern that acetaminophen is nephrotoxic when used at the recommended doses (110). Urinary retention studies for acetaminophen and its metabolites in combination with renal functional tests have not shown significant differences between healthy and renal-deficient patients (111, 112). Acetaminophen has been recommended by the National Kidney Foundation as an appropriate analgesic for patients with renal disease, especially in patients who are at higher risk for hemorrhaging (113).

4.3. Calorie Restricted Patients

Some healthcare providers believe that patients who are fasting or on a calorie-restricted diet may be at an increased risk for acetaminophen hepatotoxicity. Caloric restriction or during times of malnutrition, the metabolic process of glucuronidation may be hindered, thus causing acetaminophen to pass through the CYP2E1 pathway more readily and result in an increase in the hepatoxic metabolite NAPQI289. In addition, caloric restriction may reduce the glutathione reservoir, the necessary component to inactivating NAPQI289 (114). However, we are unaware of a definitive study identifying caloric restriction as a risk factor for acetaminophen hepatoxicity when administered at the recommended doses (115).

4.4. HIV

The glutathione reservoir in patients infected with human immunodeficiency virus have been known to decrease with the progression of the disease and that drugs which may also deplete glutathione are not recommended (116), raising the concern that acetaminophen may deplete glutathione levels and effect the long-term survival of HIV patients.

4.5. Gilbert's Syndrome

Individuals with Gilbert's syndrome have a polymorphic defect in UDP-glucuronosyltransferase isozyme UGT1A1 (117), raising a concern that acetaminophen would predominately undergo metabolism through the CYP450 pathway in these individuals. However, glucuronidation of acetaminophen is mainly by UDP-glucuronosyltransferase isozymes UGT1A6 and UGT1A9 (118, 119) and acetaminophen metabolism by glucuronidation or glutathione conjugation has been shown to be unaffected in adults with Gilbert's syndrome (120-123).

5. ADVERSE EVENTS

5.1. Allergy and Hypersensitivity

Cases of allergic reactions and hypersensitivity to acetaminophen administration are rare and can be relieved by discontinuation. If allergic reactions take place, they normally take the form of a rash, and/or urticaria, while hypersensitivity reactions can include anaphylactic shock (124, 125).

5.2. Central Nervous System

Central Nervous System side effects, including mood changes, anxiety, dizzyness, sleep disturbance, or cognitive decline has not been documented in patients receiving therapeutic doses or greater than the recommended dose (2000 mg/70 kg) of acetaminophen. Reports of coma or other CNS side effects have been reported after ingestion of large amounts of acetaminophen alone or in combination with other CNS acting agents (126, 127).

5.3. Gastrointestinal

Current recommended doses of acetaminophen (max 4000 mg/day) for adults have been shown to have minimal effects on the gastrointestinal system (e.g., gastric irritation, gastric erosions, occult or overt gastrointestinal blood loss, or ulcers) (128, 129). When compared to other analgesics, acetaminophen has been reported to be superior to NSAIDs (130-132) or aspirin (129, 133, 134) in this regard.

5.4. Hemotologic and Hemostatic

Sporadic case reports (135-142) and alerts by a few physicians (143-148) have appeared in the literature regarding possible negative effects of acetaminophen on hemotology (e.g., agranulocytosis or thrombocytopenia), but they are not conclusive and clinical-trial data have not supported such claims (149). Acetaminophen has not been documented to present immediate or delayed hemostatic effects based on bleeding time or platelet aggregation studies and thus is considered to be safe for use in hemophiliacs (150-153).

5.5. Hepatic Toxicity

Use of acetaminophen has been associated with altering liver homeostasis and promoting liver dysfunction. Hepatotoxicity has been documented to occur primarily under conditions of overdose (7500 mg - 10,000 mg in < 8 hours). When taken as directed, hepatic dysfunction has not been reported in participants taking daily-recommended doses of acetaminophen for up to two years (78) or maximum doses (4000 mg) for up to 1 year (4, 154). It should be noted that randomized clinical trials have documented transient elevations of both alanine aminotransferase and aspartate aminotransferase levels in patients receiving therapeutic dosages of acetaminophen (≤ 4000 mg/day); however, these elevations were not associated with signs of liver injury or dysfunction and were classified as being clinically insignificant (154-156).

Hepatic toxicity is the major concern related to acetaminophen use and an extensive literature exists, the scope of which is beyond the general overview of this chapter. Multiple excellent comprehensive reviews cover the varied aspects of this very important topic (157-160).

5.6. Pregnancy and Lactation

Acetaminophen is used during pregnancy and currently bears an FDA Pregnancy Risk Factor Rating of B (Defined as no fetal risk seen in animal studies and no well—controlled human studies OR adverse effects seen in animal studies but human studies have shown no risk). When taken as directed, acetaminophen does not appear to be a risk to the mother or fetus during any trimester (161, 162). For example, a retrospective analysis of 88,142 pregnant women did not associate congential birth defects with acetaminophen use during the first trimester (163).

5.7. Renal

Even though there are some data suggesting a correlation between acetaminophen and renal toxicity(164-166), acetaminophen has not been shown to be nephrotoxic at recommended doses (4) even during long-term use (167). Studies comparing the renal effects of NSAIDs to acetaminophen also suggest acetaminophen's lack of renal toxicity (168). The National Kidney Foundation recommends acetaminophen use in pain patients with concomitant renal insufficiency or renal disease.

6. DDIs

Potential drug-drug interactions can arise with co-administration of other substances that alter the ADME of acetaminophen. Some of these substances and their effects on acetaminophen are briefly described in Table 1.

Table 1.

Pharmacokinetic Interactions (4)	
Drug	Effect
Metoclopramide	Acetaminophen absorption
Anticholinergics	Acetaminophen absorption
Alcohol	Acetaminophen metabolism (accumulation of toxic metabolite)
Isoniazid:	Acetaminophen metabolism (blocks formation of toxic metabolite)
Ascorbic Acid:	Inhibit the systemic conjugation of acetaminophen with sulfate
Ciprofloxacin:	Effects saliva concentrations of acetaminophen
Oral Contraceptives	Increase the clearance of acetaminophen
Probenecid	Increase of elimination half-life
Sulfinpyrazone	Increase clearance and decrease elimination half life
Potential Pharmacodynamic Interactions (4)	
Oral anticoagulants, furosemide, anticonvulsants (Hydantoins, Carbamazepine)	

6.1. Overdose

Generally, patients are classified as having overdosed if > 7.5 g has been ingested within 8 hours or less. An overdose can cause accumulation of acetaminophen's reactive metabolite to such a level that glutathione reserves are not available for the detoxification pathways. When this occurs, the reactive metabolite causes hepatic necrosis, hepatic dysfunction, and in severe cases, hepatic failure.

The clinical course of acetaminophen overdose generally occurs in 3 phases. Phase 1: Occurs after initial ingestion of a toxic overdose and can last 12 - 24 hours. During this time the patient may experience gastrointestinal irritability, nausea, vomiting, anorexia, diaphoresis, and pallor. Phase 2: From 24 - 48 hours after ingestion the patient may begin to feel better and many of the symptoms will subside. However, it is during this time that hepatic damage begins to take place, unnoticed by the patient. Hepatic enzymes, bilirubin, lactate, phosphate, and prothrombin time or INR values will progressively rise to dangerous levels. As the damage increases, right upper-quadrant pain may develop as the liver becomes enlarged and tender. Phase 3: The final stage of overdose usually does not develop until 3 - 5 days of overdose ingestion. Symptoms may vary depending on the severity of the liver damage and can include anorexia, nausea, general malaise, and abdominal pain in less severe cases. Patients with severe liver damage may also experience confusion, stupor, jaundice, coagulation defects, hypoglycemia, and encephalopathy, as well as renal failure and cardiomyopathy. Death can occur if treatment is not initiated promptly and correctly.

6.1.1. NAC Treatment

Oral and IV formulations of acetylcysteine (*N*-acetylcysteine, NAC) have been approved as an antidote for the treatment of acetaminophen overdose (169). NAC is a precursor of glutathione and aids in increasing glutathione conjugation of NAPQI. When used appropriately and within the early stages of overdose, NAC has been shown to reduce morbidity and mortality associated with acetaminophen overdose (169).

7. Acetaminophen Formulations

7.1. Combinations

Acetaminophen is widely used in combination products, including other OTC ingredients, such as cough and cold ingredients, and other analgesics, including opioids and NSAIDs. An up to date list of combinations have been published by the US National Library of Medicine (170).

7.2. IV Formulation

A recently-approved intravenous formulation of acetaminophen (OFIRMEV™, Cadence Pharmaceuticals, Inc., San Diego, CA, USA) has entered the market and is indicated for the treatment of pain conditions of mild to moderate intensity, for use in combination with opioids for moderate to severe pain, and for use for reduction of fever (7, 94, 95). Based on clinical experience, IV acetaminophen is a reasonably safe, effective and well-tolerated analgesic for the treatment of pain following a variety of surgical procedures including oral, cardiac, abdominal, orthopedic, and breast. A systematic review of the literature for IV acetaminophen use in postoperative pain analyzed 16 randomly-controlled trials with a total of 1464 patients and concluded that IV acetaminophen has analgesic efficacy comparable to IV parecoxib, IV metamizol, or oral ibuprofen for a variety of surgical procedures. The reported side effects associated with IV acetaminophen are similar to those for oral acetaminophen (171, 172).

Conclusion

Acetaminophen (paracetemol) is a non-opioid analgesic and antipyretic widely used as a single agent or in fixed-ratio combinations with other analgesics for a large variety of mild to moderate pain conditions in a large variety of patient populations. Although the exact mechanism of its analgesic effect is not known, it appears to involve actions on both the central and peripheral nervous systems. The side effects of acetaminophen generally are mild and transient at recommended doses. However, severe hepatic toxicity can follow overdose or use in patients with hepatic susceptibility. Accidental overdose is a concern because of the prevalence of acetaminophen in multiple over-the-counter products and the cumulative effect of ingestion. Overall, when used safely and properly, acetaminophen is a very good mild to moderate pain reliever for the general consumer and postoperative patient. It is particularly useful in situations where a nonopioid analgesic with good GI tolerability is desirable.

References

[1] Wikipedia. Paracetamol. [10/4/2011]; Available from: *http://en.wikipedia.org/wiki/Paracetamol*.

[2] Toes MJ, Jones AL, Prescott L. Drug interactions with paracetamol. *Am J Ther.* 2005 Jan-Feb;12(1):56-66.

[3] Grattan T, Hickman R, Darby-Dowman A, Hayward M, Boyce M, Warrington S. A five way crossover human volunteer study to compare the pharmacokinetics of paracetamol following oral administration of two commercially available paracetamol tablets and three development tablets containing paracetamol in combination with sodium bicarbonate or calcium carbonate. *Eur J Pharm Biopharm.* 2000 May;49(3):225-9.

[4] McNeil Consumer Healthcare. *TYLENOL® Professional Product Information.* 2011.

[5] Gelotte CK, Auiler JF, Lynch JM, Temple AR, Slattery JT. Disposition of acetaminophen at 4, 6, and 8 g/day for 3 days in healthy young adults. *Clin Pharmacol Ther.* 2007 Jun;81(6):840-8.

[6] Temple AR, Mrazik TJ. More on extended-release acetaminophen. *N Engl J Med.* 1995 Nov 30;333(22):1508-9.

[7] Cadence Pharmaceuticals. OFIRMEV (acetaminophen) *Injection.* 2010.

[8] Birmingham PK, Tobin MJ, Fisher DM, Henthorn TK, Hall SC, Cote CJ. Initial and subsequent dosing of rectal acetaminophen in children: a 24-hour pharmacokinetic study of new dose recommendations. *Anesthesiology.* 2001 Mar;94(3):385-9.

[9] Milligan TP, Morris HC, Hammond PM, Price CP. Studies on paracetamol binding to serum proteins. *Ann Clin Biochem.* 1994 Sep;31 (Pt 5):492-6.

[10] Levy G. Comparative pharmacokinetics of aspirin and acetaminophen. *Arch Intern Med.* 1981 Feb 23;141(3 Spec No):279-81.

[11] Bailey DN. Relative binding of acetaminophen, lidocaine, phenobarbital, phenytoin, quinidine, and theophylline to human tissues in vitro. *J Anal Toxicol.* 1997 Jan-Feb;21(1):1-4.

[12] Forrest JA, Clements JA, Prescott LF. Clinical pharmacokinetics of paracetamol. *Clin Pharmacokinet.* 1982 Mar-Apr;7(2):93-107.

[13] Camu F, Van de Velde A, Vanlersberghe C. Nonsteroidal anti-inflammatory drugs and paracetamol in children. *Acta Anaesthesiol Belg.* 2001;52(1):13-20.

[14] Moreau X, Le Quay L, Granry JC, Boishardy N, Delhumeau A. [Pharmacokinetics of paracetamol in the cerebrospinal fluid in the elderly]. *Therapie.* 1993 Jul-Aug;48(4):393-6.

[15] Bannwarth B, Netter P, Lapicque F, Gillet P, Pere P, Boccard E, et al. Plasma and cerebrospinal fluid concentrations of paracetamol after a single intravenous dose of propacetamol. *Br J Clin Pharmacol.* 1992 Jul;34(1):79-81.

[16] Naga Rani MA, Joseph T, Narayanan R. Placental transfer of paracetamol. *J Indian Med Assoc.* 1989 Aug;87(8):182-3.

[17] American Academy of Pediatrics. Transfer of drugs and other chemicals into human milk. *Pediatrics.* 2001 Sep;108(3):776-89.

[18] Notarianni LJ, Oldham HG, Bennett PN. Passage of paracetamol into breast milk and its subsequent metabolism by the neonate. *Br J Clin Pharmacol.* 1987 Jul;24(1):63-7.

[19] Berlin CM, Jr., Yaffe SJ, Ragni M. Disposition of acetaminophen in milk, saliva, and plasma of lactating women. *Pediatr Pharmacol* (New York). 1980;1(2):135-41.

[20] Bitzen PO, Gustafsson B, Jostell KG, Melander A, Wahlin-Boll E. Excretion of paracetamol in human breast milk. *Eur J Clin Pharmacol.* 1981;20(2):123-5.

[21] Slattery JT, McRorie TI, Reynolds R, Kalhorn TF, Kharasch ED, Eddy AC. Lack of effect of cimetidine on acetaminophen disposition in humans. *Clin Pharmacol Ther.* 1989 Nov;46(5):591-7.

[22] Andrews RS, Bond CC, Burnett J, Saunders A, Watson K. Isolation and identification of paracetamol metabolites. *J Int Med Res.* 1976;4(4 Suppl):34-9.

[23] Manyike PT, Kharasch ED, Kalhorn TF, Slattery JT. Contribution of CYP2E1 and CYP3A to acetaminophen reactive metabolite formation. *Clin Pharmacol Ther.* 2000 Mar;67(3):275-82.

[24] Sarich T, Kalhorn T, Magee S, al-Sayegh F, Adams S, Slattery J, et al. The effect of omeprazole pretreatment on acetaminophen metabolism in rapid and slow metabolizers of S-mephenytoin. *Clin Pharmacol Ther.* 1997 Jul;62(1):21-8.

[25] Mitchell JR, Thorgeirsson SS, Potter WZ, Jollow DJ, Keiser H. Acetaminophen-induced hepatic injury: protective role of glutathione in man and rationale for therapy. *Clin Pharmacol Ther.* 1974 Oct;16(4):676-84.

[26] Rawlins MD, Henderson DB, Hijab AR. Pharmacokinetics of paracetamol (acetaminophen) after intravenous and oral administration. Eur *J Clin Pharmacol.* 1977 Apr 20;11(4):283-6.

[27] Villeneuve JP, Raymond G, Bruneau J, Colpron L, Pomier-Layrargues G. [Pharmacokinetics and metabolism of acetaminophen in normal, alcoholic and cirrhotic subjects]. *Gastroenterol Clin Biol.* 1983 Nov;7(11):898-902.

[28] Forrest JA, Adriaenssens P, Finlayson ND, Prescott LF. Paracetamol metabolism in chronic liver disease. *Eur J Clin Pharmacol.* 1979 Jul;15(6):427-31.

[29] Zapater P, Lasso de la Vega MC, Horga JF, Such J, Frances R, Esteban A, et al. Pharmacokinetic variations of acetaminophen according to liver dysfunction and portal hypertension status. *Aliment Pharmacol Ther.* 2004 Jul 1;20(1):29-36.

[30] Yin OQ, Tomlinson B, Chow AH, Chow MS. Pharmacokinetics of acetaminophen in Hong Kong Chinese subjects. *Int J Pharm.* 2001 Jul 17;222(2):305-8.

[31] Babalola CP, Oladimeji FA, Femi-Oyewo MN. Pharmacokinetics and saliva secretion of paracetamol in healthy male Nigerians. *West Afr J Med.* 2004 Jan-Mar;23(1):10-4.

[32] Miners JO, Osborne NJ, Tonkin AL, Birkett DJ. Perturbation of paracetamol urinary metabolic ratios by urine flow rate. *Br J Clin Pharmacol.* 1992 Oct;34(4):359-62.

[33] Lee HS, Ti TY, Koh YK, Prescott LF. Paracetamol elimination in Chinese and Indians in Singapore. *Eur J Clin Pharmacol.* 1992;43(1):81-4.

[34] Rollins DE, von Bahr C, Glaumann H, Moldeus P, Rane A. Acetaminophen: potentially toxic metabolite formed by human fetal and adult liver microsomes and isolated fetal liver cells. *Science.* 1979 Sep 28;205(4413):1414-6.

[35] Pharmacological management of persistent pain in older persons. *J Am Geriatr Soc.* 2009 Aug;57(8):1331-46.

[36] Miners JO, Penhall R, Robson RA, Birkett DJ. Comparison of paracetamol metabolism in young adult and elderly males. *Eur J Clin Pharmacol.* 1988;35(2):157-60.

[37] Triggs EJ, Nation RL, Long A, Ashley JJ. Pharmacokinetics in the elderly. *Eur J Clin Pharmacol.* 1975;8(1):55-62.

[38] Wynne HA, Cope LH, Herd B, Rawlins MD, James OF, Woodhouse KW. The association of age and frailty with paracetamol conjugation in man. *Age Ageing.* 1990 Nov;19(6):419-24.

[39] Bannwarth B, Pehourcq F, Lagrange F, Matoga M, Maury S, Palisson M, et al. Single and multiple dose pharmacokinetics of acetaminophen (paracetamol) in polymedicated very old patients with rheumatic pain. *J Rheumatol.* 2001 Jan;28(1):182-4.

[40] Divoll M, Abernethy DR, Ameer B, Greenblatt DJ. Acetaminophen kinetics in the elderly. *Clin Pharmacol Ther.* 1982 Feb;31(2):151-6.

[41] Divoll M, Ameer B, Abernethy DR, Greenblatt DJ. Age does not alter acetaminophen absorption. *J Am Geriatr Soc.* 1982 Apr;30(4):240-4.

[42] Divoll M, Greenblatt DJ, Ameer B, Abernethy DR. Effect of food on acetaminophen absorption in young and elderly subjects. *J Clin Pharmacol.* 1982 Nov-Dec;22(11-12):571-6.

[43] Vargas R, Maneatis T, Bynum L, Peterson C, McMahon FG. Evaluation of the antipyretic effect of ketorolac, acetaminophen, and placebo in endotoxin-induced fever. *J Clin Pharmacol.* 1994 Aug;34(8):848-53.

[44] Pernerstorfer T, Schmid R, Bieglmayer C, Eichler HG, Kapiotis S, Jilma B. Acetaminophen has greater antipyretic efficacy than aspirin in endotoxemia: a randomized, double-blind, placebo-controlled trial. *Clin Pharmacol Ther.* 1999 Jul;66(1):51-7.

[45] Bachert C, Chuchalin AG, Eisebitt R, Netayzhenko VZ, Voelker M. Aspirin compared with acetaminophen in the treatment of fever and other symptoms of upper respiratory tract infection in adults: a multicenter, randomized, double-blind, double-dummy, placebo-controlled, parallel-group, single-dose, 6-hour dose-ranging study. *Clin Ther.* 2005 Jul;27(7):993-1003.

[46] Maron JJ, Ickes AC. The antipyretic effectiveness of acetaminophen suppositories versus tablets: a double-blind study. *Curr Ther Res Clin Exp.* 1976 Jul;20(1):45-52.

[47] Kauffman RE, Sawyer LA, Scheinbaum ML. Antipyretic efficacy of ibuprofen vs acetaminophen. *Am J Dis Child.* 1992 May;146(5):622-5.

[48] Hunter J. Study of antipyretic therapy in current use. *Arch Dis Child.* 1973 Apr;48(4):313-5.

[49] Brewer EJ, Jr. A comparative evaluation of indomethacin, acetaminophen and placebo as antipyretic agents in children. *Arthritis Rheum.* 1968 Oct;11(5):645-51.

[50] Simila S, Keinanen S, Kouvalainen K. Oral antipyretic therapy: evaluation of benorylate, an ester of acetylsalicylic acid and paracetamol. *Eur J Pediatr.* 1975 Dec 9;121(1):15-20.

[51] Steele RW, Young FS, Bass JW, Shirkey HC. ORAL ANTIPYRETIC THERAPY. Evaluation of aspirin-acetaminophen combination. *Am J Dis Child.* 1972 Mar;123(3):204-6.

[52] Tarlin L, Landrigan P, Babineau R, Alpert JJ. A comparison of the antipyretic effect of acetaminophen and aspirin. Another approach to poison prevention. *Am J Dis Child.* 1972 Dec;124(6):880-2.

[53] Eden AN, Kaufman A. Clinical comparison of three antipyretic agents. *Am J Dis Child.* 1967 Sep;114(3):284-7.

[54] Walson PD, Galletta G, Chomilo F, Braden NJ, Sawyer LA, Scheinbaum ML. Comparison of multidose ibuprofen and acetaminophen therapy in febrile children. *Am J Dis Child.* 1992 May;146(5):626-32.

[55] Sheth UK, Gupta K, Paul T, Pispati PK. Measurement of antipyretic activity of ibuprofen and paracetamol in children. *J Clin Pharmacol.* 1980 Nov-Dec;20(11-12):672-5.

[56] Vauzelle-Kervroedan F, d'Athis P, Pariente-Khayat A, Debregeas S, Olive G, Pons G. Equivalent antipyretic activity of ibuprofen and paracetamol in febrile children. *J Pediatr.* 1997 Nov;131(5):683-7.

[57] Amdekar YK, Desai RZ. Antipyretic activity of ibuprofen and paracetamol in children with pyrexia. *Br J Clin Pract.* 1985 Apr;39(4):140-3.

[58] Koch-Weser J. Drug therapy. Acetaminophen. *N Engl J Med.* 1976 Dec 2;295(23):1297-300.

[59] Milton AS. Modern views on the pathogenesis of fever and the mode of action of antipyretic drugs. *J Pharm Pharmacol.* 1976 Apr;28(4 SUPPL):393-9.

[60] Ameer B, Greenblatt DJ. Acetaminophen. *Ann Intern Med.* 1977 Aug;87(2):202-9.

[61] Ivanov AI, Scheck AC, Romanovsky AA. Expression of genes controlling transport and catabolism of prostaglandin E2 in lipopolysaccharide fever. *Am J Physiol Regul Integr Comp Physiol.* 2003 Mar;284(3):R698-706.

[62] Hyllested M, Jones S, Pedersen JL, Kehlet H. Comparative effect of paracetamol, NSAIDs or their combination in postoperative pain management: a qualitative review. *British Journal of Anaesthesia.* 2002 February 1, 2002;88(2):199-214.

[63] McQuay HJ, Edwards JE, Moore RA. Evaluating analgesia: the challenges. *Am J Ther.* 2002 May-Jun;9(3):179-87.

[64] Toms L, Derry S, Moore RA, McQuay HJ. Single dose oral paracetamol (acetaminophen) with codeine for postoperative pain in adults. *Cochrane Database Syst Rev.* 2009(1):CD001547.

[65] Eade NR, Lasagna L. A comparison of acetophenetidin and acetaminophen. II. Subjective effects in healthy volunteers. *J Pharmacol Exp Ther.* 1967 Feb;155(2):301-8.

[66] Schachtel BP, Thoden WR, Baybutt RI. Ibuprofen and acetaminophen in the relief of postpartum episiotomy pain. *J Clin Pharmacol.* 1989 Jun;29(6):550-3.

[67] Schachtel BP, Fillingim JM, Thoden WR, Lane AC, Baybutt RI. Sore throat pain in the evaluation of mild analgesics. *Clin Pharmacol Ther.* 1988 Dec;44(6):704-11.

[68] Reuter SH, Montgomery WW. Aspirin Vs Acetaminophen after Tonsillectomy. A Comparative Double-Blind Clinical Study. *Arch Otolaryngol.* 1964 Aug;80:214-7.

[69] Anderson B, Kanagasundarum S, Woollard G. Analgesic efficacy of paracetamol in children using tonsillectomy as a pain model. *Anaesth Intensive Care.* 1996 Dec;24(6):669-73.

[70] Schachtel BP, Thoden WR. A placebo-controlled model for assaying systemic analgesics in children. *Clin Pharmacol Ther.* 1993 May;53(5):593-601.

[71] Moore N, Le Parc JM, van Ganse E, Wall R, Schneid H, Cairns R. Tolerability of ibuprofen, aspirin and paracetamol for the treatment of cold and flu symptoms and sore throat pain. *Int J Clin Pract.* 2002 Dec;56(10):732-4.

[72] Jordan KM, Arden NK, Doherty M, Bannwarth B, Bijlsma JW, Dieppe P, et al. EULAR Recommendations 2003: an evidence based approach to the management of knee osteoarthritis: Report of a Task Force of the Standing Committee for International Clinical Studies Including Therapeutic Trials (ESCISIT). *Ann Rheum Dis.* 2003 Dec;62(12):1145-55.

[73] Zhang W, Doherty M, Leeb BF, Alekseeva L, Arden NK, Bijlsma JW, et al. EULAR evidence based recommendations for the management of hand osteoarthritis: report of a Task Force of the EULAR Standing Committee for International Clinical Studies Including Therapeutics (ESCISIT). *Ann Rheum Dis.* 2007 Mar;66(3):377-88.

[74] Combe B, Landewe R, Lukas C, Bolosiu HD, Breedveld F, Dougados M, et al. EULAR recommendations for the management of early arthritis: report of a task force of the European Standing Committee for International Clinical Studies Including Therapeutics (ESCISIT). *Annals of the Rheumatic Diseases.* 2007 January 1, 2007;66(1):34-45.

[75] Simon LS, Lipman AG, Caudill-Slosberg M, Gill LH, Keefe FJ, Kerr KL, et al. *Guideline for the Management of Pain in Osteoarthritis, Rheumatoid Arthritis, and Juvenile Chronic Arthritis.* Glenview, IL: American Pain Society; 2002.

[76] Altman RD, Zinsenheim JR, Temple AR, Schweinle JE. Three-month efficacy and safety of acetaminophen extended-release for osteoarthritis pain of the hip or knee: a randomized, double-blind, placebo-controlled study. *Osteoarthritis Cartilage.* 2007 Apr;15(4):454-61.

[77] Bradley JD, Brandt KD, Katz BP, Kalasinski LA, Ryan SI. Comparison of an antiinflammatory dose of ibuprofen, an analgesic dose of ibuprofen, and acetaminophen in the treatment of patients with osteoarthritis of the knee. *N Engl J Med.* 1991 Jul 11;325(2):87-91.

[78] Williams HJ, Ward JR, Egger MJ, Neuner R, Brooks RH, Clegg DO, et al. Comparison of naproxen and acetaminophen in a two-year study of treatment of osteoarthritis of the knee. *Arthritis Rheum.* 1993 Sep;36(9):1196-206.

[79] Recommendations for the medical management of osteoarthritis of the hip and knee: 2000 update. American College of Rheumatology Subcommittee on Osteoarthritis Guidelines. *Arthritis Rheum.* 2000 Sep;43(9):1905-15.

[80] Zhang W, Moskowitz RW, Nuki G, Abramson S, Altman RD, Arden N, et al. OARSI recommendations for the management of hip and knee osteoarthritis, Part II: OARSI evidence-based, expert consensus guidelines. *Osteoarthritis Cartilage.* 2008 Feb;16(2):137-62.

[81] Pincus T, Koch G, Lei H, Mangal B, Sokka T, Moskowitz R, et al. Patient Preference for Placebo, Acetaminophen (paracetamol) or Celecoxib Efficacy Studies (PACES): two randomised, double blind, placebo controlled, crossover clinical trials in patients with knee or hip osteoarthritis. *Ann Rheum Dis.* 2004 Aug;63(8):931-9.

[82] Shamoon M, Hochberg MC. The role of acetaminophen in the management of patients with osteoarthritis. *The American Journal of Medicine.* 2001;110(3, Supplement 1):46-9.

[83] Ruoff G, Urban G. *Treatment of Primary Headache: Episodic Tension-Type Headache.* Chicago, IL: National Headache Foundation; 2004.

[84] Steiner TJ, Lange R, Voelker M. Aspirin in episodic tension-type headache: placebo-controlled dose-ranging comparison with paracetamol. *Cephalalgia.* 2003 Feb;23(1):59-66.

[85] Peters BH, Fraim CJ, Masel BE. Comparison of 650 mg aspirin and 1,000 mg acetaminophen with each other, and with placebo in moderately severe headache. *Am J Med.* 1983 Jun 14;74(6A):36-42.

[86] Packman B, Packman E, Doyle G, Cooper S, Ashraf E, Koronkiewicz K, et al. Solubilized ibuprofen: evaluation of onset, relief, and safety of a novel formulation in the treatment of episodic tension-type headache. *Headache*. 2000 Jul-Aug;40(7):561-7.

[87] Migliardi JR, Armellino JJ, Friedman M, Gillings DB, Beaver WT. Caffeine as an analgesic adjuvant in tension headache. *Clin Pharmacol Ther*. 1994 Nov;56(5):576-86.

[88] Schachtel BP, Furey SA, Thoden WR. Nonprescription ibuprofen and acetaminophen in the treatment of tension-type headache. *J Clin Pharmacol*. 1996 Dec;36(12):1120-5.

[89] Steiner TJ, Lange R. Ketoprofen (25 mg) in the symptomatic treatment of episodic tension-type headache: double-blind placebo-controlled comparison with acetaminophen (1000 mg). *Cephalalgia*. 1998 Jan;18(1):38-43.

[90] Schachtel BP, Thoden WR, Konerman JP, Brown A, Chaing DS. Headache pain model for assessing and comparing the efficacy of over-the-counter analgesic agents. *Clin Pharmacol Ther*. 1991 Sep;50(3):322-9.

[91] Association of Women's Health Obstetric and Neonatal Nurses. *Cyclic Perimenstrual Pain and Discomfort: Nursing Management. Evidence-Based Clinical Practice Guideline*. Washington, DC: Association of Women's Health Obstetric and Neonatal Nurses (AWHONN); 2003.

[92] Chou R, Qaseem A, Snow V, Casey D, Cross JT, Jr., Shekelle P, et al. Diagnosis and treatment of low back pain: a joint clinical practice guideline from the American College of Physicians and the American Pain Society. *Ann Intern Med*. 2007 Oct 2;147(7):478-91.

[93] Smith HS. Potential analgesic mechanisms of acetaminophen. *Pain Physician*. 2009 Jan-Feb;12(1):269-80.

[94] Toussaint K, Yang XC, Zielinski MA, Reigle KL, Sacavage SD, Nagar S, et al. What do we (not) know about how paracetamol (acetaminophen) works? *Journal of Clinical Pharmacy and Therapeutics*. 2010;35(6):617-38.

[95] Pergolizzi JV, Raffa RB, Tallarida R, Taylor R, Labhsetwar SA. Continuous Multimechanistic Postoperative Analgesia: A Rationale for Transitioning from Intravenous Acetaminophen and Opioids to Oral Formulations. *Pain Pract*. 2011 Jun 16.

[96] Raffa RB. Acetaminophen and Metabolite: Lack of Effect on Nitric Oxide Synthase (Constitutive or Inducible). *Headache: The Journal of Head and Face Pain*. 2002;42(3):237-8.

[97] Raffa RB, Codd EE. Lack of binding of acetaminophen to 5-HT receptor or uptake sites (or eleven other binding/uptake assays). *Life Sci*. 1996;59(2):PL37-40.

[98] Raffa RB, Stone DJ, Tallarida RJ. Discovery of "Self-Synergistic" Spinal/Supraspinal Antinociception Produced by Acetaminophen (Paracetamol). *Journal of Pharmacology and Experimental Therapeutics*. 2000 October 1, 2000;295(1):291-4.

[99] Poulsen HE, Ranek L, Andreasen PB. The hepatic glutathione content in liver diseases. *Scand J Clin Lab Invest*. 1981 Oct;41(6):573-6.

[100] Rumack BH. Acetaminophen hepatotoxicity: the first 35 years. *J Toxicol Clin Toxicol*. 2002;40(1):3-20.

[101] Schoene B, Fleischmann RA, Remmer H, von Oldershausen HF. Determination of drug metabolizing enzymes in needle biopsies of human liver. *Eur J Clin Pharmacol*. 1972 Mar;4(2):65-73.

[102] Siegers CP, Bossen KH, Younes M, Mahlke R, Oltmanns D. Glutathione and glutathione-S-transferases in the normal and diseased human liver. *Pharmacol Res Commun.* 1982 Jan;14(1):61-72.
[103] Gabrielle L, Leterrier F, Molinie C, Essioux H, Cristau P, Laverdant C. [Determination of human liver cytochrome P-450 by a micromethod using the electron paramagnetic resonance. Study of 141 liver biopsies (author's transl)]. *Gastroenterol Clin Biol.* 1977 Oct;1(10):775-82.
[104] Jorup-Ronstrom C, Beermann B, Wahlin-Boll E, Melander A, Britton S. Reduction of paracetamol and aspirin metabolism during viral hepatitis. *Clin Pharmacokinet.* 1986 May-Jun;11(3):250-6.
[105] Benson GD. Hepatotoxicity following the therapeutic use of antipyretic analgesics. *Am J Med.* 1983 Nov 14;75(5A):85-93.
[106] Benson GD. Acetaminophen in chronic liver disease. *Clin Pharmacol Ther.* 1983 Jan;33(1):95-101.
[107] Arnman R, Olsson R. Elimination of paracetamol in chronic liver disease. *Acta Hepatogastroenterol* (Stuttg). 1978 Aug;25(4):283-6.
[108] Andreasen PB, Hutters L. Paracetamol (acetaminophen) clearance in patients with cirrhosis of the liver. *Acta Med Scand Suppl.* 1979;624:99-105.
[109] Benson GD, Koff RS, Tolman KG. The therapeutic use of acetaminophen in patients with liver disease. *Am J Ther.* 2005 Mar-Apr;12(2):133-41.
[110] Bailie GR, Mason NA, Bragg-Gresham JL, Gillespie BW, Young EW. Analgesic prescription patterns among hemodialysis patients in the DOPPS: potential for underprescription. *Kidney Int.* 2004 Jun;65(6):2419-25.
[111] Prescott LF, Speirs GC, Critchley JA, Temple RM, Winney RJ. Paracetamol disposition and metabolite kinetics in patients with chronic renal failure. *Eur J Clin Pharmacol.* 1989;36(3):291-7.
[112] Berg KJ, Djoseland O, Gjellan A, Hundal O, Knudsen ER, Rugstad HE, et al. Acute effects of paracetamol on prostaglandin synthesis and renal function in normal man and in patients with renal failure. *Clin Nephrol.* 1990 Dec;34(6):255-62.
[113] Henrich WL, Agodoa LE, Barrett B, Bennett WM, Blantz RC, Buckalew VM, Jr., et al. Analgesics and the kidney: summary and recommendations to the Scientific Advisory Board of the National Kidney Foundation from an Ad Hoc Committee of the National Kidney Foundation. *Am J Kidney Dis.* 1996 Jan;27(1):162-5.
[114] Zenger F, Russmann S, Junker E, Wuthrich C, Bui MH, Lauterburg BH. Decreased glutathione in patients with anorexia nervosa. Risk factor for toxic liver injury? *Eur J Clin Nutr.* 2004 Feb;58(2):238-43.
[115] Whitcomb DC, Block GD. Association of Acetaminophen Hepatotoxicity With Fasting and Ethanol Use. *JAMA: The Journal of the American Medical Association.* 1994 December 21, 1994;272(23):1845-50.
[116] Herzenberg LA, De Rosa SC, Dubs JG, Roederer M, Anderson MT, Ela SW, et al. Glutathione deficiency is associated with impaired survival in HIV disease. *Proc Natl Acad Sci U S A.* 1997 Mar 4;94(5):1967-72.
[117] Radu P, Atsmon J. Gilbert's syndrome--clinical and pharmacological implications. *Isr Med Assoc J.* 2001 Aug;3(8):593-8.

[118] Bock KW, Forster A, Gschaidmeier H, Bruck M, Munzel P, Schareck W, et al. Paracetamol glucuronidation by recombinant rat and human phenol UDP-glucuronosyltransferases. *Biochem Pharmacol.* 1993 May 5;45(9):1809-14.
[119] Court MH, Duan SX, von Moltke LL, Greenblatt DJ, Patten CJ, Miners JO, et al. Interindividual variability in acetaminophen glucuronidation by human liver microsomes: identification of relevant acetaminophen UDP-glucuronosyltransferase isoforms. *J Pharmacol Exp Ther.* 2001 Dec;299(3):998-1006.
[120] Rauchschwalbe SK, Zuhlsdorf MT, Wensing G, Kuhlmann J. Glucuronidation of acetaminophen is independent of UGT1A1 promotor genotype. *Int J Clin Pharmacol Ther.* 2004 Feb;42(2):73-7.
[121] Schmid R, Hammaker L. Glucuronide formation in patients with constitutional hepatic dysfunction (Gilbert's disease). *N Engl J Med.* 1959 Jun 25;260(26):1310-4.
[122] Ullrich D, Sieg A, Blume R, Bock KW, Schroter W, Bircher J. Normal pathways for glucuronidation, sulphation and oxidation of paracetamol in Gilbert's syndrome. *Eur J Clin Invest.* 1987 Jun;17(3):237-40.
[123] Esteban A, Perez-Mateo M. Heterogeneity of paracetamol metabolism in Gilbert's syndrome. *Eur J Drug Metab Pharmacokinet. 1*999 Jan-Mar;24(1):9-13.
[124] Daghfous R, El Aidli S, Jday A, Kastalli S, Klouz A, Srairi S, et al. [Allergic reactions to paracetamol]. *Therapie.* 2005 Sep-Oct;60(5):523-6.
[125] Bachmeyer C, Vermeulen C, Habki R, Blay F, Leynadier F. Acetaminophen (paracetamol)-induced anaphylactic shock. *South Med J.* 2002 Jul;95(7):759-60.
[126] Flanagan RJ, Mant TG. Coma and metabolic acidosis early in severe acute paracetamol poisoning. *Hum Toxicol.* 1986 May;5(3):179-82.
[127] Zezulka A, Wright N. Severe metabolic acidosis early in paracetamol poisoning. *Br Med J* (Clin Res Ed). 1982 Sep 25;285(6345):851-2.
[128] Bannwarth B. Gastrointestinal safety of paracetamol: is there any cause for concern? *Expert Opin Drug Saf.* 2004 Jul;3(4):269-72.
[129] Hoftiezer JW, O'Laughlin JC, Ivey KJ. Effects of 24 hours of aspirin, Bufferin, paracetamol and placebo on normal human gastroduodenal mucosa. *Gut.* 1982 Aug;23(8):692-7.
[130] Lanza FL, Codispoti JR, Nelson EB. An endoscopic comparison of gastroduodenal injury with over-the-counter doses of ketoprofen and acetaminophen. *Am J Gastroenterol.* 1998 Jul;93(7):1051-4.
[131] Begaud B, Chaslerie A, Carne X, Bannwarth B, Laporte JR, Sorbette F, et al. Upper gastrointestinal bleeding associated with analgesics and NSAID use: a case-control study. *J Rheumatol.* 1993 Aug;20(8):1443-4.
[132] Laporte JR, Carne X, Vidal X, Moreno V, Juan J. Upper gastrointestinal bleeding in relation to previous use of analgesics and non-steroidal anti-inflammatory drugs. Catalan Countries Study on Upper Gastrointestinal Bleeding. *Lancet.* 1991 Jan 12;337(8733):85-9.
[133] Muller P, Simon B, Weise D, Dammann HG. [Endoscopic studies on the gastric tolerance of paracetamol and acetylsalicylic acid. A placebo-controlled, double-blind study in healthy volunteers]. *Arzneimittelforschung.* 1990 Mar;40(3):316-8.
[134] Levy M, Miller DR, Kaufman DW, Siskind V, Schwingl P, Rosenberg L, et al. Major upper gastrointestinal tract bleeding. Relation to the use of aspirin and other nonnarcotic analgesics. *Arch Intern Med.* 1988 Feb;148(2):281-5.

[135] Jouet JP, Huart JJ, Bauters F, Goudemand M. [Paracetamol, an unrecognized cause of acute, drug-induced agranulocytosis]. *Nouv Presse Med.* 1980 Apr 26;9(19):1386-7.
[136] Obel AO. Presumed analgesic-induced agranulocytosis. *East Afr Med J.* 1983 Apr;60(4):273-7.
[137] Benkirane-Agoumi N, Belkhadir J, Cherkaoui O, Dadi-el Fassi Fihri O, Bensouda JD. [Apropos of a case of agranulocytosis caused by paracetamol]. *Maroc Med.* 1986 Dec;8(4):470-4.
[138] Duhamel G, Najman A, Gorin NC, Stachowiak. [Current aspects of agranulocytosis (15 cases)]. *Ann Med Interne* (Paris). 1977 Mar;128(3):303-6.
[139] Gursoy M, Haznedaroglu IC, Celik I, Sayinalp N, Ozcebe OI, Dundar SV. Agranulocytosis, plasmacytosis, and thrombocytosis followed by a leukemoid reaction due to acute acetaminophen toxicity. *Ann Pharmacother.* 1996 Jul-Aug;30(7-8):762-5.
[140] Hirsch JF, Pichard S, Flottes P, Negellen JL. [Agranulocytosis and hyperbilirubinemia during prolonged treatment with paracetamol]. *Therapie.* 1982 Sep-Oct;37(5):593-4.
[141] Maraninchi D, Gastaut JA, Sebahoun G, Carcassonne Y. [Agranulocytosis caused by taking paracetamol? Value of the in vitro granulocyte progenitor test]. *Nouv Presse Med.* 1981 Jan 10;10(1):41.
[142] Lloyd TW. Agranulocytosis associated with paracetamol. *Lancet.* 1961 Jan 14;1(7168):114-5.
[143] Kornberg A, Polliack A. Paracetamol-induced thrombocytopenia and haemolytic anaemia. Lancet. 1978 Nov 25;2(8100):1159.
[144] Scheinberg IH. Thrombocytopenic reaction to aspirin and acetaminophen. *N Engl J Med.* 1979 Mar 22;300(12):678.
[145] Shoenfeld Y, Shaklai M, Livni E, Pinkhas J. Thrombocytopenia from acetaminophen. *N Engl J Med.* 1980 Jul 3;303(1):47.
[146] Skokan JD, Hewlett JS, Hoffman GC. Thrombocytopenic purpura associated with ingestion of acetaminophen (Tylenol). *Cleve Clin Q.* 1973 Summer;40(2):89-91.
[147] Bougie D, Aster R. Immune thrombocytopenia resulting from sensitivity to metabolites of naproxen and acetaminophen. *Blood.* 2001 June 15, 2001;97(12):3846-50.
[148] Font J, Nomdedeu B, Martinez-Orozco F, Ingelmo M, Balcells A. Amegakaryocytic thrombocytopenia and an analgesic. *Ann Intern Med.* 1981 Dec;95(6):783.
[149] Risks of agranulocytosis and aplastic anemia. A first report of their relation to drug use with special reference to analgesics. The International Agranulocytosis and Aplastic Anemia Study. *JAMA.* 1986 Oct 3;256(13):1749-57.
[150] Mielke CH, Heiden D, Britten AF, Ramos J, Flavell P. Hemostasis, Antipyretics, and Mild Analgesics. *JAMA: The Journal of the American Medical Association.* 1976 February 9, 1976;235(6):613-6.
[151] Seymour RA, Williams FM, Oxley A, Ward A, Fearns M, Brighan K, et al. A comparative study of the effects of aspirin and paracetamol (acetaminophen) on platelet aggregation and bleeding time. *Eur J Clin Pharmacol.* 1984;26(5):567-71.
[152] Kasper CK, Rapaport SI. Bleeding times and platelet aggregation after analgesics in hemophilia. *Ann Intern Med.* 1972 Aug;77(2):189-93.
[153] Mielke CH, Jr. Comparative Effects of Aspirin and Acetaminophen on Hemostasis. Arch Intern Med. 1981 February 23, 1981;141(3):305-10.
[154] Temple AR, Benson GD, Zinsenheim JR, Schweinle JE. Multicenter, randomized, double-blind, active-controlled, parallel-group trial of the long-term (6-12 months)

safety of acetaminophen in adult patients with osteoarthritis. *Clin Ther.* 2006 Feb;28(2):222-35.

[155] Watkins PB, Kaplowitz N, Slattery JT, Colonese CR, Colucci SV, Stewart PW, et al. Aminotransferase elevations in healthy adults receiving 4 grams of acetaminophen daily: a randomized controlled trial. *JAMA.* 2006 Jul 5;296(1):87-93.

[156] Kuffner EK, Temple AR, Cooper KM, Baggish JS, Parenti DL. Retrospective analysis of transient elevations in alanine aminotransferase during long-term treatment with acetaminophen in osteoarthritis clinical trials. *Curr Med Res Opin.* 2006 Nov;22(11):2137-48.

[157] Chun LJ, Tong MJ, Busuttil RW, Hiatt JR. Acetaminophen hepatotoxicity and acute liver failure. *J Clin Gastroenterol.* 2009 Apr;43(4):342-9.

[158] Amar PJ, Schiff ER. Acetaminophen safety and hepatotoxicity--where do we go from here? *Expert Opin Drug Saf.* 2007 Jul;6(4):341-55.

[159] Hinson JA, Roberts DW, James LP. Mechanisms of acetaminophen-induced liver necrosis. *Handb Exp Pharmacol.* 2010(196):369-405.

[160] Larson AM. Acetaminophen hepatotoxicity. *Clin Liver Dis.* 2007 Aug;11(3):525-48, vi.

[161] Scialli AR, Ang R, Breitmeyer J, Royal MA. A review of the literature on the effects of acetaminophen on pregnancy outcome. *Reprod Toxicol.* 2010 Dec;30(4):495-507.

[162] Briggs G, Freeman R, Yaffe S. *Acetaminophen. Drugs in Pregnancy and Lactation. 7th ed.* Philadelphia, PA: Lippincott Williams and Wilkins; 2005.

[163] Rebordosa C, Kogevinas M, Horvath-Puho E, Norgard B, Morales M, Czeizel AE, et al. Acetaminophen use during pregnancy: effects on risk for congenital abnormalities. *Am J Obstet Gynecol.* 2008 Feb;198(2):178 e1-7.

[164] Murray TG, Stolley PD, Anthony JC, Schinnar R, Hepler-Smith E, Jeffreys JL. Epidemiologic study of regular analgesic use and end-stage renal disease. *Arch Intern Med.* 1983 Sep;143(9):1687-93.

[165] Perneger TV, Whelton PK, Klag MJ. Risk of kidney failure associated with the use of acetaminophen, aspirin, and nonsteroidal antiinflammatory drugs. *N Engl J Med.* 1994 Dec 22;331(25):1675-9.

[166] Sandler DP, Smith JC, Weinberg CR, Buckalew VM, Jr., Dennis VW, Blythe WB, et al. Analgesic use and chronic renal disease. *N Engl J Med.* 1989 May 11;320(19):1238-43.

[167] Edwards OM, Edwards P, Huskisson EC, Taylor RT. Paracetamol and renal damage. *Br Med J.* 1971 Apr 10;2(5753):87-9.

[168] Prescott LF, Mattison P, Menzies DG, Manson LM. The comparative effects of paracetamol and indomethacin on renal function in healthy female volunteers. *Br J Clin Pharmacol.* 1990 Apr;29(4):403-12.

[169] Cumberland Pharmaceuticals Inc. *Acetadote Prescribing Information.* Nashville, TN2011.

[170] US National Library of Medicine. Acetaminophen. Bethesda, MD: US National Library of Medicine; 2011 [October, 2011]; Available from: *http://www.ncbi.nlm.nih.gov/pubmedhealth/PMH0000521/.*

[171] Candiotti KA, Bergese SD, Viscusi ER, Singla SK, Royal MA, Singla NK. Safety of multiple-dose intravenous acetaminophen in adult inpatients. *Pain Med.* 2010 Dec;11(12):1841-8.

[172] Gregoire N, Hovsepian L, Gualano V, Evene E, Dufour G, Gendron A. Safety and pharmacokinetics of paracetamol following intravenous administration of 5 g during the first 24 h with a 2-g starting dose. *Clin Pharmacol Ther.* 2007 Mar;81(3):401-5.

In: Acetaminophen: Properties, Clinical Uses
Editors: Atash Javaherian and Pasha Latifpour
ISBN: 978-1-61942-374-9

Chapter 2

Clinical and Experimental Relevance of Hypothermia in Acetaminophen Hepatotoxicity

***José I. Fortea*[1], *Javier Vaquero*[1], *and Roger F. Butterworth*[2*]**

[1]Laboratorio de Investigación en Hepatología y Gastroenterología del Hospital Gregorio Marañón-CIBERehd, Madrid, Spain

[2]Neuroscience Research Unit, Hôpital Saint-Luc (CHUM), University of Montreal, Montreal, QC, Canada

Abstract

Acetaminophen (APAP) overdose frequently results in the development of severe liver injury in both humans and experimental animals. In humans, APAP-induced hepatotoxicity is currently the main cause of acute liver failure in the Western world. APAP-induced hepatotoxicity in the mouse is an extensively used experimental paradigm for dissecting the mechanisms of drug-induced liver injury. Even though a decrease of body temperature is a well-known effect of APAP, body temperature has rarely been measured in experimental studies of APAP-hepatotoxicity. Importantly, active maintenance of body temperature by external warming has been shown to decrease survival and to worsen the development of liver injury in the mouse with APAP-hepatotoxicity, suggesting that body temperature should be carefully monitored in order to adequately interpret results from this model. Induction of mild hypothermia is a potentially effective therapeutic approach for controlling episodes of intracranial hypertension in patients with APAP-induced acute liver failure.

* Correspondence:Roger F. Butterworth Ph.D., D.Sc., Neuroscience Research Unit, Hôpital Saint-Luc (C.H.U.M.), 1058 St. Denis street, Montreal, QC, H2X 3J4, Canada, Phone: 1-514-890 8000 (Ext. 35759), Fax: 1-514-412 7314, Email: roger.butterworth@umontreal.ca

1. Introduction

Acetaminophen (APAP) was first approved in the mid-50's as an analgesic and antipyretic medication (as Tylenol® in the US and as Panadol® in the United Kingdom). Its use, however, did not become widespread until the 80's, when several reports linking the ingestion of aspirin with Reye's syndrome promoted the use of APAP as a safer alternative (1). Since then, the number of cases of hepatotoxicity due to APAP has progressively increased becoming the most common cause of acute liver failure (ALF) in most countries of the Western world (2-4). The administration of APAP to a diversity of animal species is also a major experimental paradigm for investigating mechanisms of drug-induced liver injury. In these experimental animals, the administration of APAP may result in a frequently overlooked reduction of body temperature. The present manuscript reviews the relevance of the development of hypothermia in APAP hepatotoxicity from both clinical and experimental perspectives.

2. APAP-Induced Hepatotoxicity in Patients with ALF

ALF is a syndrome characterized by a rapid deterioration of liver function that results in coagulopathy and altered mentation in individuals without prior history of liver disease (5). In children, the definition of ALF is based mainly on the presence of coagulopathy secondary to liver failure, as encephalopathy may be absent or appear late in the course of the illness (4). Depending on the time between jaundice and encephalopathy, ALF may be subdivided into hyperacute (< 7 days), acute (7-21 days) or subacute (21 days to 26 weeks) (6, 7), with most of the cases of ALF due to APAP hepatotoxicity falling into the hyperacute category.

The incidence of ALF secondary to APAP overdose has progressively increased during the last 30 years, being currently the most frequent cause of ALF in the US and in many European countries. In a recent series from the US, APAP overdose accounts for 39% to 46% of all cases of ALF (4, 8). APAP intoxication also causes about 20% of pediatric cases of ALF in the US, a significant number considering that the cause of ALF remains unidentified in up to 50% of children (4, 9, 10). Several studies suggest that the importance of APAP as a cause of ALF is underestimated. For example, a sensitive assay was able to detect APAP-protein adducts in 19% of adult (11) and 12.5% of pediatric patients with ALF of indeterminate etiology (4, 12). The pattern of APAP ingestion leading to ALF differs among countries, with up to 92% of ALF due to APAP in England being associated with single overdoses in suicidal attempts (13) and as much as 61% of cases in the US being accidental overdoses usually following repeated ingestion of several medications containing APAP (8, 10). Encouraged by the successful reduction of APAP-induced ALF in the United Kingdom after the limitation in package size enacted by the UK Parliament in 1998 (14), the Food and Drug Administration (FDA) has considered several measures for reducing the cases of unintentional APAP overdose in the US, including explicit package warnings in APAP-containing medications and lowering the recommended therapeutic dose of APAP (1).

ALF due to APAP hepatotoxicity characteristically follows a hyperacute course that may be grossly divided into 4 phases (15). Patients initially present non-specific gastrointestinal symptoms such as anorexia, nausea, and vomiting (first 24 hours after APAP overdose), followed by a second phase (24 to 72 hours) during which symptoms may improve or disappear and biochemical abnormalities become evident. From 72 to 96 hours after the overdose, nausea and vomiting reappear together with malaise, jaundice, confusion, somnolence or coma. This phase usually corresponds to the peak of liver injury, and may be accompanied by other systemic complications such as renal failure, intracranial hypertension, and death. If the patient survives these first days, improvement of liver tests and resolution of liver damage may be seen starting 4 days after the APAP overdose.

The diagnosis of APAP hepatotoxicity is usually based on a compatible anamnesis, a detailed recollection of drug history, and laboratory testing. Characteristically, lactate dehydrogenase (LDH) and transaminases are highly elevated (AST > 10,000 IU/L, ALT > 1,000 IU/L), whereas the increase in bilirubin is generally mild. Coagulopathy, particularly the prolongation of prothrombin time, is considered the best indicator of liver damage. Common alterations that may also reflect the severity of damage include hypophosphatemia (16), hypoglycaemia and lactic acidosis (17, 18). The toxicity of APAP is dose-dependent, and the plasma levels of APAP in the first 24 hours after ingestion can be used to predict the probability of developing hepatotoxicity (Rumack-Matthew nomogram) (19). Plasma levels of APAP, however, are frequently undetectable by the time the patient seeks help.

Since the landmark study by Prescott and co-workers (20), the administration of N-acetylcysteine remains the antidote of choice for treating APAP overdose. If given early after the overdose, N-acetylcysteine may completely prevent the occurrence of hepatotoxicity (20, 21), but it also has beneficial effects when administered later in the course of the disease (22, 23). The oral and the intravenous routes of N-acetylcysteine administration appear to be equally effective (24).

The prognosis of ALF due to APAP overdose is better than that of ALF from other causes, with an overall mortality rate of 28% (4, 8). The development of brain edema leading to high intracranial pressure (ICP) and brain herniation is a major cause of death in these patients (25). The induction of mild hypothermia is attracting increasing attention for treating intracranial hypertension in patients with ALF, particularly those with episodes of high ICP that are refractory to conventional measures (26, 27).

3. APAP-Induced Hepatotoxicity in Experimental Models

Experimental animal models of ALF are important for increasing our understanding of pathophysiologic mechanisms and developing better therapies. Several requirements have been proposed for the ideal model of ALF, but none of the currently available models fulfils all criteria (28-30). Because of its clinical relevance, the minimal hazard to personnel and the dose-dependent production of liver injury, the administration of APAP to animals is frequently used for investigating mechanisms of drug-induced liver injury. APAP hepatotoxicity has been induced in a wide variety of species, including pigs, dogs, rabbits, hamsters, rats and mice (29, 30).

3.a. Determinants of APAP-Induced Hepatotoxicity in Experimental Animal Models

A wide range of APAP doses have been used in diverse species of experimental animals and even within the same species (from 150 mg/kg bw to more than 1000 mg/kg bw). A poor reproducibility together with a lack of a standard protocol determining the optimal drug dose, route of administration and monitoring measures are important caveats that complicate the interpretation of findings from experimental models of APAP hepatotoxicity (29, 30). In addition to inter-species differences, the sensitivity to APAP hepatotoxicity within a same species may be strain-dependent (31, 32). Gender and age are also known to influence the development of APAP hepatotoxicity in experimental animals (33, 34).

The hepatotoxicity of APAP largely relies on its biotransformation by cytochrome P450 to toxic and highly reactive metabolites, particularly N-acetyl-p-benzoquinone imine (NAPQI) (35, 36). Variations in APAP metabolism partially explain the poor reproducibility of this model (37). For example, the biotransformation of APAP is enhanced in hamsters and mice, species that are highly sensitive to APAP hepatotoxicity, compared with rats, rabbits or guinea pigs, species in which the metabolism of APAP is less active (37). Its biotransformation, however, is not the only determinant of the sensitivity to APAP, as young mice were noted to be more resistant to APAP hepatotoxicity than older mice despite showing an enhanced cytochrome P450 activity (33). The rate of detoxification of APAP and its metabolites is also an important determinant of hepatotoxicity, with hamsters presenting the slowest detoxification processes (37). In addition to the overall amount of toxic metabolites, variation in the pattern of proteins modified by APAP may also determine the degree of hepatotoxicity (38). In order to improve the reproducibility, the potentiation of APAP hepatotoxicity by the depletion of cellular glutathione levels (via fasting (39) or pharmacologically (40)) and/or by the induction of cytochrome P450 systems (41, 42) has been tested with variable success. The development of methemoglobinemia and refractory anemia, particularly in large animals, and the toxicity to other organs such as the kidney are additional problems associated with experimental models of APAP hepatotoxicity (29).

3.b. Histopathology

The main histological feature of APAP hepatotoxicity is the development of hepatocellular necrosis with a characteristic centrilobular distribution within the hepatic lobule (Figure 1) (43, 44). This histological appearance is similar across all animal species, including humans (40, 45). In mice, endocytic vacuolation along sinusoidal and lateral margins of centrilobular hepatocytes can be observed at light microscopy as early as 60-90 minutes after APAP overdose in mice (44). This early change is confirmed by electron microscopy, together with other fine alterations such as loss of microvilli from bile canaliculi and sinusoidal margins, dilation of bile canaliculi and endoplasmic reticulum, disaggregation of polyribosomes, and abnormal mitochondria. Endothelial cells lining the hepatic sinusoids are also early targets of APAP toxicity (46), and rapidly develop large pores with initial preservation of intercellular junctions (43). The severity of all these changes increases progressively, leading to enlargement of Disse space due to erythrocyte accumulation with subsequent sinusoidal collapse, centrilobular congestion and features of hepatocellular necrosis in the pericentral region by 3 hours after APAP overdose. Some hours later, bridges of hepatocellular necrosis between centrilobular areas may become apparent, with increased hemorrhagic congestion (43). Even though features of hepatocellular apoptosis can be observed, detailed studies show that oncotic necrosis is generally the predominant final mode of hepatocyte death (47, 48).

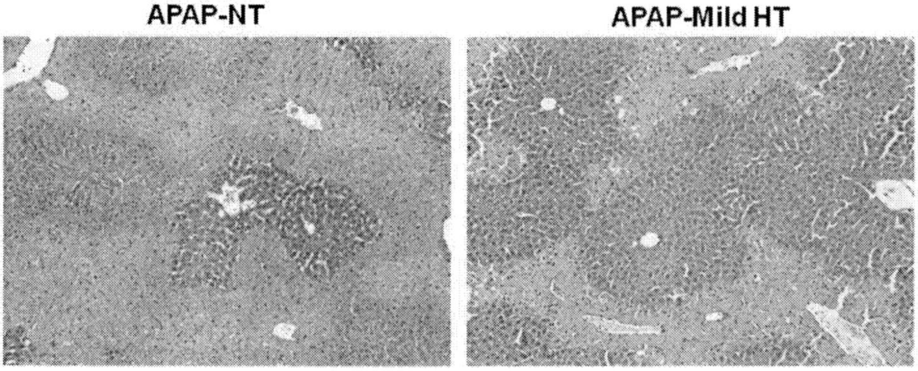

Figure 1. Representative sections of paraffin-embedded liver tissue from mice administered APAP (300 mg/kg bw i.p.) that were either maintained normothermic (APAP-NT, left panel) or allowed to develop mild hypothermia (APAP-Mild HT, right panel). Mice were euthanized 24 h after the administration of APAP. Mice maintained normothermic showed large areas of hepatocyte necrosis and haemorrhagic congestion in which only the hepatocytes closest to the portal areas of the hepatic lobule were spared. Mice allowed to develop mild hypothermia (32-35 °C) showed smaller areas of necrosis affecting the hepatocytes surrounding the central veins. Sections were stained with hematoxylin-phloxine-saffron and digitally captured at 100X magnification.

4. Mechanisms of APAP-Induced Liver Injury

APAP causes hepatotoxicity in a dose-dependent manner (49, 50). APAP-induced hepatotoxicity rarely appears with doses of APAP lower than 125-150 mg/Kg (15, 51), and in adults, ingestions leading to ALF rarely exceed 10 g/day (52). However, severe liver injury may occur even with doses below the maximum therapeutic dose (< 4 g/day) if there are concomitant risk factors such as chronic alcohol abuse, malnutrition, and/or concurrent use of drugs that induce cytochrome P450 (53).

The mechanisms of APAP hepatotoxicity have been investigated in various experimental models, but the mouse with APAP-induced hepatotoxicity has been the most frequently used. Under normal conditions, more than 90 % of APAP is detoxified in the liver by glucuronidation and sulfation (54, 55). Of the remaining APAP, about 2 % is excreted in the urine unchanged, and a small fraction of APAP (5 to 10 %) undergoes metabolism through cytochrome P-450 resulting in the formation of NAPQI, a highly reactive compound that is detoxified by conjugation with GSH (54, 56, 57). After an overdose, detoxification pathways may become saturated, diverting the metabolism of APAP to the cytochrome P450 pathway, thus increasing the production of NAPQI. The damage generally occurs when GSH levels fall below 20 % of normal (56), which results in NAPQI available to form covalent bonds with other intracellular proteins, modifying their structure and function. An early increase of cytosolic calcium (57) together with the modification of mitochondrial proteins are thought to depress mitochondrial respiration and adenosine triphosphate (ATP) synthesis (58) as well as to induce mitochondrial oxidative stress and increased production of peroxynitrite (46, 59), a potent oxidant and nitrating agent. Peroxynitrite and reactive oxygen species may induce the membrane permeability transition pore (60), causing the collapse of mitochondrial membrane potential, disruption of ATP synthesis, release of mitochondrial proteins into the cell cytoplasm, DNA damage and oncotic necrosis of hepatocytes (15, 59). Recent studies suggest that the activation of c-jun N-terminal kinase (JNK) is critical for the development of APAP hepatotoxicity (61, 62). The activation of JNK is thought to be mediated by the activation of apoptosis signal-regulated kinase 1 (ASK1), which results from its dissociation from thioredoxin in a process that involves oxidative stress induced by APAP (63). Other potential mechanisms implicated in APAP hepatotoxicity are: i) increased circulating catecholamines leading to compromised hepatic perfusion (64), ii) activation of the innate immune system, including natural killer and natural killer T cells (65), macrophages and neutrophils (66-68), although their role has been questioned and may be limited to aggravation of hepatotoxicity in certain circumstances (48, 69), and iii) toxicity to sinusoidal endothelial cells (SEC) leading to hepatic congestion. Overall, the majority of experimental evidence points toward intracellular signalling mechanisms in hepatocytes as the main cause of liver damage (59).

5. Body Temperature, APAP and the Liver

Together with its analgesic properties, the prevention and reduction of fever is one of the most common indications for the use of APAP. In addition, APAP is known to induce hypothermia in animals and, more rarely, in human beings. The mechanisms by which APAP exerts its antipyretic effects, and whether they are the same ones by which it induces hypothermia, have not been fully elucidated. Importantly, APAP is thought to potently inhibit cyclooxygenase (COX) activity and prostaglandin synthesis in the central nervous system, which is in contrast to its weak inhibitory effects on prostaglandin synthesis in the periphery (70). Indeed, the blood-brain barrier is permeable to APAP, and high levels of APAP occur in brain tissue soon after its oral administration in rodents (71, 72). In a recent study in mice, Ayoub et al. proposed that a decreased prostaglandin E2 production in the brain secondary to the inhibition of COX-3, a variant of the COX-1 gene (*Pghs1*), could be responsible for the antipyretic action of APAP (73), but a role of COX-3 could not be confirmed in a subsequent study using *Pghs1* deficient mice (74).

5.a. Reduction of Body Temperature Due to APAP in Humans

The reduction of body temperature by therapeutic doses of APAP has been anecdotally reported in adults and children (75, 76). Several studies have shown that the administration of a high (6 g/day) but not of a medium (3 g/day) dose of APAP is associated with small reductions (0.3 ºC to 0.4 ºC) of body temperature in patients with acute stroke, including those that were initially normothermic or subfebrile (77, 78). These studies suggest that APAP induces hypothermia in a dose-dependent manner in humans.

A reduction of body temperature could be a common feature in cases of APAP toxicity but body temperature has not been systematically documented in clinical studies of APAP hepatotoxicity and the development of hypothermia has only been reported anecdotally (79, 80). Noteworthy, body temperature at admission may not be representative because patients are likely to have undergone manouvers to preserve a normal body temperature (covering with blanket and others) by the time they are admitted to an intensive care unit. Block et al. reported a case of a 24 year-old female who was admitted to the emergency department in coma and profoundly hypothermic (19 °C) more than 18 hours after APAP (> 30 g) overdose (80). In this case, a low environmental temperature and ingestion of other drugs probably contributed to the induction of hypothermia. Interestingly, liver function tests always remained remarkably normal despite the enormous amount of APAP ingested, and the authors suggested that hypothermia could have prevented APAP hepatotoxicity.

5.b. Reduction of Body Temperature in Experimental Animal Models of Liver Injury

A reduction of body temperature may readily develop in experimental animal models of liver injury. This is not surprising since the liver plays an important role in normal thermoregulation as a major heat-producing organ as well as by providing metabolic substrates for other organs and tissues (81). Accordingly, the development of hypothermia is a major feature in surgical models involving hepatic devascularisation or total hepatectomy in small as well as in large animal species (82-84).

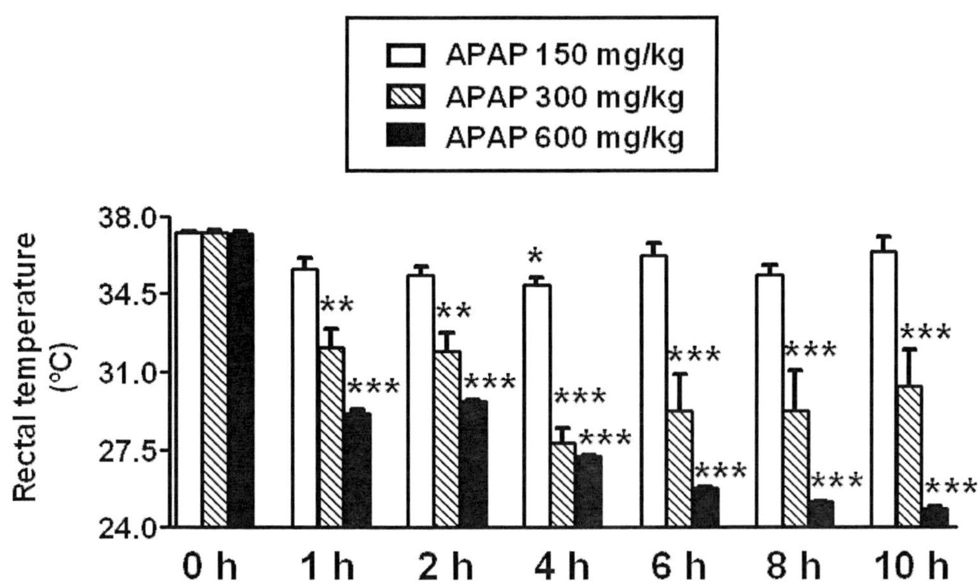

Figure 2. Effects of APAP administration on mouse body temperature. Male C57Bl6 mice (8-10 wk-old) received an i.p. injection of either 150 mg/kg bw, 300 mg/kg bw or 600 mg/kg bw of APAP. A thermometer was used to measure the rectal temperature at the indicated time points after the administration of APAP. * $p< 0.05$ vs. 0 h, ** $p< 0.01$ vs. 0 h, $p< 0.001$ vs. 0 h (Repeated measures ANOVA with Dunnett's multiple comparison test).

The development of hypothermia is a well-known phenomenon in rat and mouse models of APAP hepatotoxicity (39, 71, 85, 86). As discussed earlier, APAP is not commonly used in larger animals due to the development of methemoglobinemia, but APAP-induced hypothermia may also occur (87). In rats and mice, the reduction of body temperature occurs rapidly after APAP administration in a dose-dependent manner (Figure 2) (74, 88-90), and it seems dependent on APAP itself and not on its toxic metabolites (71). Even within mice receiving the same dose of APAP, body temperatures may differ by several deg.C (89). In addition to its pharmacological actions (71, 73), the effects of APAP on the body temperature of mice are strongly influenced by other common circumstances such as the restriction of food in the hours preceding the administration of APAP (39, 91), the inflammatory response (92), the development of liver injury, hepatic congestion and hypovolemia (93). External and technical factors, such as ambient temperature or the mode of drug administration, also influence thermoregulatory responses to APAP in mice (94). Despite its established role in multiple physiological and cellular processes, the monitoring and control of body temperature has been generally disregarded in the majority of published studies of rodent models of APAP hepatotoxicity, a factor that could seriously limit the interpretation of findings from these studies (89).

6. Relevance of Body Temperature for APAP-Induced ALF

From a clinical perspective, the induction of mild hypothermia may be a valuable approach for controlling brain edema and high ICP hypertension in APAP-induced ALF, particularly for bridging to liver transplantation in patients with ICP surges that cannot be controlled by conventional therapies (26, 27). In experimental ALF, the strict control of body temperature is important for the interpretation of studies investigating the cerebral complications of ALF (82) as well as for adequately evaluating mechanisms of APAP-induced liver injury or attributing effects to specific manipulations (95, 96).

6.1. Effects of Hypothermia on the Development of Brain Edema and Intracranial Hypertension in ALF

The development of brain edema and high ICP is a frequent complication in patients with ALF particularly in those with a short interval between the first symptoms and the appearance of hepatic encephalopathy, which is generally the case in APAP intoxication. Conventional therapies, such as osmotherapy, hyperventilation, sedating agents or hemofiltration, are initially able to control most episodes of high ICP, but relapses may occur in up to 80% of the cases, and brain herniation remains a major cause of death in ALF (97, 98). Several small clinical studies performed in patients with ALF suggest that the induction of hypothermia (32-34 ºC) is an effective approach for controlling episodes of high ICP that are refractory to conventional therapies (26, 27, 99). In the initial studies, early rewarming consistently resulted in a rapid rebound of uncontrolled intracranial hypertension and in the demise of the patients shortly thereafter (26). In contrast, ICP remained within normal values in the majority of patients (> 95%) in whom hypothermia was maintained until a donor organ was available and during liver transplantation (26, 27, 98). Occasional increases of ICP were observed in a few of these patients (~ 25%) during hypothermia, but they were generally controlled with additional boluses of mannitol. As a result, most patients were bridged to liver transplantation with global survival approaching 75%.

A number of studies have explored the mechanisms by which hypothermia prevents the cerebral complications of ALF, providing an ample rationale for its clinical use (100-102). The remarkable influence of the development of hypothermia for preventing or delaying brain edema and intracranial hypertension in experimental ALF was clearly shown in 1989 by Dr. Blei's group in a landmark study using rats with hepatic devascularisation (82). In particular, all rats that were allowed to become hypothermic showed a significant delay in the onset of encephalopathy and an abrogation of the increase in brain water content compared with rats that were maintained normothermic. This observation has consistently been confirmed in subsequent studies using both surgical and toxic models of ALF and hyperammonemia in rats and mice (83, 103-105). None of these studies was performed in APAP-treated animals, as brain edema and intracranial hypertension have not been consistently demonstrated in this experimental model. This is in contrast to clinical studies, in which most patients presented ALF secondary to APAP hepatotoxicity (26, 27, 99).

The efficacy of hypothermia for controlling the cerebral complications of ALF probably lies in its ability to influence many of the pathogenetic factors (reviewed in (100, 101)), particularly for decreasing the concentration of ammonia in blood and brain (27, 105, 106), and for reducing cerebral blood flow and preventing cerebral hyperemia (99, 104, 107). The attenuation of the alterations of brain glucose metabolism observed in ALF, particularly the increased glycolytic flux of glucose that results in increased de novo synthesis of brain lactate, is another major mechanism of hypothermia that may explain its beneficial effects (103, 108). Other major pathogenetic factors that are prevented or attenuated by hypothermia in ALF include the increase of glutamate and other amino acids in the brain extracellular fluid (83, 100), the increase of brain cytokine production and microglial activation (27, 109), the increase of pro-inflammatory cytokines in the systemic circulation (27, 109, 110), and the development of oxidative/nitrosative stress (110, 111). An increased synthesis of glutamine leading to an osmotic load inside astrocytes is a major event that has been proposed to drive the increase of brain water content in ALF and hyperammonemic conditions (112, 113). Despite ameliorating some of the alterations in other organic osmolytes such as myo-inositol and taurine, hypothermia has not been shown to prevent the accumulation of brain glutamine in rodent models of ALF or hyperammonemia (103, 104). The induction of hypothermia also corrected the altered expression of many different genes in the brains of animals with ALF, some of which are implicated in the pathogenesis of encephalopathy and brain edema in ALF such as the peripheral-type benzodiazepine receptor (114) or endothelial nitric oxide synthase (115).

6.2. Effects of Hypothermia on the Progression of Liver Injury

The hepato-protective effects of hypothermia against liver injury induced by ischemia/reperfusion have been consistently demonstrated in large- and small- animal models. In this condition, hypothermia decreases the metabolic demands of liver tissue during ischemia and attenuates the inflammatory cascade and free radical production during reperfusion which results in improved sinusoidal endothelial cell function, sinusoidal perfusion, and recovery of bile production, attenuates liver damage and improved survival (116-118).

The effects of hypothermia on liver injury induced by causes other than ischemia/reperfusion havenot received the same attention. Nonetheless a number of studies suggest that a reduction of body temperature strongly influences the progression of liver injury induced by APAP and other toxins. In a recent report (95), mice with APAP hepatotoxicity that were allowed to develop mild hypothermia (32-35 ºC) showed significantly increased survival and concomitant attenuation of liver damage compared with mice that were maintained normothermic (Figure 3). Importantly, hypothermia did not affect the bioactivation of APAP in this experimental preparation, as assessed by the amount of APAP-protein adducts and the depletion of glutathione in liver tissue. Potential hepato-protective mechanisms of hypothermia against APAP hepatotoxicity observed in this study included a significant attenuation of the hepatic hemorrhagic congestion and a rapid recovery of hepatic glycogen stores probably reflecting, respectively, improved preservation of hepatic microcirculation and reduction of energy demands from the liver itself as well as from peripheral tissues (95). Hypothermia also reduced the number of hepatocytes undergoing apoptosis, as assessed by terminal deoxynucleotidyl transferase-mediated deoxyuridine triphosphate nick-end labelling (TUNEL) staining and by the proteolytic processing of poly-(ADP-ribose) polymerase. This observation is in accordance with the suppression of apoptosis mediated by mild hypothermia (32 ºC) in primary cultures of mouse hepatocytes exposed to diverse apoptotic stimuli, including agonistic Fas antibodies (119). Interestingly, mild hypothermia suppressed cytochrome C release and caspase-9 activation, but not caspase-8 activation or Bid cleavage, pointing to mitochondria as a major site of hypothermia's anti-apoptotic effects.

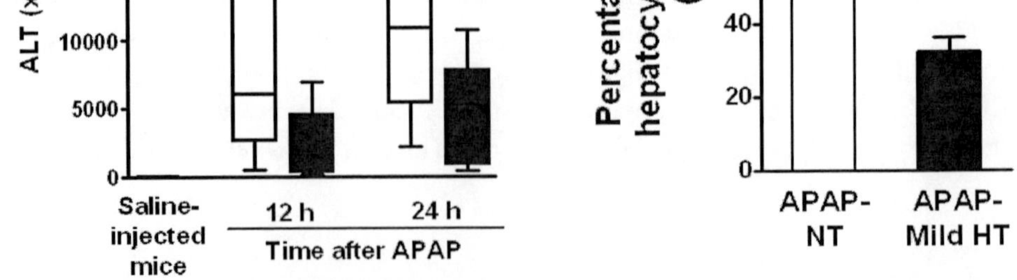

Figure 3. Effect of hypothermia on liver injury in mice with APAP hepatotoxicity, assessed by A) the plasma ALT level and B) the extent of hepatocyte necrosis in paraffin-embedded liver sections stained with hematoxylin-phloxine-saffron. Male C57Bl6 mice received an injection of saline or APAP (300 mg/kg bw i.p.) and were either maintained normothermic by external warming (APAP-NT) or allowed to develop a mild degree of hypothermia (32-35 ºC), being euthanized 24 h after the administration of APAP. * $p < 0.05$ NT vs. Mild-HT, ** $p < 0.01$ NT vs. Mild-HT.

Studies investigating mechanisms of liver injury should also take into account the effects that specific interventions may have on the body temperature of experimental animals. For example, the protection afforded by trifluoroperazine against APAP hepatotoxicity in mice has been attributed to the enhancement of hypothermia and not to specific pharmacological actions of the drug (96). Similarly, mild decreases of body temperature have been reported in rats with acute liver injury induced by carbon tetrachloride (CCl_4). In these rats, spinal cord transection and the administration of chlorpromazine were interventions that attenuated CCl_4-induced liver injury, but they were also shown to induce profound hypothermia and to reduce the bioactivation of CCl_4 (120, 121). Remarkably, the hepato-protective effects of these interventions were lost when the animals were maintained normothermic.

Conclusions

APAP hepatotoxicity is a major cause of ALF in many developed countries and serves as one of the experimental models most frequently used for studying mechanisms of acute liver injury and its complications. The administration of APAP induces variable reductions of body temperature in a dose-dependent manner in rodents, but reports examining the spontaneous evolution of body temperature in patients with APAP hepatotoxicity are scarce. In patients with ALF, including those secondary to APAP intoxication, the induction of mild hypothermia affords a potentially promising new therapy for controlling brain edema and intracranial hypertension refractory to conventional measures.

In rodent models of APAP hepatotoxicity, the development of hypothermia significantly influences survival and the degree of liver injury and, therefore, body temperature should be strictly controlled in experimental studies of APAP hepatotoxicity for an adequate interpretation of results. This observation also suggests that the benefits of mild hypothermia in ALF may not be limited to its effects on the brain. Further studies of the effects of hypothermia on APAP hepatotoxicity are both scientifically and clinically warranted.

References

[1] Lee WM. Acetaminophen toxicity: changing perceptions on a social/medical issue. *Hepatology* 2007;46:966-970.

[2] Larsen FS, Kirkegaard P, Rasmussen A, Hansen BA. The Danish liver transplantation program and patients with serious acetaminophen intoxication. *Transplant Proc* 1995;27:3519-3520.

[3] Bernal W. Changing patterns of causation and the use of transplantation in the United kingdom. *Semin Liver Dis* 2003;23:227-237.

[4] Lee WM, Squires RH, Jr., Nyberg SL, Doo E, Hoofnagle JH. Acute liver failure: Summary of a workshop. *Hepatology* 2008;47:1401-1415.

[5] Trey C, Davidson CS. The management of fulminant hepatic failure. *Prog Liver Dis* 1970;3:282-298.

[6] Bernuau J, Rueff B, Benhamou JP. Fulminant and subfulminant liver failure: definitions and causes. *Semin Liver Dis* 1986;6:97-106.

[7] O'Grady JG, Schalm SW, Williams R. Acute liver failure: redefining the syndromes. *Lancet* 1993;342:273-275.

[8] Ostapowicz G, Fontana RJ, Schiodt FV, Larson A, Davern TJ, Han SH, McCashland TM, et al. Results of a prospective study of acute liver failure at 17 tertiary care centers in the United States. *Ann Intern Med* 2002;137:947-954.

[9] Squires RH, Jr., Shneider BL, Bucuvalas J, Alonso E, Sokol RJ, Narkewicz MR, Dhawan A, et al. Acute liver failure in children: the first 348 patients in the pediatric acute liver failure study group. *J Pediatr* 2006;148:652-658.

[10] Bower WA, Johns M, Margolis HS, Williams IT, Bell BP. Population-based surveillance for acute liver failure. *Am J Gastroenterol* 2007;102:2459-2463.

[11] Davern TJ, 2nd, James LP, Hinson JA, Polson J, Larson AM, Fontana RJ, Lalani E, et al. Measurement of serum acetaminophen-protein adducts in patients with acute liver failure. *Gastroenterology* 2006;130:687-694.

[12] James LP, Alonso EM, Hynan LS, Hinson JA, Davern TJ, Lee WM, Squires RH, et al. Detection of acetaminophen protein adducts in children with acute liver failure of indeterminate cause. *Pediatrics* 2006;118:e676-681.

[13] Makin AJ, Wendon J, Williams R. A 7-year experience of severe acetaminophen-induced hepatotoxicity (1987-1993). *Gastroenterology* 1995;109:1907-1916.

[14] Bernal W, Auzinger G, Dhawan A, Wendon J. Acute liver failure. *Lancet* 2010;376:190-201.

[15] Chun LJ, Tong MJ, Busuttil RW, Hiatt JR. Acetaminophen hepatotoxicity and acute liver failure. *J Clin Gastroenterol* 2009;43:342-349.

[16] Jones AF, Harvey JM, Vale JA. Hypophosphataemia and phosphaturia in paracetamol poisoning. *Lancet* 1989;2:608-609.

[17] O'Grady JG, Alexander GJ, Hayllar KM, Williams R. Early indicators of prognosis in fulminant hepatic failure. *Gastroenterology* 1989;97:439-445.

[18] Bernal W, Donaldson N, Wyncoll D, Wendon J. Blood lactate as an early predictor of outcome in paracetamol-induced acute liver failure: a cohort study. *Lancet* 2002;359:558-563.

[19] Rumack BH, Matthew H. Acetaminophen poisoning and toxicity. *Pediatrics* 1975;55:871-876.

[20] Prescott LF, Illingworth RN, Critchley JA, Stewart MJ, Adam RD, Proudfoot AT. Intravenous N-acetylcysteine: the treatment of choice for paracetamol poisoning. *Br Med J* 1979;2:1097-1100.

[21] Rumack BH, Peterson RC, Koch GG, Amara IA. Acetaminophen overdose. 662 cases with evaluation of oral acetylcysteine treatment. *Arch Intern Med* 1981;141:380-385.

[22] Harrison PM, Keays R, Bray GP, Alexander GJ, Williams R. Improved outcome of paracetamol-induced fulminant hepatic failure by late administration of acetylcysteine. *Lancet* 1990;335:1572-1573.

[23] Keays R, Harrison PM, Wendon JA, Forbes A, Gove C, Alexander GJ, Williams R. Intravenous acetylcysteine in paracetamol induced fulminant hepatic failure: a prospective controlled trial. *Bmj* 1991;303:1026-1029.

[24] Brok J, Buckley N, Gluud C. Interventions for paracetamol (acetaminophen) overdose. *Cochrane Database Syst Rev* 2006:CD003328.

[25] Ware AJ, D'Agostino AN, Combes B. Cerebral edema: a major complication of massive hepatic necrosis. *Gastroenterology* 1971;61:877-884.

[26] Jalan R, Damink SW, Deutz NE, Lee A, Hayes PC. Moderate hypothermia for uncontrolled intracranial hypertension in acute liver failure. *Lancet* 1999;354:1164-1168.

[27] Jalan R, Olde Damink SW, Deutz NE, Hayes PC, Lee A. Moderate hypothermia in patients with acute liver failure and uncontrolled intracranial hypertension. *Gastroenterology* 2004;127:1338-1346.

[28] Terblanche J, Hickman R. Animal models of fulminant hepatic failure. *Dig Dis Sci* 1991;36:770-774.

[29] Newsome PN, Plevris JN, Nelson LJ, Hayes PC. Animal models of fulminant hepatic failure: a critical evaluation. *Liver Transpl* 2000;6:21-31.

[30] Belanger M, Butterworth RF. Acute liver failure: a critical appraisal of available animal models. *Metab Brain Dis* 2005;20:409-423.

[31] Casley WL, Menzies JA, Girard M, Larocque L, Mousseau N, Whitehouse LW, Moon TW. Differences in caffeine 3-demethylation activity among inbred mouse strains: a comparison of hepatic Cyp1a2 gene expression between two inbred strains. *Fundam Appl Toxicol* 1997;40:228-237.

[32] DeLeve LD, Wang X, Kaplowitz N, Shulman HM, Bart JA, van der Hoek A. Sinusoidal endothelial cells as a target for acetaminophen toxicity. Direct action versus requirement for hepatocyte activation in different mouse strains. *Biochem Pharmacol* 1997;53:1339-1345.

[33] Adamson GM, Papadimitriou JM, Harman AW. Postnatal mice have low susceptibility to paracetamol toxicity. *Pediatr Res* 1991;29:496-499.

[34] Tarloff JB, Khairallah EA, Cohen SD, Goldstein RS. Sex- and age-dependent acetaminophen hepato- and nephrotoxicity in Sprague-Dawley rats: role of tissue accumulation, nonprotein sulfhydryl depletion, and covalent binding. *Fundam Appl Toxicol* 1996;30:13-22.

[35] Dahlin DC, Miwa GT, Lu AY, Nelson SD. N-acetyl-p-benzoquinone imine: a cytochrome P-450-mediated oxidation product of acetaminophen. *Proc Natl Acad Sci U S A* 1984;81:1327-1331.

[36] Lee SS, Buters JT, Pineau T, Fernandez-Salguero P, Gonzalez FJ. Role of CYP2E1 in the hepatotoxicity of acetaminophen. *J Biol Chem* 1996;271:12063-12067.

[37] Gregus Z, Madhu C, Klaassen CD. Species variation in toxication and detoxication of acetaminophen in vivo: a comparative study of biliary and urinary excretion of acetaminophen metabolites. *J Pharmacol Exp Ther* 1988;244:91-99.

[38] Beierschmitt WP, Brady JT, Bartolone JB, Wyand DS, Khairallah EA, Cohen SD. Selective protein arylation and the age dependency of acetaminophen hepatotoxicity in mice. *Toxicol Appl Pharmacol* 1989;98:517-529.

[39] Walker RM, Massey TE, McElligott TF, Racz WJ. Acetaminophen toxicity in fed and fasted mice. *Can J Physiol Pharmacol* 1982;60:399-404.

[40] Kelly JH, Koussayer T, He DE, Chong MG, Shang TA, Whisennand HH, Sussman NL. An improved model of acetaminophen-induced fulminant hepatic failure in dogs. *Hepatology* 1992;15:329-335.

[41] Miller DJ, Hickman R, Fratter R, Terblanche J, Saunders SJ. An animal model of fulminant hepatic failure: a feasibility study. *Gastroenterology* 1976;71:109-113.

[42] Rahman TM, Selden AC, Hodgson HJ. A novel model of acetaminophen-induced acute hepatic failure in rabbits. *J Surg Res* 2002;106:264-272.

[43] Walker RM, Racz WJ, McElligott TF. Acetaminophen-induced hepatotoxicity in mice. *Lab Invest* 1980;42:181-189.

[44] Walker RM, Racz WJ, McElligott TF. Scanning electron microscopic examination of acetaminophen-induced hepatotoxicity and congestion in mice. *Am J Pathol* 1983;113:321-330.

[45] Portmann B, Talbot IC, Day DW, Davidson AR, Murray-Lyon IM, Williams R. Histopathological changes in the liver following a paracetamol overdose: correlation with clinical and biochemical parameters. *J Pathol* 1975;117:169-181.

[46] Knight TR, Kurtz A, Bajt ML, Hinson JA, Jaeschke H. Vascular and hepatocellular peroxynitrite formation during acetaminophen toxicity: role of mitochondrial oxidant stress. *Toxicol Sci* 2001;62:212-220.

[47] Gujral JS, Knight TR, Farhood A, Bajt ML, Jaeschke H. Mode of cell death after acetaminophen overdose in mice: apoptosis or oncotic necrosis? *Toxicol Sci* 2002;67:322-328.

[48] Jaeschke H. Innate immunity and acetaminophen-induced liver injury: why so many controversies? *Hepatology* 2008;48:699-701.

[49] Henne-Bruns D, Artwohl J, Broelsch C, Kremer B. Acetaminophen-induced acute hepatic failure in pigs: controversical results to other animal models. *Res Exp Med* (Berl) 1988;188:463-472.

[50] Kofman AV, Morgan G, Kirschenbaum A, Osbeck J, Hussain M, Swenson S, Theise ND. Dose- and time-dependent oval cell reaction in acetaminophen-induced murine liver injury. *Hepatology* 2005;41:1252-1261.

[51] Makin AJ, Williams R. Acetaminophen-induced hepatotoxicity: predisposing factors and treatments. *Adv Intern Med* 1997;42:453-483.

[52] Schiodt FV, Rochling FA, Casey DL, Lee WM. Acetaminophen toxicity in an urban county hospital. *N Engl J Med* 1997;337:1112-1117.

[53] Larson AM, Polson J, Fontana RJ, Davern TJ, Lalani E, Hynan LS, Reisch JS, et al. Acetaminophen-induced acute liver failure: results of a United States multicenter, prospective study. *Hepatology* 2005;42:1364-1372.

[54] Nelson SD. Molecular mechanisms of the hepatotoxicity caused by acetaminophen. *Semin Liver Dis* 1990;10:267-278.

[55] Larson AM. Acetaminophen hepatotoxicity. *Clin Liver Dis* 2007;11:525-548, vi.

[56] Mitchell JR, Jollow DJ, Potter WZ, Gillette JR, Brodie BB. Acetaminophen-induced hepatic necrosis. IV. Protective role of glutathione. *J Pharmacol Exp Ther* 1973;187:211-217.

[57] Ray SD, Kamendulis LM, Gurule MW, Yorkin RD, Corcoran GB. Ca2+ antagonists inhibit DNA fragmentation and toxic cell death induced by acetaminophen. *Faseb J* 1993;7:453-463.

[58] Meyers LL, Beierschmitt WP, Khairallah EA, Cohen SD. Acetaminophen-induced inhibition of hepatic mitochondrial respiration in mice. *Toxicol Appl Pharmacol* 1988;93:378-387.

[59] Jaeschke H, Bajt ML. Intracellular signaling mechanisms of acetaminophen-induced liver cell death. *Toxicol Sci* 2006;89:31-41.

[60] Masubuchi Y, Suda C, Horie T. Involvement of mitochondrial permeability transition in acetaminophen-induced liver injury in mice. *J Hepatol* 2005;42:110-116.

[61] Gunawan BK, Liu ZX, Han D, Hanawa N, Gaarde WA, Kaplowitz N. c-Jun N-terminal kinase plays a major role in murine acetaminophen hepatotoxicity. *Gastroenterology* 2006;131:165-178.

[62] Henderson NC, Pollock KJ, Frew J, Mackinnon AC, Flavell RA, Davis RJ, Sethi T, et al. Critical role of c-jun (NH2) terminal kinase in paracetamol- induced acute liver failure. *Gut* 2007;56:982-990.

[63] Nakagawa H, Maeda S, Hikiba Y, Ohmae T, Shibata W, Yanai A, Sakamoto K, et al. Deletion of apoptosis signal-regulating kinase 1 attenuates acetaminophen-induced liver injury by inhibiting c-Jun N-terminal kinase activation. *Gastroenterology* 2008;135:1311-1321.

[64] Randle LE, Sathish JG, Kitteringham NR, Macdonald I, Williams DP, Park BK. alpha(1)-Adrenoceptor antagonists prevent paracetamol-induced hepatotoxicity in mice. *Br J Pharmacol* 2008;153:820-830.

[65] Liu ZX, Govindarajan S, Kaplowitz N. Innate immune system plays a critical role in determining the progression and severity of acetaminophen hepatotoxicity. *Gastroenterology* 2004;127:1760-1774.

[66] Laskin DL, Gardner CR, Price VF, Jollow DJ. Modulation of macrophage functioning abrogates the acute hepatotoxicity of acetaminophen. *Hepatology* 1995;21:1045-1050.

[67] Michael SL, Pumford NR, Mayeux PR, Niesman MR, Hinson JA. Pretreatment of mice with macrophage inactivators decreases acetaminophen hepatotoxicity and the formation of reactive oxygen and nitrogen species. *Hepatology* 1999;30:186-195.

[68] Liu ZX, Han D, Gunawan B, Kaplowitz N. Neutrophil depletion protects against murine acetaminophen hepatotoxicity. *Hepatology* 2006;43:1220-1230.

[69] Masson MJ, Carpenter LD, Graf ML, Pohl LR. Pathogenic role of natural killer T and natural killer cells in acetaminophen-induced liver injury in mice is dependent on the presence of dimethyl sulfoxide. *Hepatology* 2008;48:889-897.

[70] Clissold SP. Paracetamol and phenacetin. *Drugs* 1986;32 Suppl 4:46-59.

[71] Massey TE, Walker RM, McElligott TF, Racz WJ. Acetaminophen-induced hypothermia in mice: evidence for a central action of the parent compound. *Toxicology* 1982;25:187-200.

[72] Courad JP, Besse D, Delchambre C, Hanoun N, Hamon M, Eschalier A, Caussade F, et al. Acetaminophen distribution in the rat central nervous system. *Life Sci* 2001;69:1455-1464.

[73] Ayoub SS, Botting RM, Goorha S, Colville-Nash PR, Willoughby DA, Ballou LR. Acetaminophen-induced hypothermia in mice is mediated by a prostaglandin endoperoxide synthase 1 gene-derived protein. *Proc Natl Acad Sci U S A* 2004;101:11165-11169.

[74] Li S, Dou W, Tang Y, Goorha S, Ballou LR, Blatteis CM. Acetaminophen: antipyretic or hypothermic in mice? In either case, PGHS-1b (COX-3) is irrelevant. *Prostaglandins Other Lipid Mediat* 2008;85:89-99.

[75] Van Tittelboom T, Govaerts-Lepicard M. Hypothermia: an unusual side effect of paracetamol. *Vet Hum Toxicol* 1989;31:57-59.

[76] Denes E, Amaniou M, Rogez JP, Weinbreck P, Merle L. [Acetaminophen-induced hypothermia, an AIDS related side-effect? About 4 cases*]. Ann Med Interne* (Paris) 2002;153:411-413.

[77] Dippel DW, van Breda EJ, van Gemert HM, van der Worp HB, Meijer RJ, Kappelle LJ, Koudstaal PJ. Effect of paracetamol (acetaminophen) on body temperature in acute ischemic stroke: a double-blind, randomized phase II clinical trial. *Stroke* 2001;32:1607-1612.
[78] Dippel DW, van Breda EJ, van der Worp HB, van Gemert HM, Kappelle LJ, Algra A, Koudstaal PJ. Timing of the effect of acetaminophen on body temperature in patients with acute ischemic stroke. *Neurology* 2003;61:677-679.
[79] Lieh-Lai MW, Sarnaik AP, Newton JF, Miceli JN, Fleischmann LE, Hook JB, Kauffman RE. Metabolism and pharmacokinetics of acetaminophen in a severely poisoned young child. *J Pediatr* 1984;105:125-128.
[80] Block R, Jankowski JA, Lacoux P, Pennington CR. Does hypothermia protect against the development of hepatitis in paracetamol overdose? *Anaesthesia* 1992;47:789-791.
[81] Stoner HB. The role of the liver in non-shivering thermogenesis in the rat. *J Physiol* 1973;232:285-296.
[82] Traber P, DalCanto M, Ganger D, Blei AT. Effect of body temperature on brain edema and encephalopathy in the rat after hepatic devascularization. *Gastroenterology* 1989;96:885-891.
[83] Rose C, Michalak A, Pannunzio M, Chatauret N, Rambaldi A, Butterworth RF. Mild hypothermia delays the onset of coma and prevents brain edema and extracellular brain glutamate accumulation in rats with acute liver failure. *Hepatology* 2000;31:872-877.
[84] Arkadopoulos N, Chen SC, Khalili TM, Detry O, Hewitt WR, Lilja H, Kamachi H, et al. Transplantation of hepatocytes for prevention of intracranial hypertension in pigs with ischemic liver failure. *Cell Transplant* 1998;7:357-363.
[85] Walker RM, Massey TE, McElligott TF, Racz WJ. Acetaminophen-induced hypothermia, hepatic congestion, and modification by N-acetylcysteine in mice. *Toxicol Appl Pharmacol* 1981;59:500-507.
[86] Briyal S, Gulati A. Endothelin-A receptor antagonist BQ123 potentiates acetaminophen induced hypothermia and reduces infarction following focal cerebral ischemia in rats. *Eur J Pharmacol* 2010;644:73-79.
[87] Anvik JO. Acetaminophen toxicosis in a cat. Can Vet J 1984;25:445-447.
[88] Stolar MH, Siegel F, Morris RW. Influence of dosage form on antipyretic activity of acetaminophen administered intraperitoneally in the rat. *J Pharm Sci* 1973;62:338-339.
[89] Vaquero J, Belanger M, Blei AT, Butterworth RF. Lack of assessment of body temperature in mice with acetaminophen toxicity. *Hepatology* 2006;44:279-280.
[90] Corley G, Rawls SM. Opioid, cannabinoid CB1 and NOP receptors do not mediate APAP-induced hypothermia in rats. *Pharmacol Biochem Behav* 2009;92:503-507.
[91] Kersten S, Seydoux J, Peters JM, Gonzalez FJ, Desvergne B, Wahli W. Peroxisome proliferator-activated receptor alpha mediates the adaptive response to fasting. *J Clin Invest* 1999;103:1489-1498.
[92] Blazka ME, Wilmer JL, Holladay SD, Wilson RE, Luster MI. Role of proinflammatory cytokines in acetaminophen hepatotoxicity. *Toxicol Appl Pharmacol* 1995;133:43-52.
[93] Walker RM, Racz WJ, McElligott TF. Acetaminophen-induced hepatotoxic congestion in mice. *Hepatology* 1985;5:233-240.
[94] Rudaya AY, Steiner AA, Robbins JR, Dragic AS, Romanovsky AA. Thermoregulatory responses to lipopolysaccharide in the mouse: dependence on the dose and ambient temperature. *Am J Physiol Regul Integr Comp Physiol* 2005;289:R1244-1252.

[95] Vaquero J, Belanger M, James L, Herrero R, Desjardins P, Cote J, Blei AT, et al. Mild hypothermia attenuates liver injury and improves survival in mice with acetaminophen toxicity. *Gastroenterology* 2007;132:372-383.
[96] Yamamoto H. Antagonism of acetaminophen-induced hepatocellular destruction by trifluoperazine in mice. *Pharmacol Toxicol* 1990;67:115-119.
[97] Hoofnagle JH, Carithers RL, Jr., Shapiro C, Ascher N. Fulminant hepatic failure: summary of a workshop. *Hepatology* 1995;21:240-252.
[98] Jalan R. Intracranial hypertension in acute liver failure: pathophysiological basis of rational management. *Semin Liver Dis* 2003;23:271-282.
[99] Jalan R, Olde Damink SW, Deutz NE, Davies NA, Garden OJ, Madhavan KK, Hayes PC, et al. Moderate hypothermia prevents cerebral hyperemia and increase in intracranial pressure in patients undergoing liver transplantation for acute liver failure. *Transplantation* 2003;75:2034-2039.
[100] Vaquero J, Rose C, Butterworth RF. Keeping cool in acute liver failure: rationale for the use of mild hypothermia. *J Hepatol* 2005;43:1067-1077.
[101] Jalan R, Rose C. Hypothermia in acute liver failure. *Metab Brain Dis* 2004;19:215-221.
[102] Vaquero J, Blei AT. Cooling the patient with acute liver failure. *Gastroenterology* 2004;127:1626-1629.
[103] Chatauret N, Zwingmann C, Rose C, Leibfritz D, Butterworth RF. Effects of hypothermia on brain glucose metabolism in acute liver failure: a H/C-nuclear magnetic resonance study. *Gastroenterology* 2003;125:815-824.
[104] Cordoba J, Crespin J, Gottstein J, Blei AT. Mild hypothermia modifies ammonia-induced brain edema in rats after portacaval anastomosis. *Gastroenterology* 1999;116:686-693.
[105] Belanger M, Cote J, Butterworth RF. Neurobiological characterization of an azoxymethane mouse model of acute liver failure. *Neurochem Int* 2006;48:434-440.
[106] Schenker S, Warren KS. Effect of temperature variation on toxicity and metabolism of ammonia in mice. *J Lab Clin Med* 1962;60:291-301.
[107] Jalan R, Olde Damink SW, Deutz NE, Hayes PC, Lee A. Restoration of cerebral blood flow autoregulation and reactivity to carbon dioxide in acute liver failure by moderate hypothermia. *Hepatology* 2001;34:50-54.
[108] Chatauret N, Rose C, Therrien G, Butterworth RF. Mild hypothermia prevents cerebral edema and CSF lactate accumulation in acute liver failure. *Metab Brain Dis* 2001;16:95-102.
[109] Jiang W, Desjardins P, Butterworth RF. Direct evidence for central proinflammatory mechanisms in rats with experimental acute liver failure: protective effect of hypothermia. *J Cereb Blood Flow Metab* 2009;29:944-952.
[110] Bemeur C, Desjardins P, Butterworth RF. Antioxidant and anti-inflammatory effects of mild hypothermia in the attenuation of liver injury due to azoxymethane toxicity in the mouse. *Metab Brain Dis* 2010;25:23-29.
[111] Jiang W, Desjardins P, Butterworth RF. Hypothermia attenuates oxidative/nitrosative stress, encephalopathy and brain edema in acute (ischemic) liver failure. *Neurochem Int* 2009;55:124-128.
[112] Swain M, Butterworth RF, Blei AT. Ammonia and related amino acids in the pathogenesis of brain edema in acute ischemic liver failure in rats. *Hepatology* 1992;15:449-453.

[113] Takahashi H, Koehler RC, Brusilow SW, Traystman RJ. Inhibition of brain glutamine accumulation prevents cerebral edema in hyperammonemic rats. *Am J Physiol* 1991;261:H825-829.

[114] Belanger M, Desjardins P, Chatauret N, Rose C, Butterworth RF. Mild hypothermia prevents brain edema and attenuates up-regulation of the astrocytic benzodiazepine receptor in experimental acute liver failure. *J Hepatol* 2005;42:694-699.

[115] Sawara K, Desjardins P, Chatauret N, Kato A, Suzuki K, Butterworth RF. Alterations in expression of genes coding for proteins of the neurovascular unit in ischemic liver failure. *Neurochem Int* 2009;55:119-123.

[116] Biberthaler P, Luchting B, Massberg S, Teupser D, Langer S, Leiderer R, Messmer K, et al. The influence of organ temperature on hepatic ischemia-reperfusion injury: a systematic analysis. *Transplantation* 2001;72:1486-1490.

[117] Kato A, Singh S, McLeish KR, Edwards MJ, Lentsch AB. Mechanisms of hypothermic protection against ischemic liver injury in mice. *Am J Physiol Gastrointest Liver Physiol* 2002;282:G608-616.

[118] Heijnen BH, Straatsburg IH, Gouma DJ, van Gulik TM. Decrease in core liver temperature with 10 degrees C by in situ hypothermic perfusion under total hepatic vascular exclusion reduces liver ischemia and reperfusion injury during partial hepatectomy in pigs. *Surgery* 2003;134:806-817.

[119] Fu T, Blei AT, Takamura N, Lin T, Guo D, Li H, O'Gorman MR, et al. Hypothermia inhibits Fas-mediated apoptosis of primary mouse hepatocytes in culture. *Cell Transplant* 2004;13:667-676.

[120] Larson RE, Plaa GL, Crews LM. The Effect of Spinal Cord Transection on Carbon Tetrachloride Hepatotoxicity. *Toxicol Appl Pharmacol* 1964;103:154-162.

[121] Marzi A, de Toranzo EG, Castro JA. Mechanism of chlorpromazine prevention of carbon tetrachloride-induced liver necrosis. *Toxicol Appl Pharmacol* 1980;52:82-88.

In: Acetaminophen: Properties, Clinical Uses
Editors: Atash Javaherian and Pasha Latifpour
ISBN: 978-1-61942-374-9

Chapter 3

NOVEL APPLICATIONS OF ACETAMINOPHEN

Eric R. Blough1,2,3,4,5 and Miaozong Wu[1,2,3,6,*]
[1]Center for Diagnostic Nanosystems
[2]Department of Biological Sciences
[3]Department of Exercise Science, Sport and Recreation,
College of Education and Human Services
[4]Department of Pharmacology, Physiology and Toxicology
[5]Department of Cardiology
[6]Department of Internal Medicine, Joan C. Edwards School of Medicine,
Marshall University, Huntington, WV, US

ABSTRACT

Acetaminophen (N-Acetyl-4-aminophenol), also known as APAP or paracetamol, is one of the most widely used analgesics (pain reliever) and antipyretics (fever reducer). According to the U.S. Food and Drug Administration (FDA), currently there are 221 approved prescription and over-the-counter drug products containing acetaminophen as an active ingredient. When used as directed, acetaminophen is very safe and effective; however when taken in excess or ingested with alcohol hepatotoxicity and irreversible liver damage can arise. In addition to well-known clinical application as pain relief and fever reduction, recent laboratory and pre-clinical studies have demonstrated that acetaminophen may also have beneficial effects on blood glucose control, skeletal muscle function, and potential use as cardioprotective and neuroprotective agents. Extensive laboratory and pre-clinical studies have revealed that these off-label applications may be derived from the ability of acetaminophen to function as an antioxidant. Using our recent work as a reference point (Blough ER and Wu M. (2011). Acetaminophen: beyond pain and fever-relieving. Front Pharmacol. 2:72. Doi:10.3389/fphar.2011.00072), herein, we will highlight these novel applications of acetaminophen, and attempt, where possible, to highlight how these findings may lead to new directions of inquiry and clinical relevance of other disorders.

---

* Correspondence: Dr. Miaozong Wu - Translational Research Division, Center for Diagnostic Nanosystems, Marshall University, Rm. 217 BBSC, 1700 3rd Avenue, Huntington, WV, USA 25755. E-mail: wum@marshall.edu.

Keywords: Acetaminophen; antioxidant; hyperglycemia; skeletal muscle; cardiac protection

INTRODUCTION

Acetaminophen also known as "APAP" or "paracetamol" is one of the most widely used medicines in the United States. According to the data from IMS Health, ~24.6 billion doses of acetaminophen were sold in 2008. The market demand for acetaminophen is growing. Recent data has demonstrated a 28% growth in the market sales of acetaminophen between 2004 and 2008 with sales approaching approximately $2.6 billion in 2008 alone (Data from IMS Health).

Table 1. Approved drug products containing acetaminophen as an active ingredient (December 2011)

	Approved Drugs	Companies
Prescription Drug Products (Rx)	199	30
Over-the-Counter Drug Products (OTC)	22	9
Discontinued Drug Products	260	65
Total	481	104

Data source: the Orange Book from FDA. Modified from (Blough and Wu, 2011).

Table 2. Over-the-Counter drug products (OTC) containing acetaminophen (December 2011)

Company Name	Drug Name
Actavis Mid Atlantic	Infants' Feverall; Acetaminophen.
G and W Labs	Acephen
McNeil Consumer Healthcare	Tylenol
Novartis	Excedrin (Migraine); Tavist Allergy/sinus/headache.
Ohm Labs	Acetaminophen
Perrigo	Acetaminophen; Acetaminophen, Aspirin and Caffeine.
Polymedica	Neopap
Ranbaxy	Acetaminophen
Schering Plough	Drixoral Plus

Data source: the Orange Book from FDA. Modified from (Blough and Wu, 2011).

Acetaminophen exhibits both analgesic and antipyretic properties and has been widely used as an active ingredient in many approved drugs. According to the U.S. Food and Drug Administration (FDA), 481 drugs contain acetaminophen (Table 1). As of December 2011, 221 out of the 481 acetaminophen-containing drugs exhibit active approval status, which include 199 prescription drug products owned by 30 companies and 22 over the counter (OTC) drug products produced by 9 companies (Tables 1, 2). Given its wide use and easy availability, scientists have recently begun to examine acetaminophen for off-label applications. Herein, we will investigate these potential applications, and attempt, where possible, to highlight how these findings may lead to new directions of inquiry and clinical relevance of other disorders.

2. Chronic Acetaminophen Ingestion Can Improve Blood Glucose Control

Although a toxic dose of acetaminophen (three hours following 500 mg APAP / kg body weight) can rapidly induce hyperglycemia (Hinson et al., 1984) can rapidly induce hyperglycemia (Hinson et al., 1984) and acute liver failure secondary to clinical acetaminophen overdose can further impair the peripheral uptake of glucose (Clark et al., 2001), recent animal studies have demonstrated that acetaminophen, when taken at lower dosages (20-30 mg/kg body weight) exhibits an ability to lower blood glucose levels in several animal disease models, including diabetes, high-fat diet-induced obesity and aging.

Using a streptozotocin (STZ)-induced diabetic mice model, Shertzer and colleagues showed that acetaminophen at 20 mg / kg body weight is able to normalize STZ-induced increases in blood glucose levels (Shertzer et al., 2008). This effect appears to be associated with protection against STZ-induced destruction of pancreatic beta-cells given that acetaminophen treatment appears to be associated with the maintenance of pancreatic insulin synthesis (Shertzer et al., 2008). Like that observed in the STZ model, acetaminophen at 20 or 30 mg / kg body weight has also been reported to prevent hyperglycemia in animals fed a high-fat (HF) diet (Shertzer et al., 2008; Shertzer et al., 2010). In addition to preventing hyperglycemia, acetaminophen ingestion is also associated with the restoration of fasting insulin levels, improvements in glucose tolerance, and an increased ability of the HF-fed mice to boost blood insulin levels after a glucose challenge (Shertzer et al., 2008; Shertzer et al., 2010). Although the exact mechanism(s) responsible for these findings remain unclear, it is thought that these effects, like that seen in the rat STZ model, may be related to improvements in pancreatic insulin synthesis / secretion.

Research using both humans and animal models have demonstrated that the incidence of insulin resistance increases with age (Houmard et al., 1995; Wu et al., 2009a). Wu and co-workers using Fisher 344 x Brown Norway (F344BN) aging rat model have shown that age-associated increases in blood glucose can be corrected by chronic acetaminophen treatment at a dosage of 30 mg /kg body weight (Wu et al., 2009a). It has been postulated that this effect was predicated, at least in part, on the ability of acetaminophen to diminish age-related losses in amount of muscle glucose transporter-4 (Glut4) expression (Wu et al., 2009a). Further study demonstrated that acetaminophen treatment was also associated with an attenuation of muscle reactive oxygen species (ROS) levels and in the amount of proteins that become oxidatively modified (Wu et al., 2009a). It has been shown that prolonged MAPK activation is associated with decreased Glut4 expression (Fujishiro et al., 2001; Carlson et al., 2003) and Glut4 translocation in response to insulin (Bandyopadhyay et al., 2001; Izawa et al., 2005; D'Alessandris et al., 2007). Supporting this contention, Wu and colleagues showed that acetaminophen treatment was also associated with diminished aging-associated increases in p38- and ERK-mitogen activated protein kinase (MAPK) activation (Wu et al., 2009a). Taken together, these findings suggests that acetaminophen might function to improve blood glucose levels by employing multiple mechanisms including decreases in intracellular ROS levels, diminished aging-associated MAPK hyperphosphorylation and by increasing muscle Glut4 expression (Wu et al., 2009a).

3. Long Term Acetaminophen Ingestion Can Improve Skeletal Muscle Structure and Function

In addition to the beneficial effect of acetaminophen on relieving muscle soreness and pain (Prior et al., 2011), recent studies have suggested that acetaminophen can improve aged skeletal muscle structure and function (sarcopenia). Wu and colleagues reported that chronic acetaminophen treatment at 30 mg /kg body weight is able to decrease the aging-associated myocyte apoptosis and decreases in myocyte size (muscle fiber cross sectional area) with this latter effect occurring most likely due to acetaminophen-associated increases in myosin and actin expression (Wu et al., 2009b). These effects are believed to be mediated, at least in part, via reductions in the amount of oxidative and nitrosative stress as acetaminophen intervention lowers the amount of superoxide and the abundance of oxidatively modified proteins (Wu et al., 2009a). It also appears that acetaminophen treatment reduces the phosphorylation of eukaryotic initiation factor 2a (eIF2a) (Wu et al., 2010), a key protein translational factor which when phosphorylated in response to stress leads to the inhibition of protein translational initiation (Kimball, 1999). Other data has demonstrated that acetaminophen can decrease muscle reactive nitrogen species (RNS) as evidenced by reduced expression of inducible NOS (iNOS) and S-nitrosylation of Akt (Wu et al., 2009b). The Akt / protein kinase B is critical regulator of cellular homeostasis and functions to control cellular anabolism (protein synthesis, glucose uptake and metabolism) and cell fate (proliferation, apoptosis) (Wu et al., 2011). Akt S-nitrosylation impairs Akt kinase activity (Carvalho-Filho et al., 2005; Yasukawa et al., 2005; Wu et al., 2009b), which if not corrected can lead to a dysregulation of Akt signaling. Importantly, the restoration of Akt function by acetaminophen is associated with improvements in protein translational signaling (increased phosphorylation / activation of S6 ribosomal protein (Ser235/236) and translation initiation factor eIF4E (Ser209)), increases in the amount of muscle Glut4, myosin and actin, along with a decrease in myocyte apoptosis and the prevention of age-associated hyperglycemia (Wu et al., 2009a; Wu et al., 2009b; Wu et al., 2010).

The positive effects of acetaminophen on skeletal muscle structure and function have also been shown in other experimental settings. Shertzer et al. reported that acetaminophen is able to prevent high-fat diet induced decreases in lean muscle volume and body water retention (Shertzer et al., 2008). Trappe et al. demonstrated during 12 weeks of knee extensor progressive resistance exercise training that acetaminophen (4 g/day) can increase exercise-induced muscle (quadriceps) hypertrophy and strength in older adults when compared to that seen with placebo, although muscle (vastus lateralis) protein content, muscle water content, and myosin heavy chain distribution did not increase (Trappe et al., 2011). Interestingly, increased muscle volume and strength by acetaminophen does not appear to be mediated by cyclooxygenase (COX), as the expression of COX-1 and COX-2 was not changed with acetaminophen consumption (Trappe et al., 2011). Importantly, acetaminophen at 4 g/day for

12 wks when used in combination with resistance training did not alter blood creatinine and ALT levels (Trappe et al., 2011), a finding which suggests that this dosage does not cause liver or kidney damage. Interestingly, the effect of combining acetaminophen and exercise appears dependent on the type of exercise as acetaminophen has been reported to suppress the protein synthesis in skeletal muscle after eccentric resistance exercise (Trappe et al., 2002). Mauger et al. reported that ingestion of acetaminophen (1.5 g) can improve the performance of a 10-mile cycle time trial (TT) with no difference in exertion or perceived pain, and that cyclists who ingested acetaminophen had a higher mean power output and heart rate (Mauger et al., 2010). Whether a similar finding exists for other types of exercise modalities is currently unclear.

4. Acetaminophen Possesses Cardioprotective and Neuroprotective Properties

Clinical studies have suggested that the risk for major cardiovascular events is increased if acetaminophen is taken frequently ($\geq$ 22 days / month) or at high doses (15 tablets / week) (Chan et al., 2006). Nonetheless, when used properly, acetaminophen has been shown to exhibit remarkable cardioprotective effects. Using an isolated guinea pig heart model, studies have shown that acetaminophen (0.35 mM) can increase coronary vascular resistance and positive inotropy (Merrill et al., 2001), attenuate ischemia-reduced monophasic action potentials (Merrill and Goldberg, 2001), and improve left ventricular contractility (rate of developed pressure) during postischemia-reperfusion (Merrill et al., 2001; Merrill, 2002). Further examination using electron microscopy has suggested that acetaminophen can preserve left ventricular myofibrillar ultrastructure in the reperfused myocardium, including protection against ischemia/reperfusion-induced diffused and blurred Z lines, the presence of contraction bands, and swollen, sparsely packed mitochondria (Merrill et al., 2001). Using two dog models of ventricular arrhythmias induced by regional myocardial ischemia / reperfusion or ouabain (25 μg/kg), Merrill et al. demonstrated an anti-arrhythmic effect for acetaminophen, and found that acetaminophen (15 mg / kg, i.v.) significantly reduced the number of ventricular ectopic beats during ischemia and reperfusion, the amount of ouabain-induced ventricular premature beats, ventricular salvo, ventricular bigeminy and nonsustained ventricular arrhythmia (Merrill et al., 2007). In the iron-overloaded gerbil, Walker and colleagues have demonstrated that acetaminophen is able to prevent iron overload-induced cardiac structural and functional changes, including alterations in cardiac rhythm, ventricular distension, reductions in left ventricular ejection fraction, decreases in fractional shortening and decreases in mortality (Walker et al., 2007; Walker et al., 2009). Merrill et al. using a myocardial infarction dog model showed that acetaminophen at 30 mg/kg body weight is able to decrease infarct size (Merrill et al., 2004). These researchers also showed acetaminophen treatment can reduce cardiac damage, including swollen mitochondria and fragmented nucleus (Merrill et al., 2004). Conversely, others using different animal models have failed to show beneficial effects of acetaminophen treatment on infarct size in non-preconditioned rats (Dai and Kloner, 2003) or in coronary artery occlusion/reperfusion in rabbits (Hale and Kloner, 2004), however all suggest that acetaminophen is a safe drug in the postmyocardial infarction setting (Dai and Kloner, 2003; Hale and Kloner, 2004; Leshnower et al., 2006).

Further studies defining detailed conditions are needed to verify the protective effect of acetaminophen on infarct size.

It has also been reported that acetaminophen has neuroprotective effects. Maharaj et al. reported that acetaminophen (0.25 – 1 mM) treatment *ex vivo* can inhibit cyanide-induced superoxide anion generation and lipid peroxidation in rat brain homogenates (Maharaj et al., 2004). Further animal study has suggested the acetaminophen (100 mg / kg / day, i.p.) can inhibit quinolinic acid (QA)-induced lipid peroxidation, superoxide anion generation, and cell damage in the rat hippocampus (Maharaj et al., 2006). Naziroğlu et al. also reported that acetaminophen (5 to 100 mg / kg) can reduce brain and microsomal lipid peroxidation, while it also increases brain vitamin E levels and microsomal glutathione peroxidase (GSH-Px) activity (Naziroglu et al., 2009). In addition, Bisaglia et al. used rat primary hippocampal neurons and rat pheochromocytoma cells demonstrated that acetaminophen (100 μM) can protect against amyloid beta-fragment-induced impairment of mitochondrial redox activity, increases in phospholipid peroxidation and apoptotic nuclear fragmentation (Bisaglia et al., 2002), suggesting a possible therapeutic effect of acetaminophen on Alzheimer's disease.

5. Acetaminophen Exhibits Potent Antioxidant Activity

It is well known that acetaminophen overdose can lead to oxidative stress and induce hepatic and renal damage (Ghosh et al., 2010; Agarwal et al., 2011). Acetaminophen is initially metabolized in the liver, and generates the toxic metabolite, N-acetyl-p-benzoquinone imine (NAPQI). Under normal conditions, NAPQI can be efficiently detoxified by glutathione (GSH) however, during an overdose, intracellular glutathione can become depleted within 1-4 hours (Al-Turk and Stohs, 1981; Porubek et al., 1987; Lores Arnaiz et al., 1995), resulting in accumulation of intracellular reactive oxygen and nitrogen species (ROS/RNS), and increased oxidative / nitrosative stress. In addition, excessive NAPQI can also covalently bind to the cysteinyl thiol groups of cellular proteins and form protein-(cystein-S-yl)-APAP adducts (Hoffmann et al., 1985), which may impair protein function. Given this mechanism, antioxidant therapy using N-acetylcysteine (NAC) is commonly used to attenuate acetaminophen-induced hepatotoxicity.

Interestingly, extensive animal and *in vitro* studies have suggested that acetaminophen possesses remarkable antioxidant properties when used within the therapeutic dosage. Acetaminophen is phenolic in structure with a substituent at the para position relative to the hydroxyl group (Figure 1) which allows it to react with reactive species (Dinis et al., 1994; Shertzer et al., 2008). For example, Shertzer et al. using cell-free assay systems demonstrated that acetaminophen is directly scavenge reactive oxygen (Shertzer et al., 2008). Nam and colleagues found that acetaminophen has higher reactivity with peroxyl radicals than many widely-used phenolic antioxidants, including ubiquitous butylated hydroxytoluene (BHT) (Nam et al., 2009). Other *in vitro* studies showed that acetaminophen can significantly inhibit hemoprotein-induced lipid peroxidation by its ability to reducing ferryl heme to its ferric state and the quenching globin radicals (Boutaud et al., 2010). Acetaminophen has also be shown to reduce the degree of low-density lipoproteins (LDL) hydroperoxides induced by Cu^{2+} ions (Ozsoy and Pabuccuoglu, 2007) or myeloperoxidase in presence of nitrite and hydrogen peroxide (Chou and Greenspan, 2002). Several studies have also demonstrated that acetaminophen can directly scavenge peroxynitrite (Van Dyke et al., 1998; Rork et al., 2006; Schildknecht et al., 2008), a highly reactive oxidant and nitrating agent that can oxidize lipids, proteins and nucleic acids. Nam and colleagues showed that when nitrogen is incorporated into the phenolic ring the antioxidant activity of acetaminophen is greatly reduced and that this finding seems to be associated with increased O–H bond dissociation enthalpy (Nam et al., 2009). However, this structural change increases the efficacy of acetaminophen to act as an inhibitor of lipid hydroperoxide biosynthesis by soybean LOX-1 (sLOX-1) (Nam et al., 2009) suggesting that altered acidity of the phenolic O–H may lead to chelation of the catalytic non-heme iron atom in sLOX-1 (Nam et al., 2009). Taken together, it appears that the structure of the acetaminophen phenolic ring is critical for its pharmacological and antioxidant properties.

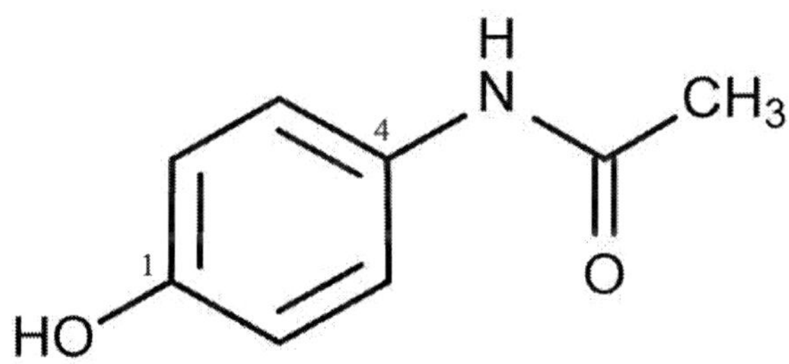

Figure 1. Structure of acetaminophen (N-Acetyl-4-aminophenol). The phenolic structure with a substituent at the para position relative to the hydroxyl group allows acetaminophen to react with reactive species and possesses antioxidant activity. Cited from (Blough and Wu, 2011).

Ex vivo and *in vivo* animal studies have suggested that acetaminophen can effectively reduce ROS/RNS in multiple tissue types. DuBois and colleagues (1983) reported that acetaminophen had antioxidant effects in the rat liver (DuBois et al., 1983). Shertzer et al. also showed that acetaminophen (20 mg / kg) can decrease liver mitochondrial H_2O_2 formation in both control and high-fat diet fed mice (Shertzer et al., 2008). Wu and colleagues demonstrated that acetaminophen treatment at 30 mg / kg for 6 months can attenuate aging-related increases in skeletal muscle ROS content, the amount of proteins that are oxidatively modified, and protein S-nitrosylation, suggesting acetaminophen can decrease oxidative / nitrosative stress during aging (Wu et al., 2009a; Wu et al., 2009b; Wu et al., 2010). Using a rhabdomyolysis-induced renal failure animal model, Boutaud and colleagues showed that acetaminophen (100 mg/kg, i.p.) can significantly decrease myoglobin-derived radical species and that this finding was associated with reduced renal damage and improved renal function (Boutaud et al., 2010). Using a high-fat fed animal model, Shertzer et al. demonstrated that acetaminophen (30 mg / kg / day) was able to inhibit production of reactive oxygen species (at least partially via inhibition of NADPH oxidase activity) and lipid peroxidation in white adipose tissue (WAT) and that these findings were associated with improved glucose tolerance and insulin sensitivity in HF animals (Shertzer et al., 2010).

Although not yet well understood, the cardioprotective effects of acetaminophen appears to be related to its ability to act as an antioxidant (Merrill et al., 2001; Merrill and Goldberg, 2001; Merrill, 2002; Rork et al., 2006; Hadzimichalis et al., 2007; Walker et al., 2007; Walker et al., 2009; Kakarla et al., 2010). Using Langendorff-perfused guinea pig hearts, Hadzimichalis and colleagues reported that acetaminophen (0.35 mM) can reduce mitochondrial swelling, and inhibit the mitochondrial permeability transition pore-induced apoptotic pathway and mitochondrial cytochrome C release in heart with induced low-flow global myocardial ischemia (Hadzimichalis et al., 2007). Merrill et al. demonstrated that acetaminophen can significantly attenuate the burst of hydroxyl radicals during the first 10 min of reperfusion, and block 3-morpholinosydnominine (SIN-1)-induced peroxynitrite generation (Merrill et al., 2001). Kakarla and co-workers have found that chronic acetaminophen treatment at 30 mg/kg body weight is able to attenuate aging-associated increases in cardiac oxidative (superoxide) and nitrosative (protein nitrotyrosylation) stresses, caspase-3 activation and apoptosis in F344BN rats (Kakarla et al., 2010). Rork et al. reported that acetaminophen (0.35 mM) can reduce peroxynitrite in the isolated guinea pig myocardium and that this finding was associated with an attenuated activation of MMP-2 and decreased cleavage of troponin I (TnI) following ischemia/reperfusion (Rork et al., 2006). Therefore, cardioprotective effects of acetaminophen are at least partially mediated by reducing tissue reactive oxygen and nitrogen species.

CONCLUSIONS AND PERSPECTIVES

Recent experimental data suggests that acetaminophen may have several remarkable effects other than its well-known analgesic/antipyretic properties. Thus far, acetaminophen has been shown to improve blood glucose control, improve skeletal muscle structure and function in the aged, and that this agent exhibits cardioprotective and neuroprotective effects (Figure 2). Current laboratory and pre-clinical studies have revealed that many of these findings can be linked to its incredible antioxidant properties. It is also worth noting that since acetaminophen overdose or ingestion with alcohol can cause hepatotoxicity and death, well controlled clinical studies must be conducted to ensure the safety and efficiency of acetaminophen before its clinical application for off-label applications.

Therapeutic effects of acetaminophen

1. Well-known (clinically proven):

    Analgesics (pain reliever)
    Antipyretics (fever reducer)

2. Unexpected (laboratory and pre-clinical studies):

    Control of hyperglycemia (aging and diabetic models)
    Improvement of skeletal muscle structure and function
    Cardioprotective
    Neuroprotective

Figure 2. Summary of acetaminophen therapeutic effects. In addition to the clinically-proven analgesic/antipyretic properties, laboratory and pre-clinical studies demonstrated that acetaminophen has other beneficial effects that would increase clinical application of acetaminophen. However, clinical studies are needed to ensure its safety, efficiency and proper dosage. Cited from (Blough and Wu, 2011).

Conflict of Interest Statement

The authors declare that the manuscript was conducted in the absence of any commercial or financial relationships that could be construed as a potential conflict of interest.

Acknowledgments

The authors would like to acknowledge the support of the Huntington VA Medical Center for laboratory space and equipment.

References

[1] Agarwal, R., Macmillan-Crow, L.A., Rafferty, T.M., Saba, H., Roberts, D.W., Fifer, E.K., James, L.P., and Hinson, J.A. (2011). Acetaminophen-induced hepatotoxicity in mice occurs with inhibition of activity and nitration of mitochondrial manganese superoxide dismutase. *J. Pharmacol. Exp. Ther.* 337, 110-116.

[2] Al-Turk, W.A., and Stohs, S.J. (1981). Hepatic glutathione content and aryl hydrocarbon hydroxylase activity of acetaminophen-treated mice as a function of age. *Drug Chem. Toxicol.* 4, 37-48.

[3] Bandyopadhyay, G., Sajan, M.P., Kanoh, Y., Standaert, M.L., Quon, M.J., Reed, B.C., Dikic, I., and Farese, R.V. (2001). Glucose activates protein kinase C-zeta /lambda through proline-rich tyrosine kinase-2, extracellular signal-regulated kinase, and phospholipase D: a novel mechanism for activating glucose transporter translocation. *J. Biol. Chem.* 276, 35537-35545.

[4] Bisaglia, M., Venezia, V., Piccioli, P., Stanzione, S., Porcile, C., Russo, C., Mancini, F., Milanese, C., and Schettini, G. (2002). Acetaminophen protects hippocampal neurons and PC12 cultures from amyloid beta-peptides induced oxidative stress and reduces NF-kappaB activation. *Neurochem. Int.* 41, 43-54.

[5] Blough, E.R., and Wu, M. (2011). Acetaminophen: Beyond Pain and Fever-Relieving. *Front Pharmacol.* 2, 72.

[6] Boutaud, O., Moore, K.P., Reeder, B.J., Harry, D., Howie, A.J., Wang, S., Carney, C.K., Masterson, T.S., Amin, T., Wright, D.W., Wilson, M.T., Oates, J.A., and Roberts, L.J., 2nd (2010). Acetaminophen inhibits hemoprotein-catalyzed lipid peroxidation and attenuates rhabdomyolysis-induced renal failure. *Proc. Natl. Acad. Sci. U S A* 107, 2699-2704.

[7] Carlson, C.J., Koterski, S., Sciotti, R.J., Poccard, G.B., and Rondinone, C.M. (2003). Enhanced basal activation of mitogen-activated protein kinases in adipocytes from type 2 diabetes: potential role of p38 in the downregulation of GLUT4 expression. *Diabetes* 52, 634-641.

[8] Carvalho-Filho, M.A., Ueno, M., Hirabara, S.M., Seabra, A.B., Carvalheira, J.B., De Oliveira, M.G., Velloso, L.A., Curi, R., and Saad, M.J. (2005). S-nitrosation of the insulin receptor, insulin receptor substrate 1, and protein kinase B/Akt: a novel mechanism of insulin resistance. *Diabetes* 54, 959-967.

[9] Chan, A.T., Manson, J.E., Albert, C.M., Chae, C.U., Rexrode, K.M., Curhan, G.C., Rimm, E.B., Willett, W.C., and Fuchs, C.S. (2006). Nonsteroidal antiinflammatory drugs, acetaminophen, and the risk of cardiovascular events. *Circulation* 113, 1578-1587.

[10] Chou, T.M., and Greenspan, P. (2002). Effect of acetaminophen on the myeloperoxidase-hydrogen peroxide-nitrite mediated oxidation of LDL. *Biochim. Biophys. Acta* 1581, 57-63.

[11] Clark, S.J., Shojaee-Moradie, F., Croos, P., Seed, P.T., Umpleby, A.M., Wendon, J.A., and Miell, J. (2001). Temporal changes in insulin sensitivity following the development of acute liver failure secondary to acetaminophen. *Hepatology* 34, 109-115.

[12] D'alessandris, C., Lauro, R., Presta, I., and Sesti, G. (2007). C-reactive protein induces phosphorylation of insulin receptor substrate-1 on Ser307 and Ser 612 in L6 myocytes, thereby impairing the insulin signalling pathway that promotes glucose transport. *Diabetologia* 50, 840-849.

[13] Dai, W., and Kloner, R.A. (2003). Effects of acetaminophen on myocardial infarct size in rats. *J. Cardiovasc. Pharmacol. Ther.* 8, 277-284.

[14] Dinis, T.C., Maderia, V.M., and Almeida, L.M. (1994). Action of phenolic derivatives (acetaminophen, salicylate, and 5-aminosalicylate) as inhibitors of membrane lipid peroxidation and as peroxyl radical scavengers. *Arch. Biochem. Biophys.* 315, 161-169.

[15] Dubois, R.N., Hill, K.E., and Burk, R.F. (1983). Antioxidant effect of acetaminophen in rat liver. *Biochem. Pharmacol.* 32, 2621-2622.

[16] Fujishiro, M., Gotoh, Y., Katagiri, H., Sakoda, H., Ogihara, T., Anai, M., Onishi, Y., Ono, H., Funaki, M., Inukai, K., Fukushima, Y., Kikuchi, M., Oka, Y., and Asano, T. (2001). MKK6/3 and p38 MAPK pathway activation is not necessary for insulin-induced glucose uptake but regulates glucose transporter expression. *J. Biol. Chem.* 276, 19800-19806.

[17] Ghosh, J., Das, J., Manna, P., and Sil, P.C. (2010). Acetaminophen induced renal injury via oxidative stress and TNF-alpha production: therapeutic potential of arjunolic acid. *Toxicology* 268, 8-18.

[18] Hadzimichalis, N.M., Baliga, S.S., Golfetti, R., Jaques, K.M., Firestein, B.L., and Merrill, G.F. (2007). Acetaminophen-mediated cardioprotection via inhibition of the mitochondrial permeability transition pore-induced apoptotic pathway. *Am J Physiol Heart Circ Physiol* 293, H3348-3355.

[19] Hale, S.L., and Kloner, R.A. (2004). Acetaminophen and experimental acute myocardial infarction. *Cardiovasc. Drugs Ther.* 18, 121-125.

[20] Hinson, J.A., Han-Hsu, H., Mays, J.B., Holt, S.J., Mclean, P., and Ketterer, B. (1984). Acetaminophen-induced alterations in blood glucose and blood insulin levels in mice. *Res. Commun. Chem. Pathol. Pharmacol.* 43, 381-391.

[21] Hoffmann, K.J., Streeter, A.J., Axworthy, D.B., and Baillie, T.A. (1985). Identification of the major covalent adduct formed in vitro and in vivo between acetaminophen and mouse liver proteins. *Mol. Pharmacol.* 27, 566-573.

[22] Houmard, J.A., Weidner, M.D., Dolan, P.L., Leggett-Frazier, N., Gavigan, K.E., Hickey, M.S., Tyndall, G.L., Zheng, D., Alshami, A., and Dohm, G.L. (1995). Skeletal muscle GLUT4 protein concentration and aging in humans. *Diabetes* 44, 555-560.

[23] Izawa, Y., Yoshizumi, M., Fujita, Y., Ali, N., Kanematsu, Y., Ishizawa, K., Tsuchiya, K., Obata, T., Ebina, Y., Tomita, S., and Tamaki, T. (2005). ERK1/2 activation by angiotensin II inhibits insulin-induced glucose uptake in vascular smooth muscle cells. *Exp. Cell Res.* 308, 291-299.

[24] Kakarla, S.K., Fannin, J.C., Keshavarzian, S., Katta, A., Paturi, S., Nalabotu, S.K., Wu, M., Rice, K.M., Manzoor, K., Walker, E.M., Jr., and Blough, E.R. (2010). Chronic acetaminophen attenuates age-associated increases in cardiac ROS and apoptosis in the Fischer Brown Norway rat. *Basic Res. Cardiol.* 105, 535-544.

[25] Kimball, S.R. (1999). Eukaryotic initiation factor eIF2. *Int. J. Biochem. Cell Biol.* 31, 25-29.

[26] Leshnower, B.G., Sakamoto, H., Zeeshan, A., Parish, L.M., Hinmon, R., Plappert, T., Jackson, B.M., Gorman, J.H., 3rd, and Gorman, R.C. (2006). Role of acetaminophen in acute myocardial infarction. *Am. J. Physiol. Heart Circ. Physiol.* 290, H2424-2431.

[27] Lores Arnaiz, S., Llesuy, S., Cutrin, J.C., and Boveris, A. (1995). Oxidative stress by acute acetaminophen administration in mouse liver. *Free Radic. Biol. Med.* 19, 303-310.

[28] Maharaj, D.S., Saravanan, K.S., Maharaj, H., Mohanakumar, K.P., and Daya, S. (2004). Acetaminophen and aspirin inhibit superoxide anion generation and lipid peroxidation, and protect against 1-methyl-4-phenyl pyridinium-induced dopaminergic neurotoxicity in rats. *Neurochem. Int.* 44, 355-360.

[29] Maharaj, H., Maharaj, D.S., and Daya, S. (2006). Acetylsalicylic acid and acetaminophen protect against oxidative neurotoxicity. *Metab. Brain Dis.* 21, 189-199.

[30] Mauger, A.R., Jones, A.M., and Williams, C.A. (2010). Influence of acetaminophen on performance during time trial cycling. *J. Appl. Physiol.* 108, 98-104.

[31] Merrill, G., Mcconnell, P., Vandyke, K., and Powell, S. (2001). Coronary and myocardial effects of acetaminophen: protection during ischemia-reperfusion. *Am. J. Physiol. Heart Circ. Physiol.* 280, H2631-2638.

[32] Merrill, G.F. (2002). Acetaminophen and low-flow myocardial ischemia: efficacy and antioxidant mechanisms. *Am. J. Physiol. Heart Circ. Physiol.* 282, H1341-1349.

[33] Merrill, G.F., and Goldberg, E. (2001). Antioxidant properties of acetaminophen and cardioprotection. *Basic Res. Cardiol.* 96, 423-430.

[34] Merrill, G.F., Merrill, J.H., Golfetti, R., Jaques, K.M., Hadzimichalis, N.S., Baliga, S.S., and Rork, T.H. (2007). Antiarrhythmic properties of acetaminophen in the dog. *Exp. Biol. Med. (Maywood)* 232, 1245-1252.

[35] Merrill, G.F., Rork, T.H., Spiler, N.M., and Golfetti, R. (2004). Acetaminophen and myocardial infarction in dogs. *Am. J. Physiol. Heart Circ. Physiol.* 287, H1913-1920.

[36] Nam, T.G., Nara, S.J., Zagol-Ikapitte, I., Cooper, T., Valgimigli, L., Oates, J.A., Porter, N.A., Boutaud, O., and Pratt, D.A. (2009). Pyridine and pyrimidine analogs of acetaminophen as inhibitors of lipid peroxidation and cyclooxygenase and lipoxygenase catalysis. *Org. Biomol. Chem.* 7, 5103-5112.

[37] Naziroglu, M., Uguz, A.C., Kocak, A., and Bal, R. (2009). Acetaminophen at different doses protects brain microsomal Ca2+-ATPase and the antioxidant redox system in rats. *J. Membr. Biol.* 231, 57-64.

[38] Ozsoy, M.B., and Pabuccuoglu, A. (2007). The effect of acetaminophen on oxidative modification of low-density lipoproteins in hypercholesterolemic rabbits. *J. Clin. Biochem. Nutr.* 41, 27-31.

[39] Porubek, D.J., Rundgren, M., Harvison, P.J., Nelson, S.D., and Moldeus, P. (1987). Investigation of mechanisms of acetaminophen toxicity in isolated rat hepatocytes with the acetaminophen analogues 3,5-dimethylacetaminophen and 2,6-dimethylacetaminophen. *Mol. Pharmacol.* 31, 647-653.

[40] Prior, M.J., Lavins, B.J., and Cooper, K. (2011). A Randomized, Placebo-controlled Trial of Acetaminophen Extended Release for Treatment of Post-marathon Muscle Soreness. *Clin. J. Pain.*

[41] Rork, T.H., Hadzimichalis, N.M., Kappil, M.A., and Merrill, G.F. (2006). Acetaminophen attenuates peroxynitrite-activated matrix metalloproteinase-2-mediated troponin I cleavage in the isolated guinea pig myocardium. *J. Mol. Cell Cardiol.* 40, 553-561.

[42] Schildknecht, S., Daiber, A., Ghisla, S., Cohen, R.A., and Bachschmid, M.M. (2008). Acetaminophen inhibits prostanoid synthesis by scavenging the PGHS-activator peroxynitrite. *Faseb. J.* 22, 215-224.

[43] Shertzer, H.G., Kendig, E.L., Nasrallah, H.A., Johansson, E., and Genter, M.B. (2010). Protection from olanzapine-induced metabolic toxicity in mice by acetaminophen and tetrahydroindenoindole. *Int. J. Obes. (Lond)* 34, 970-979.

[44] Shertzer, H.G., Schneider, S.N., Kendig, E.L., Clegg, D.J., D'alessio, D.A., and Genter, M.B. (2008). Acetaminophen normalizes glucose homeostasis in mouse models for diabetes. *Biochem. Pharmacol.* 75, 1402-1410.

[45] Trappe, T.A., Carroll, C.C., Dickinson, J.M., Lemoine, J.K., Haus, J.M., Sullivan, B.E., Lee, J.D., Jemiolo, B., Weinheimer, E.M., and Hollon, C.J. (2011). Influence of acetaminophen and ibuprofen on skeletal muscle adaptations to resistance exercise in older adults. *Am. J. Physiol. Regul. Integr. Comp. Physiol.* 300, R655-662.

[46] Trappe, T.A., Fluckey, J.D., White, F., Lambert, C.P., and Evans, W.J. (2001). Skeletal muscle PGF(2)(alpha) and PGE(2) in response to eccentric resistance exercise: influence of ibuprofen acetaminophen. *J. Clin. Endocrinol. Metab.* 86, 5067-5070.

[47] Trappe, T.A., White, F., Lambert, C.P., Cesar, D., Hellerstein, M., and Evans, W.J. (2002). Effect of ibuprofen and acetaminophen on postexercise muscle protein synthesis. *Am. J. Physiol. Endocrinol. Metab.* 282, E551-556.

[48] Van Dyke, K., Sacks, M., and Qazi, N. (1998). A new screening method to detect water-soluble antioxidants: acetaminophen (Tylenol) and other phenols react as antioxidants and destroy peroxynitrite-based luminol-dependent chemiluminescence. *J. Biolumin. Chemilumin.* 13, 339-348.

[49] Walker, E.M., Jr., Epling, C.P., Parris, C., Cansino, S., Ghosh, P., Desai, D.H., Morrison, R.G., Wright, G.L., Wehner, P., Mangiarua, E.I., Walker, S.M., and Blough, E.R. (2007). Acetaminophen protects against iron-induced cardiac damage in gerbils. *Ann. Clin. Lab. Sci.* 37, 22-33.

[50] Walker, E.M., Jr., Morrison, R.G., Dornon, L., Laurino, J.P., Walker, S.M., Studeny, M., Wehner, P.S., Rice, K.M., Wu, M., and Blough, E.R. (2009). Acetaminophen combinations protect against iron-induced cardiac damage in gerbils. *Ann. Clin. Lab. Sci.* 39, 378-385.

[51] Wu, M., Desai, D.H., Kakarla, S.K., Katta, A., Paturi, S., Gutta, A.K., Rice, K.M., Walker, E.M., Jr., and Blough, E.R. (2009a). Acetaminophen prevents aging-associated hyperglycemia in aged rats: effect of aging-associated hyperactivation of p38-MAPK and ERK1/2. *Diabetes Metab. Res. Rev.* 25, 279-286.

[52] Wu, M., Falasca, M., and Blough, E.R. (2011). Akt/protein kinase B in skeletal muscle physiology and pathology. *J. Cell Physiol.* 226, 29-36.

[53] Wu, M., Katta, A., Gadde, M.K., Liu, H., Kakarla, S.K., Fannin, J., Paturi, S., Arvapalli, R.K., Rice, K.M., Wang, Y., and Blough, E.R. (2009b). Aging-associated dysfunction of akt/protein kinase B: s-nitrosylation and acetaminophen intervention. *PLoS One* 4, e6430.

[54] Wu, M., Liu, H., Fannin, J., Katta, A., Wang, Y., Arvapalli, R.K., Paturi, S., Karkala, S.K., Rice, K.M., and Blough, E.R. (2010). Acetaminophen improves protein translational signaling in aged skeletal muscle. *Rejuvenation Res.* 13, 571-579.

[55] Yasukawa, T., Tokunaga, E., Ota, H., Sugita, H., Martyn, J.A., and Kaneki, M. (2005). S-nitrosylation-dependent inactivation of Akt/protein kinase B in insulin resistance. *J. Biol. Chem.* 280, 7511-7518.

In: Acetaminophen: Properties, Clinical Uses
Editors: Atash Javaherian and Pasha Latifpour
ISBN: 978-1-61942-374-9

Chapter 4

ADVANCED METHODS FOR THE REMOVAL OF ACETAMINOPHEN FROM WATER

***Ana P. Carvalho*[1], *Ana S. Mestre*[1], *Marta Haro*[2], and *Conchi O. Ania*[2]**

[1]Departamento de Química e Bioquímica and CQB, Faculdade de Ciências da Universidade de Lisboa, Ed. C8, Campo Grande, 1749-016 Lisboa, Portugal

[2]Department of Chemical Processes in Energy and Environment, Instituto Nacional del Carbón, CSIC, Apdo. 73, 33011 Oviedo, Spain

ABSTRACT

During the last decades, the scientific community has become increasingly concerned about the potential public health impact of new environmental contaminants originating from industrial, agricultural and human activities. These compounds, known as emergent pollutants, include prescription and non-prescription human and veterinary pharmaceutical compounds, personal care products, household chemicals, pesticides, fertilizers and so forth. Among them, the occurrence of pharmaceuticals in water represents an outstanding environmental issue due to their therapeutic and/or biological activity, even at trace levels. The development of analytical techniques with low detection limits and high sensibility has enabled undertaking ambient monitoring studies to control the occurrence and fate of these emergent pollutants. Acetaminophen, a non-prescription analgesic widely consumed worldwide, is among the six pharmaceutical ingredients most often detected in drinking water. This is a direct consequence of the low efficiency of conventional water treatment processes for the removal/degradation of these compounds, along with their continuous discharge in the environment. To overcome the emergent environmental challenge associated with the occurrence and persistence of pharmaceuticals in water and wastewater, novel advanced water treatment techniques are currently being extensively investigated. In this chapter, a comprehensive review of recent advances on the development of new strategies to improve the water quality is made; special emphasis is paid to methods based on adsorption and degradation processes including adsorption, photo- and electro-assisted degradation techniques, etc.

1. INTRODUCTION

"There is no life without water.
It is a treasure indispensable to all human activity"
Article 1, 2 European Water Charter
Proclaimed in Strasbourg, 6th May 1968

Water is the most important compound for life in our planet, not only for all the ecosystems but also for the development of anthropogenic (human) activities that determine the socio-economic development of regions and countries. Indeed, the International Human Rights Declaration recognizes the fundamental right of all humans themselves and their families to an adequate standard of living, including food, clothing, housing and free access to clean freshwater [1, 2].

Thus, for a sustainable development of human societies—as defined in the Rio de Janeiro Declaration on Environment and Development in 1987—it is essential to guarantee water availability and quality; this brings together two fundamental aspects of society: the need to improve people's living conditions (in present generations) while protecting the environment and without compromising future generations to meet their needs [3].

Despite the fact that water is the most abundant natural compound on Earth, most of it is not directly available for human purposes (domestic, industry, and agriculture uses) due to the high salinity of main water resources (oceans and seas) and availability restrictions. Total global freshwater constitutes only *ca.* 2.7% of the overall water mass, and most of it is located in polar icecaps, glaciers and permanent snow. Only *ca.* 0.7% of freshwater, contained in rivers, lakes and groundwater, can be directly used by humans. Besides water shortage, worldwide demand for freshwater is growing at an alarming rate, and water scarcity is becoming a critical issue in many populated areas. In addition to drought impacts, overexploitation of water resources in some areas, especially for agriculture, increases the risk of water deficits and also the environmental hazards associated with water management and disposal. Therefore, it is essential to guarantee the access to clean freshwater and to promote integrated strategies to control water management and disposal in order to protect the population from sanitary and environmental risks.

Albeit water is in a continuous movement in nature, and thus removal of certain compounds in solution occurs to some extent in the hydrologic cycle (evaporation and condensation, filtration in soil); however, this natural water purification process is usually not enough to remove the wide variety of undesirable chemical species (i.e., pesticides, solvents, pharmaceutical compounds, household chemicals and so forth) that can be found in all sorts of water [4, 5].

In this regard, the occurrence of chemical compounds with therapeutic and/or biological activity in aquatic environments—including drinking water [5]—has become an outstanding environmental issue in the last decades; since then, the scientific community has devoted much research effort to develop advanced techniques to detect these compounds (usually present at extremely low concentrations) and more efficient technologies to remove them before discharge to the treated water effluent.

It should be mentioned that these compounds pose a potential risk to public health due to their biological activity, and little is currently known on the long-term exposure to these pollutants (and their mixtures) [6]. Even thought their concentration is usually low (trace levels, ca. μg L^{-1} and ng L^{-1}) and seldom exceeds water quality standards (when regulation applies), most of these compounds are continually introduced in the environment due to their high worldwide consumption; consequently, the levels in the environment are very high and almost constant [7, 8], for which high concentrations may appear; this is the case, for instance, of peak concentrations of pesticides in surface water during run-off in agricultural areas soon after application or in urban areas due to abusive household chemical uses. In some other cases (such as pharmaceuticals), they have acute toxicity, their side effects on human health are unknown, or simply their presence on water is not yet regulated.

Summarizing, quite extensive research has been done in the last years on the occurrence and removal of emergent pollutants, including pharmaceuticals, detected in water [4, 5, 9]. The purpose of this chapter is to provide a global view on the particular case of acetaminophen, one of the most worldwide consumed analgesics that has been frequently found in all sorts of water [4, 5]. An overview of the results available on the literature concerning acetaminophen occurrence in the aquatic environment and its fate in conventional and advanced water treatment technologies will be presented and discussed.

2. Pharmaceuticals as Emergent Pollutants

The control of water pollution by industrial activities was first considered in USA in 1972, in the "Federal Water Pollution Control Act Amendments" in which the Congress established a national system of unloading and elimination of pollutants [10]. Major amendments to the pristine document ("Clean Water Act" and "Water Quality Act") were enacted in 1977 and 1987. In Europe, the Water Framework Directive (2000/60/EC) and its amendments and transpositions into the national legislation of the European Community members regulate integrated pollution and control [11].

Today's society is increasing its use of a variety of chemicals (synthetic or natural products), which are being found in water systems. These compounds, known as emergent pollutants, are mainly originated from industrial, agricultural and human activities and include pesticides, industrial chemicals, pharmaceutical and personal care products (PPCPs), household chemicals, and so forth. As mentioned above, the main challenge of these compounds is their continuous discharge in the environment due to their high worldwide consumption and the potential impact on human health due to the therapeutic and/or biological activity of some of them. Moreover, many of these compounds are not regulated by international or national environmental legislation, thus they are infrequently measured or controlled as environmental markers in water pollution.

The presence of a wide variety of emergent pollutants in the aquatic environment has been frequently reported in the literature for the last decades after the early findings of Stumm-Zollinger and Fair (1965) and Hignite and Azarnoff (1977) [12-18]. However, little attention has been paid to these pollutants until toxicological impacts in fish [19-24] were linked to the occurrence of trace pollutants in the ecosystem. The high incidence of intersexuality in river fish throughout United Kingdom was demonstrated in the study published in 1998, by Jobling et al. [21], and more recently, in Potomac River (USA) [25]. The results presented in 1994, by Stan et al. [26] showing the presence of clofibric acid (metabolite of the blood lipid regulators, also used as pesticide) in 64 drinking water samples taken in Berlin (Germany) were also fundamental in drawing the attention of the scientific community towards the importance of undertaking monitoring studies of emergent pollutants. Since then, the occurrence of small concentrations of PPCP has been associated with chronic toxicity, endocrine disruption, development of pathogen resistance, alterations in development, reproduction and metabolisms, as well as genetic toxicity leading to malformations. The presence of micropollutants also endangers the reuse of treated wastewater, a strategy envisaged nowadays to achieve a sustainable water cycle management [27].

However, although available data are now much more abundant, still little is known about the occurrence, fate, synergistic, and long-term effects of PPCPs and their metabolites in water environments following their end-use [28-32]. Despite the fact that this source of water pollution is considered an important and emerging issue in water quality, there are few coordinated efforts concerning the monitoring or remediation of water and wastewater to confront the presence of these chemicals. The lack of specific regulation that controls the occurrence and effects of these emergent water pollutants is another challenge in most developed countries. A precise control of water quality is essential in order to protect the population from sanitary and environmental risks associated with water pollution.

One of the key emergent pollutants are pharmaceuticals and personal care products, firstly addressed as water pollutants by Daughton and Ternes in 1999 [33]. This group of substances comprises a large class of chemicals such as human and veterinary pharmaceuticals (over-the-counter and prescription medicines), and also other substances commonly used in daily life (i.e. household-cleaning chemicals, fragances, disinfectants, etc.). Current estimates on their presence in water are still being gathered; a few studies investigating the occurrence and most likely pollution pathways of these chemicals in water resources in different countries [25, 34-45] have reported that water bodies may contain some antibiotics, steroids and hormones, and other chemicals for personal care. It has been estimated that about six million of commercial PPCPs are available in the world, and the use of pharmaceuticals is increasing *ca.* 3-4% every year [46].

Due to their therapeutic activity, the issue of pharmaceutical residues in the water supply is nowadays considered a major environmental and human health threat. Developed to promote human health and well-being, a variety of pharmaceuticals including painkillers, tranquilizers, anti-depressants, antibiotics, birth control pills, chemotherapy agents, etc., are finding their way into the environment via human and animal excreta from disposal into the sewage system and from landfill leachate that may impact groundwater supplies. Moreover, their control results very difficult due to the diversity of pollution sources (see Figure 1). Pharmaceutical industries, hospitals and other medical facilities are obvious sources, but agricultural practices and householders also contribute to a large extent. The agricultural sector is a major antibiotic consumer through their use as growth enhancers to livestock. People often dispose of unused medicines by flushing them down toilets, and human excreta can also contain varied incompletely metabolized medicines; all these compounds end up in the streams in water treatment facilities [47-52]. From this stage, contamination of rivers, lakes, aquifers and groundwater is a considerably high risk [4, 53].

Another challenge is that these drugs can pass intact through conventional sewage treatment facilities (STP) into waterways, lakes and even aquifers. Further, discarded pharmaceuticals often end up at dumps and landfills, posing a threat to underlying groundwater. Since pharmaceuticals may have long half-lives in the environment, they can accumulate reaching biologically active levels [33]. For instance, it has been reported that the environmental persistence of several commonly used pharmaceuticals such has erythromycin, naproxen, or sulfametoxazol is longer than one year; in the case of clofibric acid, this is estimated to persist for several years [54-56].

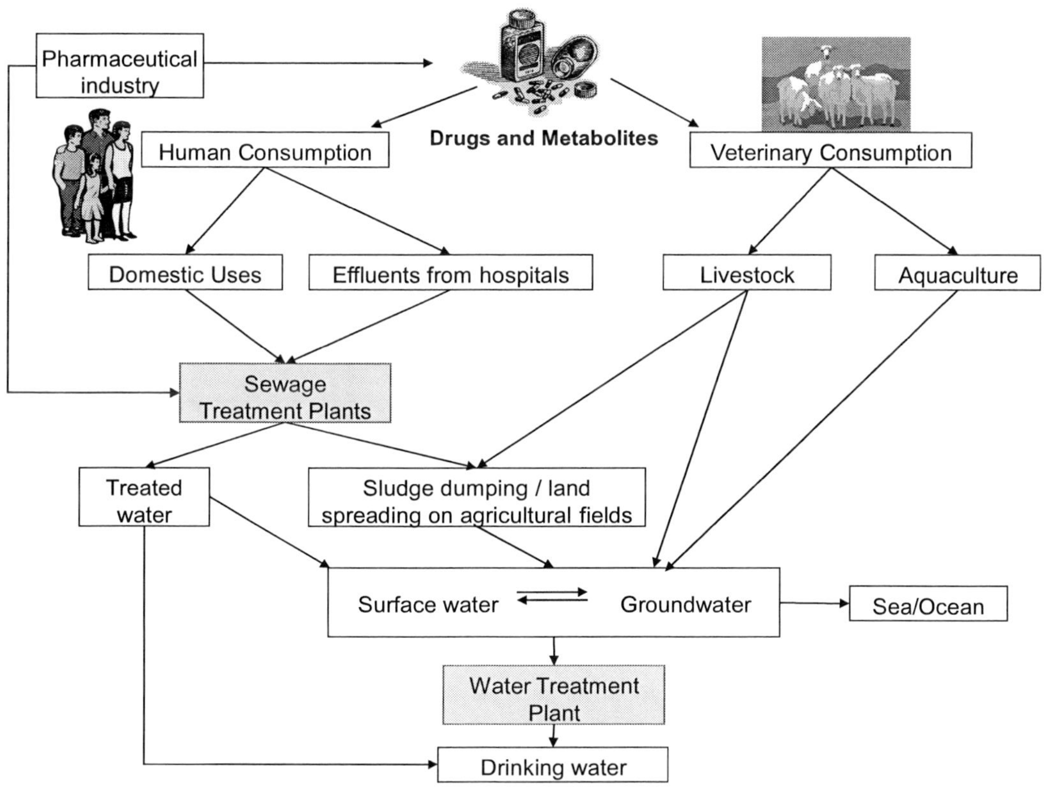

Figure 1. Scheme of main routes of water bodies pollution by pharmaceutical compounds and their metabolites.

Despite the number of studies on the topic, still little is known about the effects of pharmaceuticals and their metabolites when they are discharged to the environment [57]. Moreover, once entered in the food chain, these pollutants can easily reach humans. Although no direct effects of pharmaceutical pollution of water streams have been observed in human health [4, 58], some threats to public health associated with interactive effects from complex mixtures of drug compounds (such as development of mutations, antibiotic bacteria resistance and allergies) have been considered [59-64]. As an example, Goñi-Urizza et al. [65] have found a correlation between the presence of antibiotic-resistant bacteria and the occurrence of pharmaceuticals in influent waters from sewage treatment plan. Some other studies have revealed that the presence of low traces of pharmaceuticals have harmful effects in aquatic organisms as seaweeds and crustaceans [66, 67] and on earth fertility due to the destruction of soil microorganisms [68, 69].

The enormous diversity of chemical composition of these pollutants in waters requires a coherent strategy for reversing this threat and achieving sustainability management and quality of water. In this regard, the US-EPA has recently included a series of pharmaceuticals in the drinking water Contaminant Candidate List (CCL), in an effort to prioritize research and data collection that helps to determine whether these unregulated pollutants should be considered as specific water contaminants [70, 71].

As mentioned above, another challenge of pharmaceutical pollution in water is that many of these substances escape to conventional wastewater treatments, which allows them to reach surface waters and distribute in the environment [9, 54, 72, 73]. Indeed, PPCPs (either metabolised or not) represent a rising part of the trace pollutants found in urban and domestic wastewaters that reach sewage treatment plants [74]. Recent studies have demonstrated that conventional wastewater treatments plants (WWTP) are not generally effective to eliminate and/or degrade the majority of these compounds. This is the case of biological treatment, by far the most widely applied and cost-effective water treatment method. Unfortunately, this technology cannot deal with the non-biodegradable pollutants present in wastewater, which in addition are very often inhibitors of the biological processes. Consequently, pharmaceuticals often remain in treated water, making WWTP discharges a significant source of these substances to the aquatic environment; they have even been found to accumulate in drinking (tap) water [25, 34, 35, 75-82].

Alternatives for their removal are not yet sufficiently developed and thus have not been implemented on a large scale. Reverse osmosis, ion-exchange resins and adsorption on activated carbons are among the most utilized [83]. Their major drawbacks are a poor economic feasibility, a limited applicability and effectiveness, and a short lifetime due to low regeneration capacities. For instance, membranes for reverse osmosis are subjected to degradation by oxidants (free chlorine), reducing dramatically their performance and lifetime. Ion exchange resins are limited in applicability and effectiveness by fouling (oil, grease, suspended solids), oxidation and low regeneration capacities. Oxidation treatments, used in water potabilization such as ozonization and chlorination, have also been reported with relative success [81, 84-86]. For example, ClO_2 is only effective to oxidize sulphonamide and macrolide-derived antibiotics and estrogens [85]. In other cases, such as the chlorination of amine functionalized drugs, undesirable oxidation products might be obtained [87].

The need for developing advanced treatment technologies for water remediation that can provide safe treated effluents has resulted in a new area of research and action for water treatment systems, with many efforts directed to upgrade WWTP and to implement new competing technologies for biological degradation of emergent pollutants. Current technological alternatives with great potential in the field of water remediation focus on the development of membrane bioreactors [88] and on the advanced oxidation processes (AOP) alone [89, 90] or combined with nanofiltration or ozonation [91]. Combinations of AOP such as Fenton-based systems, heterogeneous photocatalysis, and ultraviolet or ozone-based oxidation processes have also been considered to degrade these refractory pollutants [92-94].

3. Acetaminophen in Water Resources

Acetaminophen (*N*-acetyl-4-aminophenol, *N*-(4-hydroxyphenyl)acetamide) or paracetamol is a pharmaceutical compound often detected in water resources. The molecular structure and arrangement of the atoms in space along with dimensions estimated according crystallographic data [95] are presented in Figure 2. Acetaminophen was introduced into human medicine by Von Mering in 1887 [96]; it is an analgesic and antipyretic drug regularly used for the relief of fever, headaches and some minor pains in adults and children. It is then an effective over-the-counter drug (the most used in USA [97]) that benefits millions of consumers worldwide.

Moreover, data recently gathered by several authors, reproduced in Table 1, show that the annual consumption of acetaminophen is very high in all the mentioned countries, being the first or the second most consumed pharmaceutical in the ranking of each country [98-102].

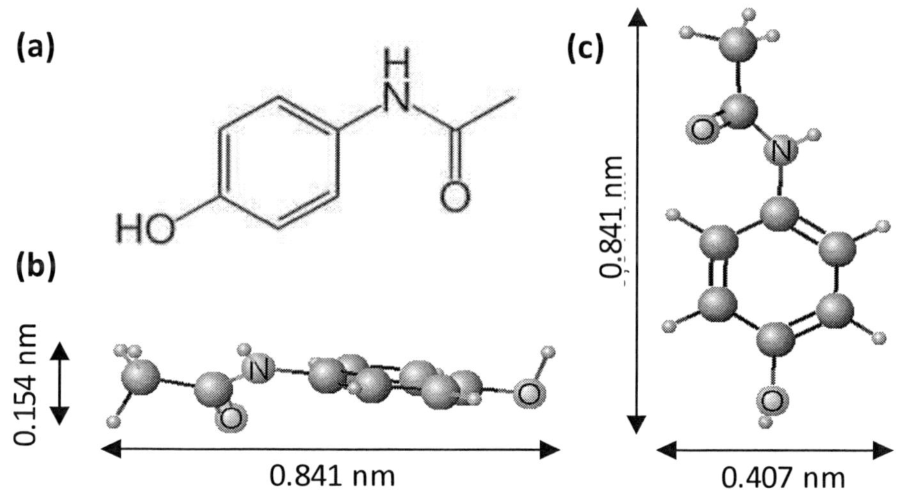

Figure 2. Molecular structure of acetaminophen. (a) General structure (b) and (c) special arrangement of the atoms with molecular dimensions.

For instance, about 3.5 billion 500 mg tablets of acetaminophen were purchased in UK in 2000 [98]; the average consumption in Europe varies widely among the countries, and for Italy it has been estimated in 9 g/person/ year [99]. However, the estimation of the overall acetaminophen consumption must take into account that this is also a co-ingredient in the formulation of other pharmaceuticals; thus the overall amount of prescribed acetaminophen becomes larger, increasing from 403 to 1135 tonnes in the case of England in the year 2000 [100].

Once ingested, acetaminophen is quickly and almost entirely absorbed from the gastrointestinal tract, whereas exceeding doses of un-metabolized acetaminophen or its metabolites are eliminated by renal excretion [103, 104] . The main metabolites formed by hepatic biotransformation are glucuronic acid and sulphate conjugates (up to 90%). Considering the above-mentioned average annual ingestion of acetaminophen in Italy (*ca.* 9 g/person/year) and the excretion rate of un-metabolized compound, *ca.* 27 tonnes would be released to water streams annually. Besides clinical uses in human medicine, another source of environmental pollution related to acetaminophen results from its use for chemical control of the brown tree snakes' population [9, 105, 106]. This leads to soil and groundwater contamination with this compound, while the result of the human consumption is mainly linked to the influents of sewage treatments plants [9, 106].

Table 1. Annual consumption of acetaminophen and its position in the ranking consumption list within a country

Country	Year	Annual consumption (t/year)	Ranking position	Ref.
Australia	1998	296	1	[101]
Austria	1997	35	2	[101]
Denmark	1997	296	1	[101]
England	2000	391	1	[101]
England	2000	403	1	[100]
Germany	2001	622	2	[101]
Switzerland	2004	95	1	[101]
USA	1997	30 000 – 35 000	1	[102]

Table 2 gathers the acetaminophen concentrations detected in various countries since late 1990s, for different sorts of waters, along with the removal efficiencies achieved depending on the water treatment process applied. The values reported for most of the STPs and WWTPs effluents are in the order of tens of ng L^{-1}. The removal efficiency of the different treatment processes was rather high in almost all cases, although acetaminophen in some treated effluents (i.e., hospitals) was still extremely high. Detected concentrations of acetaminophen in surface water, groundwater, and drinking water are of the same order of treated effluents (ng L^{-1}), and only in a reduced number of cases it was not detected or at concentrations close to the detection limit of the analytical techniques used for quantification. In Europe, the reported mean concentrations vary from not detectable to *ca.* 100 ng L^{-1} [74, 107-110]. In the USA, average concentrations of 110 ng L^{-1} with maximum values of 10000 ng L^{-1} have been reported for surface water [4], although a recent study has revealed unusual high acetaminophen concentrations in bottled water samples [111]. In Taiwan, high acetaminophen amounts have been detected in River Sindian (*ca.* 1450- 2360 ngL^{-1}) [112].

As a pharmaceutical compound, acetaminophen has an adverse drug reaction (ADR) associated with normal and excessive dosages or drug accumulation and/or the formation of chemically reactive metabolites (CRM). Acute overdose of acetaminophen is the foremost cause of acute liver failure in USA (*ca.* 80%) and Europe [145-147]. As all compounds with therapeutic activity, the potential risks of acetaminophen to both human health and the environment are estimated by the Environmental Risk Assessment (ERA) [148]. According to the European Medicines Agency (EMEA), the ERA is evaluated by means of the predicted environmental concentration of the pharmaceutical in surface water, ($PEC_{\text{surf.water}}$)[149]:

$$PEC(mg{\cdot}L^{-1})_{sur.fwater} = \frac{DOSE_{ai}{\cdot}F_{pen}}{WASTEW_{inhab}{\cdot}DILUTION} \qquad (1)$$

where $DOSE_{ai}$ is the maximum daily dose consumed per inhabitant (in mg inh^{-1} d^{-1}), F_{pen} is the market penetration fraction of the active ingredient (*ca.* 0.01 for acetaminophen), $WASTEWi_{\text{nhab}}$ is the amount of wastewater per inhabitant per day (*ca.* 200 L inh^{-1} d^{-1} according to the EU Technical Guidance Document, TGD), and *DILUTION* is the dilution factor (*ca.* 10 for acetaminophen according to TGD).

Table 2. Country-wise occurrence of acetaminophen in STPs and WWTPs influents/effluents, surface water, groundwater, and drinking water. Treatments and removal efficiencies are mentioned for the case of STPs and WWTPs

Sewage Treatment Plants (STP)						
	Sampling year	Influent (ng L^{-1})	Effluent (ng L^{-1})	Treatment	Removal (%)	Ref.
Canada	2003		5 (9000)			[113]
France (Aix-en-Provence)	2008	5200 (6700)	393 (640)	Activated sludge nitrification	93	[114]
Germany (Frankfurt/Main)	1996		n.d. (6000)	Activated sludge	98	[74]
Japan (Kumamoto City)	2009	8000 - 10000	n.d. – 1.39 g/day	Activated sludge	> 90	[115]
Spain (Almería)	2003/04	134000 (246000)	220 (4300)	Activated sludge	99	[53]
Spain	2007/08	149226 (19850)	< LOQ (30.0)	Activated sludge	> 95	[116]
Spain	2009	163-260	10.7-22.0	Diox, sand filtered, ozonated, GAC filtered	96	[117]
			1.3 – 3.8	Ultrafiltration, reverse osmosis, remineralization	99	
Spain (Madrid)		23202 (37458)	< LOD	Activated sludge	> 99	[118]
South Korea	2004	70 (260)	60 (160)	Activated sludge, coagulation, flocculation, and sedimentation	8.7	[119]
Sweden (Stockholm)	2007	34400	1700		95	[120]
Switzerland	2009	29000 (44000)	350	Activated sludge	99	[121]
Taiwan	2008		16	Activated sludge		[122]
UK	2004			Activated sludge nitrification/de-nitrification	91.93	[123]
USA (Louisiana)	2001/02		1.2	Activated sludge		[124]
USA	2004	5529 - 69570	< 20	Activated sludge		[125]
			< 20	Activated sludge and UV		

Table 2. (Continued).

	Sampling year	Influent (ng L^{-1})	Effluent (ng L^{-1})	Treatment	Removal (%)	Ref.
Sewage Treatment Plants (STP)						
USA (Georgia)	2008	80000 (130000)	< 50	Activated sludge	> 99	[73]
			< 50	Activated sludge and granular activated carbon	> 99	
			< 50	Activated sludge, GAC and ozone	> 99	
Wastewater Treatment Plants (WWTPs)						
Croatia		10194 (26090)	2101 (5990)			[126]
France (Marseille)			108.1 – 11308.9			[127]
London (UK)	2003/04		10 – 112 (281)			[110]
South Korea	2004/05	11500	9.5 (19)	Membrane bioreactor	≈ 99	[128]
Spain (Almería)			1767 (3130) hospital effluent			[129]
Spain (Almería)			16020 (29000) hospital effluents			[130]
Spain (Barcelona)	2005	≈ 18000 (≈ 22000)	< 1000	Activated sludge Membrane bioreactor	98.4 99.6	[131]
Spain (Barcelona)	2007		99000 (11400) primary effluent	Activated sludge Membrane bioreactor	99.9 99.8-99.9	[132]
Spain		1570	30	Activated sludge	98	[133]
Switzerland (Genova)	2010		300			[107]
Taiwan	2008		36950 (100433) hospital effluent			[122]
Taiwan	2008	1800 - 30967	< 200	Activated sludge and chlorination or UV	> 95	[134]
USA			6 (1060)			[135]
USA (New York City)	2005	61000	860		99	[136]
USA (Baltimore)		960	n.d.	Activated sludge, disinfection, dechlorination	> 99	[137]

Table 2. (Continued).

Surface water			
	Sampling year	Concentration (ng L^{-1})	Ref.
Canada	2003	5 (3600)	[113]
France (Marseille)		10.6 – 72.3 (Herault) 5 x10^4 – 2 x10^5 (Cortiou)	[127]
Germany (Frankfurt/Main)	1996	n.d.	[74]
Germany	2000	< LOD – 66	[109]
South Korea	2004/05	33 (73)	[128]
Spain (Barcelona)		42 (250)	[126]
Switzerland	2010	25	[107]
Taiwan	2007/08	1450 – 2360	[112]
Taiwan		14 – 1600	[134]
USA	1999/00	110 (10^4)	[4]
UK (London)	2003/04	9 – 289 (555)	[110]
USA	2001	160	[138]
USA (Iowa)	2001	n.d. – 1950	[139]
USA (Louisiana)	2001/02	n.d.	[124]
USA	2003	15	[140]
USA		684 - 1780	[135]
USA (New Jersey)		n.d. - 31	[141]
USA (Louisiana)	2004	24.7 – 65.2	[142]
Groundwater			
	Sampling year	Concentration (ng L^{-1})	
USA	2000	380	[143]

Table 2. (Continued).

Tap water / Drinking water / Bottled water			
	Sampling year	Concentration (ng L^{-1})	Ref.
Canada (Ontario)	2002	0.2	[124]
France (Marseille)		n.d. – 210.1	[127]
South Korea	2004/05	n.d.	[128]
Switzerland		160	[121]
USA	1998	detected	[144]
USA (Louisiana)	2001/02	0.1	[124]
USA	2003	300 – 3000 (2 out of 12 samples)	[140]
USA		1100 – 1300 (3 out of 10 brands of bottled water)	[111]

Values indicated alone are mean concentrations (maximum concentration).

LOQ: limit of quantification

LOD: limit of detection

n.d.: not detected

GAC: granular activated carbon

Table 3. PEC values and physico-chemical properties of the acetaminophen

Property	Value	Ref.
	15 (EMEA)	[150]
	44 (Pharmatreat)	[150]
PEC ($\mu g\ L^{-1}$)	20 (EMEA)	[110]
	7 (GREAT-ER)	[151]
	37 (CPMP, 2001)	[58]
log K_{ow}	0.46	[150]
log K_{oc}	1.79	[152]
	3.1 d	[153]
% transformation or DT_{50}(d)[a]	57%	[154]
	99%	[155]

[a] DT_{50} is the time for 50% disappearance in days

This parameter assumes that the drug is used uniformly over the time period and target area, no metabolism occurs in the patient, and that WWTPs are the main points of entry into the aqueous environment. Other models have been postulated by different organisations to evaluate the PEC parameter; thus it is important to indicate the ERA guideline used for its determination. Some examples of the PEC values for acetaminophen, reported by different organisms, are compiled in Table 3.

The values exceed the threshold bioconcentration value taken as 0.01 $\mu g\ L^{-1}$, and in general overestimate the environmental concentrations detected in different aqueous environments for different countries (see Table 2), with the exception of hospitals and STPs and WWTPs effluents.

If the aquatic PEC is > 0.01 $\mu g\ L^{-1}$ (or lower than this threshold value but the compound is suspected from special ecotoxic effects) further investigation is required. In this regard, Phase II is divided into two tiers. Tier A involves a review of physico-chemical (adsorption-desorption using batch equilibrium method, biodegradability test, etc.) and toxicological (values such as LC_{50} or EC_{50}) data of the pharmaceutical, while Tier B evaluates the bioaccumulation of the pharmaceutical compound itself and its metabolites. Some basic physico-chemical properties of acetaminophen for EMEA phase II tier A are also reported in Table 3, such as the octanol-water (K_{ow}), and the soil organic carbon-water partition coefficients (K_{oc}) that allow the evaluation of the acetaminophen-water affinity. Degradation studies are also recommended for evaluating the persistence of acetaminophen in the aqueous environment; available studies (Tables 2 and 3) suggest a rather low persistence of acetaminophen.

Concerning the ecotoxicity of acetaminophen, scarce data are available in the literature, although some results are summarized in Table 4 [154, 156, 157]. In general, there is a huge discrepancy between reported data, mainly due to the different methods used in the determination of the LC_{50} parameter. Some authors [154] suggest that standard tests (algae, Daphnia, and fish) underestimate the toxicity of acetaminophen, when compared to other well-known pharmaceuticals. Despite this, acetaminophen was classified as harmful pollutant by the European Union (Directive 93/67/EEC on the risk assessment for new notified substances) based on the LC_{50} values [158].

Besides reporting ERA parameters for individual pharmaceuticals, it has to be considered that very often mixtures of PPCPs can be present in water streams. Thus, the combined concentrations of compounds with pharmacologically similar (concentration addition) and different (response addition) modes of action should be considered to evaluate the toxicity of real complex mixtures [159]. In fact, a relatively small effect of a mixture of seven pharmaceuticals (acetaminophen among them) has been observed on crustaceans (Hyalella) [160]. The scarcity of data on ecotoxicity tests of mixture of pollutants requires further research in this area.

Table 4. Lethal Dose 50% (LC_{50}) of acetaminophen

Test	Time (h)	LC_{50} (mg/L)	Method	Ref.
Fish	96	258	ECOSAR	[161]
Daphnia	48	41	ECOSAR	[161]
Algae	48	2549	ECOSAR	[161]
Daphnia	48	20		[154]
Zebra mussel haemocytes		0.35		[162]
Bacteria	1/4	331	ISO 11348-3	[163]
Crustacean	48	50	OECD 202	[163]
Crustacean	24	56	OECD 202	[163]
Algae	96	134	OECD 201	[154]
Daphnia	48	50	OECD 201	[154]
Lumin Bacteria	1/2	650	DIN 38412	[154]
Daphnia	24	136		[164]
Daphnia	48	9		[164]
S. proboscideu	24	30		[164]

4. Acetaminophen Removal and Degradation

As mentioned above, recent studies have demonstrated that recalcitrant pharmaceutical compounds are frequently found in urban and domestic wastewaters since conventional non-oxidative water treatment processes (i.e. biological method, coagulation, flocculation, and sedimentation) do not seem to be effective to eliminate and/or degrade the majority of the active pharmaceutical ingredients [54, 72].

In the particular case of acetaminophen, relatively large removal efficiencies have been reported in the literature after conventional non-oxidative waste treatment processes (see Table 2). As an example, two different studies carried out on sewage treatment plants in United Kingdom and USA, during 2004, revealed that the use of activated sludge allowed a 90-100% removal of acetaminophen [123, 125].

However, it must be emphasized that despite such large removal efficiency, still several hundreds of ng L^{-1} were detected in the treated effluent discharged. At converse, analysis of the influents and effluents of several South Korea sewage treatment plants—also in 2004—showed an acetaminophen removal rate of *ca.* 8.7%, much lower than that of other pharmaceutical compounds (i.e., salicylic acid and ibuprofen) [119]. Even in most favourable cases, the complete removal of acetaminophen (or other compounds) using conventional water treatment process is not usually attained; other processes must be coupled to further eliminate the remaining compound and remediate the wastewater effluent. Oxidation treatments with chlorine (chlorination) are most commonly used [124], although their major drawback (besides the economic penalty to the overall processes) is linked with the formation of toxic metabolites, also classified as carcinogenic and/or mutagenic compounds [165, 166]. Chlorination of acetaminophen has been studied showing the formation of two chlorinated aromatic products (i.e., chloro-4-acetamidophenol and dichloro-4-acetamidophenol), and two quinoidal oxidation by-products (i.e., 1,4-benzoquinone and *N*-acetyl-*p*benzoquinoneimine) [167, 168]. These are toxic oxidation intermediate compounds associated with acetaminophen overdoses in humans with lethal effects [169]. It must also be mentioned that Chiron et al. [114] identified nitrophenolic transformation products of acetaminophen in effluents of full-scale WWTPs, pointing out acetaminophen nitration during the treatment with nitrifying activated sludges.

Additionally, one should bear in mind that the interpretation of the results might be very often influenced by the detection limits of the quantification method utilized to measure the pollutant concentration. In this regard, pre-concentration techniques (for instance, solid phase extraction) are recommended to improve the recovery yields for acetaminophen [128]. Some other times, important information on water pollution is left behind when the analysis is restricted to the target pharmaceutical compound, disregarding the possibility of side reactions and the formation of metabolites. In this case, besides the removal efficiency of the studied compound, it becomes extremely important to quantify the mineralization rate (using for instance Total Organic Carbon (TOC) or Dissolved Organic Carbon (DOC)) [114] and to identify the metabolites.

Hence, the search for more efficient water treatment technologies leading to effective removal and/or mineralization of pharmaceutical compounds, while avoiding the formation of by-products with equal or even more adverse effects than the pristine drug, is a continuous challenge for the scientific community. For this reason, many research efforts are being directed to implement new competing technologies for degradation of these recalcitrant pollutants with therapeutic activity. Technological alternatives with great potential focused on the development of membrane bioreactors, adsorption processes based on activated carbons or other adsorbent materials, and advanced oxidation processes. A detailed discussion of the recent literature data available on these technologies is presented in the following sections of this chapter.

4.1 Membrane Bioreactors

Membrane bioreactor technology combines biological activated sludge processes and a solid-liquid separation by membrane filtration and, according to the literature, seems to be the most promising development in microbiological wastewater treatment applied to urban and industrial effluents [88, 170]. The performance of this technology for the removal of several pharmaceutical compounds [131, 171] has been evaluated with different success depending on the nature of the drug present on solution; for instance, low efficiencies have been reported for erythromycim and diclofenac degradation [128]. More satisfactory and encouraging results have been reported for membrane bioreactor technology applied to the removal of acetaminophen, with almost complete removal efficiencies [128, 131, 132]. An interesting work developed by Radjenovic et al. [[132] reports the need and benefits of coupling several advanced treatment stages (i.e., secondary and tertiary processes) during the water treatment to remove certain refractory pharmaceutical compounds (such as acetaminophen), which are not removed after primary treatments (i.e., primary activated sludge step). This behaviour was explained by electrostatic repulsive interactions between the negatively charged groups of the activated sludge and the negatively charged drug species.

4.2 Advanced Oxidation Processes

In the last few years, a considerable amount of research has been carried out in the field of advanced oxidation processes (AOPs) or technologies (AOTs) for the removal and degradation of pharmaceutical compounds from wastewaters. This is clearly seen in the increase in the number of publications about this topic in peer-reviewed journals, as recently reviewed by Klavarioti et al. [8] and Ziylan and Ince [9]. Table 5 gathers the information concerning recently published data on AOPs for acetaminophen degradation.

AOPs can be broadly defined as aqueous phase oxidation methods based on the formation of highly reactive species such as (mainly but not exclusively) hydroxyl radicals (•OH), leading to the destruction of the target pollutants [172]. Hydroxyl radicals are non-selective and very powerful oxidizing agents that can readily attack organic molecules (by means of dehydrogenation and/or hydroxylation reactions) leading to complete mineralization of the pollutants into carbon dioxide, water, and some inorganic compounds (ammonium, nitrates, sulphates) or at least to the conversion of the organics into highly oxidized and (preferably) more innocuous products. AOPs can be classified either as homogenous or heterogeneous processes, with the former further subdivided into processes with or without the requirement of energy input (photochemical and non-photochemical). Most explored methods include Fenton's and modified Fenton's reactions, ozonation, photocatalysis, sonolysis, combinations of UV irradiation and chemical oxidants, wet oxidation processes, and so forth.

In the field of water remediation, extensive research has been carried out on the use of AOPs to treat industrial (distillery, agrochemical, kraft blending, pulp and paper, textile, metal-plating wastes) and urban effluents (hospital and slaughterhouse wastes, effluents from municipal wastewater facilities), as well as in soil remediation, odour control, etc.

These technologies can be used either alone or coupled to other physico-chemical and biological processes in order to improve the removal efficiency of the target molecules. A review of most representative results concerning the use of AOP for the removal and/or degradation of acetaminophen from aqueous media will be addressed in the following paragraphs. Figure 3 presents the main acetaminophen degradation pathways resultants from various advanced oxidation processes.

Photolysis. This is one of the simplest AOPs; it involves the interaction of irradiation (typically UV but also visible light) with the polluted water to promote the degradation of the contaminant. Irradiation under UV light has been long used in disinfection of drinking water as an alternative to chlorination to avoid the formation of harmful by-products during the reaction with chlorine [190].

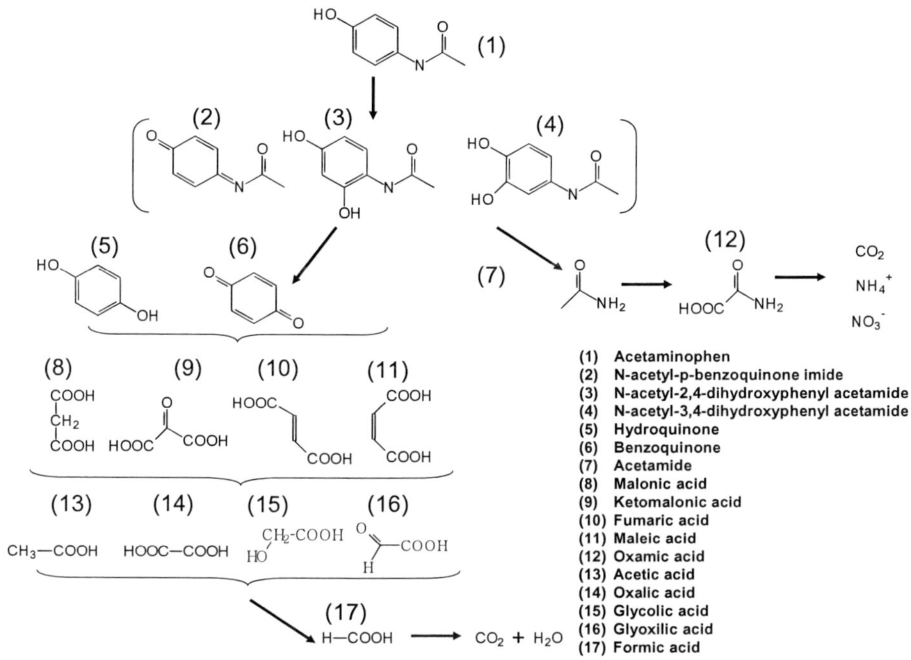

Figure 3. Main degradation pathways of acetaminophen by AOPs [93, 105, 106, 170, 173-179].

The degradation efficiency of some pharmaceutical compounds by means of direct irradiation has been investigated, and a great number of oxidation intermediates has been detected [106, 180, 190]. In the particular case of acetaminophen, direct photolysis does not seem to be efficient (degradation upon photolysis is negligible). For this reason, this technique is often used in combination with other methods such as the addition of oxidizing chemicals (hydrogen peroxide) that generate hydroxyl radicals to promote the oxidation of acetaminophen and enhance the efficiency of the degradation process [106, 190]. For instance, removal efficiency of acetaminophen is almost complete when UV irradiation is combined with H_2O_2 [106, 180] with *ca.* 40% degree of mineralization [106].

Ozonation. This is a well-known AOP for the generation of hydroxyl radicals without using light energy (non-photochemical method). Ozone is a strong oxidation agent, and its reaction with organic molecules can follow two different pathways: decomposition in water to form hydroxyl and superoxide anion radicals (even stronger oxidizing agents than ozone) or selective attack of certain functional groups of organic molecules through an electrophilic mechanism (the rate of the attack by ozone is several orders of magnitude slower than that of hydroxyl radicals) [191]. The reaction between ozone and superoxide anion radical gives rise to the formation of ozonide anion radical ($\bullet O_3^-$), which also decomposes giving $\bullet$OH radical. The main challenge of this method is the cost of electricity for ozone generation, although it is widely used in wastewater disinfection [192], drinking water treatment for odors and taste control [34].

Table 5. Treatment of acetaminophen in waters by AOPs

AOPs	Initial conc.	Experimental conditions	Measure of degradability	Summary of results	Ref.
Photolysis					
	≈ 5 ng L^{-1}	Real wastewater, UV dose of 2768 mJ/cm^2, UV 254 nm, hydraulic retention time of 5 min	Specific drug, DOC	Removal efficiency 1%	[180]
Photolysis/H_2O_2					
	≈ 5 ng L^{-1}	Real wastewater, UV dose of 923 mJ/cm^2, UV 254 nm, hydraulic retention time of 5 min	Specific drug, DOC	Removal efficiency > 90%	[180]
	10^{-5} M	Distilled water solutions, LP UV 254 nm at pH 5	Specific drug, TOC	Complete removal and 40% mineralization in one and four min, respectively. Identification of oxidation by-products.	[106]
Ozonation					
	$5x10^{-5}$ M	Distilled water solution, 10^{-5} M O_3 at pH 2-7	Specific drug, TOC	Complete removal and 30% mineralization in 20 and 120 min, respectively regardless the solution pH. Identification of oxidation by-products and postulate of degradation pathway.	[106]
	0.078–1 gL^{-1}	Distilled water, O_3 alone or O_3/UV at 300-420 nm, pH 2-6 with and without Fe^{2+} of Cu^{2+}	Specific drug, TOC	Catalysis and/or irradiation improve both degradation and mineralization by ozone. Conversion decreases with increasing [ACE] and decreasing metal loading and is pH insensitive between two and four. Iron is more active than copper. Identification of degradation by-products and pathways.	[170]

Table 5. (Continued).

Fenton and photo-Fenton				
100 µg L^{-1}	Demineralised water and standard freshwater, solar irradiation , [Fe]i = 5, 15 and 55M, $[H_2O_2]$i = 50 mg L^{-1}, pH 2.8 or unadjusted	Specific drug, DOC	Fenton was far more effective than TiO_2. Almost complete degradation of ACE is achieved within 20 min of irradiation. ACE was also degraded in dark Fenton in simulated freshwater ([Fe]= 5 mg L^{-1} without pH adjustment in demineralised water). Mineralization > 50% in the absence of bicarbonates.	[181]
0.1 mM	STP effluents, FeO_x and $Fe(NO_3)_3$ at 0.2 mmol L^{-1}, pH 2.5, UVA 320-400 nm, $[H_2O_2]$i = 1.0 to 10.0 mmol L^{-1}	Specific drug, TOC	Experimental condition tested: iron source, $[H_2O_2]_0$ and water source (synthetic and STP effluent). Removal of 98% using FeO_x, and 53% when using $Fe(NO_3)_3$, both after five min irradiation.	[182]
10 mg L^{-1}	Water and synthetic wastewater effluent, UVA and UVC, H_2O_2	TOC, COD, DBO-5	Under the optimum conditions (H_2O_2 flow rate=50 mL h^{-1}, [Fe(II)]=2 mg L^{-1}, pH 2.5 and T=40 °C) 83% of the COD, 71% of the TOC and 94% of BDO-5 are degraded in 120 min. Mineralization decreased in real water samples (120 min) from 96% to about 71%.	[183]
157 mg L^{-1} (≈ 1 mM)	pH 2.7-2.9, solar irradiation, Fe(II)	Specific drug, DOC	Acetaminophen removal after 90 min irradiation, while only 44% of organic carbon mineralization was achieved. In the optimized conditions, ([Fe(II)]= 20 mg L^{-1} and $[H_2O_2]$= 200 mg L^{-1}) in 25 min it attained the desired biocompatibility (mineralization ≥18.6%, for total ACE degradation and biodegradability > 40%).	[184]
100 µg L^{-1}	Real wastewater effluents, solar irradiation, [Fe] = 5 and 20 mg L^{-1}, pH 3, $[H_2O_2]$I = 50 mg L^{-1}	Specific drug, DOC	With [Fe] = 5 mg L^{-1}total degradation after 150 min irradiation, and using [Fe] = 20 mg L^{-1}total degradation after 50 min irradiation.	[185]
	pH 2.8	Specific drug, DOC	Best conditions for solar photo-Fenton of ACE solutions using a light path of 5 cm were 0.36 mM Fe(II), irradiance above 30W/m2 and a molar ratio H_2O_2 to DOC of around 1.65.	[186]

Table 5. (Continued).

Semiconductor photocatalysis				
2-10mM	Deionized water, suspended Degussa TiO_2, UV 254 or 365 nm at pH 3.5-11	Specific drug, TOC	UVC irradiation allows faster decomposition than UVA. Factors tested during degradation: initial drug, catalyst and oxygen concentrations, pH and light intensity. Degradation > 95% for 2 mM acetaminophen solution within 80 min. Identifies by-products.	[173]
25-100μM	Aqueous solutions, TiO_2, UV ≥ 365, pH 3.5, 6.9 and 9.5	Specific drug	After 100 min irradiation, about ≈ 95% acetaminophen is decomposed in the 1.0 g L^{-1} TiO2 aqueous solution with [ACE]i = 100 μM. Highly efficient at pH 9 (removal ≈ 100% when [ACE]i = 50μM and TiO_2 = 0.5 g L^{-1}. [ACE]i and TiO_2 dosage affect the degradation efficiency. Quantum calculations show that further oxidation of the by-products identified can breakdown their aromatic structure up to carboxylate acid and CO_2.	[187]
$1.0x10^{-4}$ M	Aqueous solutions, UV 254 nm, 0.1 g L^{-1} TiO_2,	Specific drug, TOC	Degradation of 90% after 160 min of irradiation, and only 39% of TOC removal is observed. Identification of toxic oxidation by-products.	[105]
100 μg L^{-1}	Demineralised water and standard freshwater, solar irradiation, [TiO_2] = 5 mg L^{-1}, [H_2O_2]i = 50 mg L^{-1}	Specific drug, DOC	$TiO_2$was less effective than Fenton. Almost complete degradation of ACE (< LOQ) was achieved after 145 min under illumination. The presence of bicarbonates should be avoided to assure drug concentration < LOQ.	[181]
	Deionized water, TiO_2, UV 254 nm	Specific drug,	Mineralization of 85% after 450 min of irradiation. Presents by-products and pathways.	[174]
5 mg L^{-1}	Effluent WWTP, [TiO_2]= 0.5 g L^{-1}, UV-A,	Specific drug, DOC	After 3h of irradiation [ACE] < LOD.	[133]
100 μg L^{-1}	Synthetic water and simulated effluent, solar irradiation, TiO_2 immobilized on glass spheres	Specific drug, DOC	Total ACE degradation in synthetic water and simulated effluent after, respectively, 60 and 100 min.	[188]

Table 5. (Continued).

Electrochemical oxidation					
	157 mg L^{-1}	0.05 M Na_2SO_4, pH 7.8	Specific drug, TOC	Applied current 300 mA for 360 min. Pt and BDD electrodes, 17 and 98% TOC removal for Pt and BDD electrodes, respectively.	[93]
	1 mM	0.025 M Na_2SO_4, pH 7.8	Specific drug	Applied current 200 mA for 210 min, Ti/IrO_2 and Ti/SnO_2 electrodes, 1 and 40% TOC removal for Ti/IrO_2 and Ti/SnO_2, respectively.	[175]
	1 mM	0.1 NaCl	Specific drug, TOC	Applied current 80 mA for 300 min, BDD and Ti/RuO_2 electrodes, 28 and 55% TOC removal for BDD and Ti/RuO_2 electrodes, respectively.	[176]
Electrofenton					
	157 mg L^{-1}	0.05 M Na_2SO_4, pH 3.5	Specific drug, TOC	Pt/GDE, Applied current 300 mA for 240 min, Fe^{2+} and Cu^{2+} additives. Between 59-90% TOC removal.	[177]
Fotoelectrofenton					
	157 mg L^{-1}	0.05 M Na_2SO_4, pH 3.5	Specific drug, TOC	Pt/GDE, Applied current 300 mA for 240 min+ UVA light (6 W) , Fe^{2+} and Cu^{2+} additives. Between 79-95% TOC removal.	[178]
	157 mg L^{-1}	0.05 M Na_2SO_4, pH 3.5	Specific drug, TOC	Pt/GDE (pilot plant), Solar CPC (5A) for 120 min, 0.4 mM Fe2+ additives. 6% TOC removal.	[179]
Sonolysis					
	25-150 mg L^{-1}	Aqueous solutions, 574-1134 kHz and 9-32 W	Specific drug, COD	Complete conversion and 39% mineralization after eight h of ultrasonic irradiation of [ACE]i = 25 mg L^{-1} at 574 kHz and 32 W). Efficiency improved by H_2O_2 addition.	[189]

ACE= acetaminophen

TOC = Total Organic Carbon

DOC= Dissolved Organic Carbon

COD = Chemical Oxygen Demand

However, ozonation of water containing organic compounds does not generally lead to complete oxidation of the pollutant to CO_2 and H_2O (mineralization). Very often, intermediate oxidation products remain in the solution, and completion of the oxidation reactions can also be achieved by supplementing the ozonation reaction with, for instance, UV irradiation or H_2O_2 (O_3/UV and/or O_3/H_2O_2/UV processes) [170]. The UV enhancement is based on the ability of ozone to absorb UV light at 254 nm wavelength, generating H_2O_2 as an intermediate that will further be decomposed as •OH radicals [193]. Addition of hydrogen peroxide to ozone can also initiate the decomposition cycle of ozone to form •OH radicals, increasing the degradation yield of different pollutants [194]. Another strategy to accelerate the ozonation reaction is to use heterogenous or homogenous catalysts; several metal oxides and metal ions have been explored for this purpose (Fe_2O_3, MnO_2, Ru/CeO_2, Fe^{2+}, Fe^{3+}, Mn^{2+}) with outstanding improvements in the decomposition rate and yield of the target pollutants. It is important to point out that the operating costs of the UV/O_3 or H_2O_2 systems are a key parameter to be considered depending on the wastewater flow rate, types and concentrations of pollutants present, and the degree of removal required (otherwise photolysis of ozone would simply be an expensive way to generate hydrogen peroxide).

Applied to the removal of pharmaceutical compounds, a few studies in the literature show that ozonation of acetaminophen containing effluents allows the complete removal of this drug, along with a large degree of mineralization (see Table 5).

Fenton and photo-Fenton. The Fenton reaction was reported over a hundred years ago by Fenton [195]; about forty years later, Haber-Weiss [196] demonstrated the oxidative power of Fenton's reagent (H_2O_2/Fe^{2+}) based on the generation of hydroxyl radicals (see reaction below), which can be further consumed for the degradation of the target pollutant. Since then, Fenton process has become one of the most widely studied homogenous catalytic process for water remediation. Mixtures of Fe^{3+}/H_2O_2 can also be used (Fenton-like systems) to promote the oxidation of pollutants. Although the reaction mechanism is not yet completely elucidated, the formation of hydroxyl radicals in the presence of Fenton's reagent can be very briefly described by the following reactions:

$$Fe^{2+} + H_2O_2 \rightarrow Fe^{3+} + {\bullet}OH{\cdot} + {\bullet}OH^{-} \qquad \text{reaction (1)}$$

$$Fe^{3+} + H_2O_2 \rightarrow Fe^{2+} + OOH{\bullet} + H^{+} \qquad \text{reaction (2)}$$

The rate constant of reaction (1) is very high, and once ferric ion is formed, excess amounts of hydrogen peroxide are further decomposed, generating again hydroxyl radicals according to reaction (2). Fenton reaction is very sensitive to solution pH, and it becomes operative at optimum pH values of *ca.* 2.8-3.0, where it is propagated by the catalytic behavior of the Fe^{3+}/Fe^{2+} couple. However, parasitic reactions based on the consumption of •OH by the Fenton's reagent may also occur, being one of major sources that contributes to decrease the oxidizing power of Fenton systems [197, 198]. UV and solar irradiation can also be used to increase the formation of the hydroxyl radicals (photo-Fenton reaction).

Although the Fenton processes are usually a tertiary stage of the water treatment, in the case of highly polluted effluents with pharmaceutical compounds (i.e. hospital or pharmaceutical manufacturing effluents), this technology can be applied in a very early stage since it can mineralize a substantial fraction of the polluting species increasing the efficiency of the biological post-treatment [197, 199]. The major drawbacks of this technology are related with the relatively narrow operational pH range and the need to introduce an additional step to recover iron ions after the treatment. To overcome this limitation, the immobilization of the Fenton catalyst on a heterogeneous matrix is currently being largely explored. Also, heterogeneous Fenton processes using Fe_2O_3 and α-FeOOH [198] as source of iron species have been proposed.

The usefulness of the Fe^{2+}/H_2O_2 system as a potential oxidant for degradation of pharmaceuticals (including acetaminophen) has been investigated, mainly in real water samples using the photo-Fenton process with UV and solar irradiation (see Table 5). Among them, solar photo-Fenton is a very promising strategy to decrease the costs of the process (common cornerstone of most AOPs). In this sense, several studies have been carried out in a pilot plant at the Solar Platform in Almería (southern Spain), confronting the efficiency of solar photo-Fenton and photocatalytic process using TiO_2 and UV light to treat synthetic solutions with low concentrations (*ca.* 100 $\mu g\ L^{-1}$) of different pharmaceuticals (including acetaminophen) [181].

Solar photo-Fenton has proven to be more effective than TiO_2–based processes, since lower irradiation time was needed to degrade the studied compounds at concentrations below the LOD of the analytical method. For example, ten min of solar irradiation were enough to promote the degradation of acetaminophen, compared to 145 min for the TiO_2 process to attain the same result. Some studies performed in real water samples (STP and wastewater effluents) reported removal rates near 100% after only five min of UV irradiation (see Table 5) in such complex water matrices. This is important since the mineralization rate and efficiency can be strongly controlled by other species present in the water effluent. Indeed, a decrease in the mineralization efficiency of *ca.* 30% has been reported in the presence of synthetic complex matrices [181-183, 200].

Heterogeneous catalysis. After Fujishima and Honda discovered the photocatalytic splitting of water using TiO_2 electrodes in 1972 [201], research on the heterogeneous photocatalysis has rapidly expanded in many fields, and particularly the use of semiconductor materials for environmental protection has received much attention [202-204]. Among the catalysts, titanium oxide—a direct wide-band gap semiconductor (i.e. 3.20 eV)—has been extensively studied since it is non-toxic, photostable, cheap and very efficient under ultraviolet light (UV). However, a wide range of semiconductors, other than titania, based on transition metal oxides and sulfides (such as ZnO, MgO, WO_3, Fe_2O_3, CdS) may be used for photocatalysis, some of them showing certain activity under visible light [8]. In this regard, intensive studies are in progress to develop advanced photocatalysts that can be used under solar energy (towards an efficient use of solar spectrum) [181, 188, 205]; novel synthetic strategies based on improving the photocatalytic activity of current semiconductors by immobilization on porous supports (silica, glass fibers, carbon supports) or synthesizing porous semiconductors with increased surface area are being widely explored [206-210].

Photocatalysis over a semiconductor is initiated by the absorption of a photon ($h\nu$) with energy equal to or greater than the band gap of the semiconductor. This provokes the excitation of an electron (e^-) from the valence to the conduction band; simultaneously an electron vacancy or hole (h^+) is created in the valence band of the semiconductor:

$$h\nu + \text{semiconductor} = h^+ + e^-$$

The created electron-hole (e^-/h^+) pairs migrate to the photocatalyst surface where it can either recombine producing thermal energy (with no chemical effect), or participate in redox reactions with the pollutants in the solution or gas phase in contact with the semiconductor. Despite the lifetime of e^-/h^+ pairs is a few nanoseconds, this is still long enough for promoting redox reactions [211]. The photo-generated hole is a strong oxidizing agent that can react with the pollutant itself (photo-oxidation, if the redox potential is less negative than that of the semiconductor valence band) or with water to produce hydroxyl radicals (leading to the oxidation of the pollutant through radical chain reactions); at converse, the electron in the conduction band is a strong reducing agent and can react with electron acceptors, such as dissolved oxygen to create superoxide radical, or other species with a redox potential more positive than that of the photocatalyst conduction band (photo-reduction). These reactions of the e^-/h^+pairs prevent the recombination of both species, and thus increase the photo-oxidation of the target pollutants. Compared to photolysis, the presence of a catalyst typically accelerates the rate of the degradation reactions, thereby increasing the efficiency of the process.

Photocatalysis has been used for the destruction of a variety of inorganic and organic compounds, natural organic matter into harmless products e.g., carbon dioxide, water, [212] and water disinfection to destroy bacteria and viruses [213, 214].

The degradation yields of acetaminophen after semiconductor photocatalysis with TiO_2, reported in Table 5, show that this methodology allows high degradation rates (> 90%) in both real [133] and synthetic waters samples [181, 188]. However, again the complexity of real samples matrices can determine the experimental conditions to be used for optimizing the degradation efficiency [181, 188].

Concerning acetaminophen, quite a large number of studies report the extent of mineralization and the identification of the degradation by-products formed using photocatalytic methods [105, 173, 174, 187]. In general, high mineralization rates (*ca.* 85%) are obtained from synthetic solutions, although this parameter is largely dependent on the experimental conditions (mostly the irradiation source and geometry, pH, initial concentration) [105, 174]. The main detected intermediate products are presented in Figure 3, namely, 1,4-benzoquinone, hydroquinone, acetamide and short alkyl chain organic acids such as hydroxy-acetic acid, butenedioic acid, oxamic acid and maleic acid, so forth.

Electro-assisted degradation. The use of electricity for water treatment was first suggested in 1889 [215], although its application to environmental processes is rather new and it is expanding rapidly. Considerable amount of research has been carried out in the field of direct or integrated electrochemical processes applied to environmental protection during the last years; and quite a few electrochemical technologies have been proposed as promising alternatives to conventional degradation methods, due to the freedom of choice in adjusting the electrode potential and electrode material to meet almost any demand and the coupling with low-cost renewable energy sources (solar energy) [216-221].

Compared to classical water remediation techniques, electrochemical techniques applied to wastewater remediation offer manifold advantages such as environmental compatibility (electrons are clean reagents per se), energetic efficiency, versatility (they are not selective and thus can deal with a wide variety of pollutants), low cost and easy automation (usually low temperatures and pressures are needed), and so forth. On the other hand, some challenges need still to be faced, particularly those related to the electrodes' stability, cost and erosion, lowering the cost of electricity by the coupling with solar or renewable energetic sources, and improving the efficiency of mineralization to avoid the formation of oxidation intermediates eventually toxic. Moreover, a variety of electroanalytical techniques are available (polarography, voltammetry, chronopotentiometry, chronoamperometry), which offer the possibility of performing a plethora of qualitative or quantitative determinations of pollutants in different matrices, often involving low detection limits (very attractive for the determination pollutants present at trace levels).

Electrochemical techniques can be classified as separation and oxidation technologies. Electrochemical separation technologies include membrane technologies, electro-coagulation and internal micro-electrolysis, where the pollutant is not decomposed but merely isolated. On the other hand, electrochemical oxidation (EO) techniques include direct and indirect anodic oxidation, electro-oxidation, electro-Fenton, photo-electro-Fenton and photo-electrocatalysis among most representatives [216].

A few studies have been carried out on the use of EO for the degradation of acetaminophen; most of them were focused on synthetic wastewater, although some data on real wastewaters have also been reported [179]. The success of the electrodegradation techniques depends on the operating conditions (initial concentration, solution pH) and, particularly, on the electrode materials chosen (see Table 5). For instance, anodic oxidation of acetaminophen using boron-doped diamond (BDD) anodes led to higher degree of removal in a wide pH range, where the use of Pt anodes yielded very low mineralization of the pollutant [93, 175-177]. As for the oxidation intermediates detected during acetaminophen degradation, ammonium and nitrate ions have been detected with different anodes, as well as aromatic compounds (mainly hydroquinone and 1,4-benzoquinone) and carboxylic acids (oxalic and oxamic acids). It is important to mention that the distribution of the oxidation intermediates is highly sensitive to the electrode material; for instance, the concentration of carboxylic acids decreases promptly when BDD is used as anode, as compared to Pt or Ti/SnO_2, which cannot promote the further oxidation of these compounds. This is most outstanding since some of these intermediates might present higher toxicity than acetaminophen. Some other parameters such as the inner electrolyte ($NaCl$, $NaClO_4$, Na_2SO_4) [176] are also important to control the acetaminophen using different electrodes, and cell acetaminophen mineralization extents have been achieved with BDD anodes (tendency also observed for other pharmaceuticals), which was been explained in terms of the greater concentration of hydroxyl radicals (•OH), which are formed near the BDD surface upon polarization. Acetaminophen oxidation mechanism seems to proceed via direct electron transfer to the electrode material (e.g., using Ti/RuO_2 electrodes), reaction with •OH formed at the electrode surface, and/or reaction with active chlorine species (Cl_2, $HClO$, and/or ClO^-) in chloride medium. Based on the analysis of the intermediates detected during the AOP by GCMS and HPLC, a mechanism of acetaminophen degradation has been proposed, following a pseudo-first order kinetics. The initial hydroxylation of acetaminophen renders hydroquinone and acetyl-1,4 benzoquinoneimide, both releasing acetamide, which is converted finally to oxamic acid. Further opening of the benzenic ring of 1,4-benzoquinone leads to carboxylic acids like ketomalonic, maleic and fumaric, which are further oxidized to short alkyl chain organic acids such as oxalic acid (Figure 3). Both oxalic and oxamic acids are highly stable, and their further mineralization is strongly affected by the action of catalysts [93, 177, 178, 216].

Besides anodic oxidation, better results concerning acetaminophen mineralization have been reported for electrochemical technologies based on Fenton's reaction chemistry (electro-Fenton and photo-electro-Fenton) [177, 178]. The presence of Fe^{2+} and Cu^{2+} and their mixtures as additives seems to have a synergistic effect enhancing the complete mineralization through the degradation of oxalic and oxamic acids (not attacked by •OH). Photo-electrochemical degradation of acetaminophen using a Pt/GDE cell coupled with ultraviolet light yielded much better results, with an almost complete TOC removal when Fe^{2+} and Cu^{2+} ions are also added in the catalytic cell. In such conditions, metallic complexes of oxalic and oxamic acids are formed, which catalyses their complete destruction. In contrast, acetaminophen does not seem to be degraded by direct UV irradiation (photolysis). Recently, some progress has been reported on solar –assisted electrochemical processes, and promising results were presented by Almeida et al. [179] in a flow pre-pilot plant for the degradation of acetaminophen solutions (Table 5).

As mentioned above, scarce efforts have been devoted to study the electrochemical treatment on real pharmaceutical wastewaters [222, 223]. Mostly, real hospital and pharmaceutical wastewaters have been treated by electrochemical oxidation using BDD anodes and electro-coagulation processes. Despite the excellent degradation performance of electrochemical technologies based on Fenton's reaction chemistry, these processes have not yet been applied to real wastewaters. The complexity of real wastewater matrices hinders the study of electrochemical oxidation process, since parasitic reactions can be easily produced, thereby decreasing the degradation yield of the electrodes and/or generating secondary potentially toxic by-products. Despite the promising results obtained to date with electrochemical degradation techniques, still much research needs to be done to enhance the performances of existing electrode devices (i.e., noble-metal-based oxides), without disdaining possible new electrode materials.

Sonolysis. In this process, high-intensity acoustic radiation (typically in the range of 20-1000 kHz) is applied to the aqueous medium to generate cavitation (i.e., bubbles) in the liquid followed by immediate implosion of the bubbles leading to the release of hydroxyl radicals. Sonication reactions can occur in the cavitation bubble, at the interface bubble-liquid and in the solution bulk. The application of ultrasounds in water treatment processes is very recent, and scarce data are available in the literature [189, 224, 225].

The degradation efficiency of pharmaceutical compounds upon sonolysis is similar to other AOPs, both in wastewater treatment effluents and synthetic solutions, although smaller mineralization rates have been reported [189, 225]. As for the intermediates, as in other •OH mediated reaction, hydroxylated derivates are identified at the early stages (low sonication times); in contrast, longer treatments lead to the formation of organic acids. The efficiency of the process might be improved by increasing the hydroxyl radical concentration in the medium, by combining this method with other techniques, such as, for instance, the addition of an optimized amount of H_2O_2.

4.3 Adsorption Processes

Adsorption at a solid-liquid interface can be defined as the enrichment of one or more components at an interfacial layer generated at the surface between the solid (adsorbent) and liquid (solution) phase, when these are brought into contact. The intermolecular forces involved in most solid-liquid systems are weak and non-specific interactions (mainly van der Waals), although some specific interactions (electrostatic, polarization, dipolar, covalent forces) may also arise from particular geometric and electronic properties of the adsorbent and species to be retained (adsorptive or adsorbate).

Adsorption is a well-established technique for the removal of pollutants, being activated carbons (ACs) the preferred adsorbents for the remediation of water with low pollutant concentration. Porous carbon-based materials are known to be very effective adsorbents due to their unique combination of a highly developed porous network (surface areas and pore volumes) coupled with their ability to react with other heteroatoms (that is, other than carbon) creating a variety of surface functional groups [226, 227]. The typically high values of surface areas in ACs (usually between 700-1500 m^2g^{-1}) are due to the presence of micropores (pores with openings up to 2 nm) [228], which are known as active sites of adsorption of most organic pollutants. Besides microporosity, the presence of a well-developed network of transport pores (so-called mesopores, pore width between 2 and 50 nm) is most outstanding to guarantee the diffusion and accessibility of the organic molecules towards the inner micropore structure of the adsorbent. Other advantages of activated carbons is their versatility of forms, shapes and structures (such as powders, granular, monoliths, fibers, cloths, etc.) as well as the possibility of regeneration and thus reutilization over a number of cycles.

The use of activated carbons and charcoals in the removal of pollutants from either gas and liquid phase is as old as history, and first documented applications are attributed to Hippocrates, the father of medicine, who would have used charcoals to relieve indigestion problems [227]. This application continues today for the removal of overdoses of drugs from stomachs. Charcoal was used for drinking water filtration and as medical adsorbent and purifying agent by the Egyptians [227]. Since then, carbon materials have been widely used for the removal of odours and tastes from drinking water and organic pollutants (priority persistent and emergent pollutants) from wastewater either in classical adsorption methods [227] or coupled to advanced techniques [229-232]. In developed countries with high coverage of water sanitation, activated carbons are used in the final stages of the water treatment (tertiary treatment), allowing the removal of pharmaceuticals and other emergent pollutants from the treated effluent. Thus, in areas with low coverage of water sanitation—where water treatments consist of only primary or secondary processes—most pollutants are usually not removed from the treated water. In drinking water facilities, ACs are also used to remove taste and odour compounds and to decrease dissolved organic matter (Figure 4).

Before the choice of the most adequate carbon adsorbent for the removal of a given pharmaceutical, it has to be considered that the adsorption process is complex and it strongly depends on many factors including texture (specific surface area and pore size distribution) and surface chemistry (i.e., presence of functional groups) of the activated carbon, the physico-chemical properties of the target pharmaceutical compound, and the operating conditions (such as solution pH and temperature). In this regard, solution pH is one of the most important parameters to be taken into account in most adsorption processes, since it may affect the ionization state of the adsorbate (many pharmaceutical compounds are weak electrolytes) and also the distribution of surface charges in the activated carbon (due to the dissociation of the surface functionalities). Additionally, competitive adsorption is rather common due to the occurrence of other substances (humic acids, mixtures of pollutants, suspended particles) that might compete, hinder or suppress the adsorption of target pharmaceutical compound.

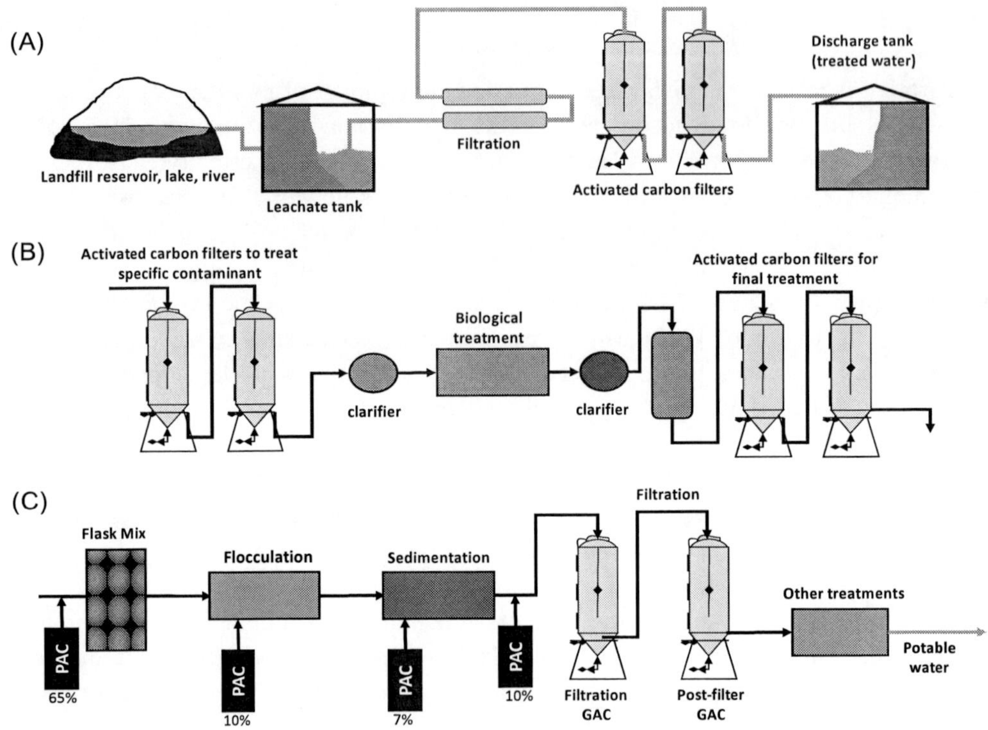

Figure 4. Simplified scheme of (a) groundwater remediation, (b) municipal wastewater treatment plants and (c) drinking water treatment plants employing powdered activated carbon (PAC). Percentages of PAC in plot (c) show an example of the likely distribution of PAC locations for taste and odor control. Adapted from references [233] and [234].

Concerning the use of activated carbons to remove pharmaceutical compounds, there are plenty of studies reporting the removal from water and wastewater [226, 227, 235-243], as well as clinical applications for the removal of drugs (i.e., acetaminophen) in stomach poisoning treatments [244-253] or *in vitro* and *in vivo* hemoperfusions [254, 255]. As an example, activated carbon has proven to efficiently remove acetaminophen without inducing loss of leucocytes and platelets in essays performed in pigs [254].

Several studies can be found in the literature reporting the use of activated carbons for the removal of pharmaceuticals from aqueous phase from real water samples [9, 34, 73, 84, 124, 128]. For instance, Ternes et al. [34] have shown that granular ACs provided a major elimination of several pharmaceuticals from German groundwater and surface water but was not effective in the case of clofibric acid. The results obtained by Kim et al. [128] on South Korean surface water and wastewater treatments demonstrated that removal efficiencies of ≈ 99% can be attained in drinking water for several pharmaceuticals and endocrine disruptors after the use of activated carbon. Similar results were observed in a USA wastewater treatment plant, where erythromycin and carbamazepine (resistant to biological treatment) were largely eliminated (efficiencies of 74 and 88%) by granular activated carbon [73].

In the case of acetaminophen, some studies report the elimination after primary clarification treatment [73] at concentrations below 50 ng L^{-1}, whereas others report the advantages of activated carbon use for its removal [9].

A number of fundamental studies investigating the mechanism of adsorption of acetaminophen on activated carbons are reported in the literature. For this purpose, acetaminophen concentrations higher than the actual levels found in real waterways are investigated; the main objective of these works is to get a deep understanding of the adsorption mechanism and to evaluate the potentialities of novel carbon materials to be used in water treatment facilities. Particularly special emphasis is paid to the use of green carbons obtained from waste-based precursors [256-259]. This is a very important issue since the implementation of activated carbons on large scale industrial processes is often limited due to a poor economic feasibility associated with manufacturing and regeneration costs [260].

For instance, activated carbons synthesized from several industrial (cork, peach stones and sisal) and municipal (plastic) wastes [256, 257] and biomass wastes [259] have shown an excellent performance for the removal of acetaminophen from solution. Acetaminophen removal efficiencies of such green carbons were, in some cases, comparable to those of commercially available activated carbons. There are studies where acetaminophen adsorption process presents an endothermic character (increasing with the temperature), which has been attributed to the formation of acetaminophen dimmers [259, 261].

Studies on the use of commercial activated carbons for oral administration in the cases of overdoses are of fundamental importance to understand the influence of the textural and surface chemistry properties of the adsorbents on the adsorption of acetaminophen [261-272]. The effect of acidic surface functionalities of carbon surfaces on the removal of acetaminophen has been reported; on the one hand, the adsorption capacity decreased for oxidized carbons due to competitive retention of water molecules for the adsorption sites [258]. On the other hand, enhanced wetability of the oxidized carbon favours a fast initial adsorption rate due to the enhanced transfer of acetaminophen from solution through the pore structure of the carbon [258].

Besides the use of wastes as precursors in the preparation of activated carbons, the study performed by Villaescusa et al. [273] revealed that vegetable wastes (grap stalk, yohimbe and cork bark) can be also used as adsorbent materials for acetaminophen removal. Despite the modest acetaminophen sorption capacities, these solids present some advantages: they can be used without any previous treatment and after use can be eliminated by controlled combustion. A possible application of these wastes behind lab-scale will obviously depend on the cost/benefit ratio.

Inorganic solid materials such as montmorillonite type clays, alumina, and silica have also been used as adsorbents for the removal of pharmaceutical compounds [274-277], including acetaminophen [278]. As a general rule, adsorption capacities of acetaminophen were lower in the inorganic adsorbents than in activated carbons. Moreover, Lorphensri et al. [278] demonstrated that solution pH is a key factor, since several assays performed at neutral pH render almost negligible adsorption of acetaminophen on alumina and silica from various organic media.

Xiao et al. [279] reported the use of polymeric nanomaterials, namely cyclodextrins (cyclic oligosaccharides with a hydrophobic cavity and two hydrophilic rims) as acetaminophen adsorbents. The authors found a structure/property relationship with the β-cyclodextrin showing high adsorption capacity for acetaminophen and other studied pharmaceuticals.

It has to be pointed out that, in general, a straightforward comparison of acetaminophen removal efficiencies using different adsorbents is not an easy task due to the differences in the operating conditions (pH, initial concentration, temperature, characteristic of the adsorbents, and so forth) and the complexity of the adsorption process, particularly when real wastewater samples are investigated. The adsorption capacities can be largely affected by the experimental parameters, thus discouraging systematic comparison of different studies. Nevertheless, good adsorption capacities are obtained in general with porous adsorbents of adequate textural and chemical features. Particularly, activated carbons seem to be excellent materials for the removal of low concentration of pharmaceuticals from different sorts of water, and coupled to STP provide treated water effluents with good quality standards.

CONCLUSION

The main objective of this chapter was to provide a comprehensive review on one of most important environmental problems of modern society, linked to water pollution by a pharmaceutical active compound—acetaminophen. Recent advances on monitoring the occurrence of acetaminophen in different sorts of waters as well as on the development of new strategies to improve water quality have been made, with special emphasis paid to degradation processes including adsorption, photo- and electro-assisted degradation techniques.

Detection of substances with therapeutic and biological activity in water is a reality that has stimulated the research on the development of advanced water treatment technologies. Recent studies have demonstrated the long-term persistence of pharmaceutical compounds in the environment, due to their continuous discharge (motivated by large consumption) and low biodegradability. In this regard, conventional water treatments are not effective to eliminate and/or degrade the majority of these compounds, which can then accumulate in drinking water. Additionally, the effects on human health associated with the continuous exposure to these chemicals are still rather unknown. The development of novel techniques aims at achieving large water remediation rates (ideally total mineralization of the target pollutants), while preventing the formation of degradation intermediates eventually more toxic that the pristine contaminant.

Acetaminophen is a widely consumed analgesic frequently found in water and wastewater. Although it may be removed by conventional biological treatment to a large extent, still large concentrations have been detected in drinking water and treated effluents (after STP and WWTP). Thus, the combination of conventional technologies with advanced processes seems to be an efficient way to meet the water quality standards.

Quite extensive research has been carried out recently on the use of advanced oxidation processes (AOPs) and adsorption technology for the removal and degradation of acetaminophen from both synthetic and real water samples and mainly at lab-scale (although some preliminary pilot scale studies can also be found). The most promising and interesting results on acetaminophen degradation are processes based on Fenton reaction (and related processes), photocatalysis and electrochemical oxidation. Although quite large acetaminophen degradation rates can be obtained in most cases, the extent of mineralization rate (fully conversion to CO_2 and H_2O without generation of intermediates) is still a major drawback. Indeed, several oxidation intermediates have been detected during the degradation processes; some of them are highly recalcitrant (short alkyl chain organic acids), for which the economic penalty associated with complete mineralization is very high. Coupling AOP with solar energy seems to be a promising alternative to face this cornerstone, although it still needs to be further explored for most investigated processes, particularly in the case of real samples. This is particularly important due to the complexity of the reactions in heterogeneous water matrices where interferences may arise, for instance, from natural organic matter or other inorganic species. As opposed to AOPs, adsorption is a well-established technology for the removal of a plethora of pollutants from water. Important advantages of adsorption are that it is non-selective method (thus providing an interesting alternative to simultaneously remove all the pollutants present in water) and the availability of a variety of adsorbents (activated carbons, zeolites, sepiolites, and so forth) with large removal capacities. The main cornerstone, however, is that the pharmaceutical compounds are not degraded, and thus the exhausted adsorbent needs to be regenerated.

Perhaps the most important idea that should be emphasized is that no single method is capable of (nor should be applied to) providing a complete water remediation to meet the required water quality standards. Very often, it is necessary to apply various techniques in tandem, so as to profit from the technological and economical advantages of each method while assuring an effective abatement of pollutants and environmental protection.

ACKNOWLEDGMENTS

The authors thank the support of the Portuguese and Spanish Ministries of Science (grants CTM2008/01556, CTM2011/23378, Acción Integrada ABI2010PT-00209 and Acção Integrada Luso-Espanhola E-11/11). ASM and MH thank the financial support of AdI – QREN Project Watercork and CSIC (JAE-Doc contract), respectively.

REFERENCES

[1] Universal Declaration of Human Rights. In *Article 25*, 10 December 1948.

[2] International Covenant on Economic, Social and Cultural Rights. In *Article 11*, 16 December 1966.

[3] Principles 3 and 4 of Rio Declaration on Environment and Development. In United Nations Conference on Envirnoment and Development (UNCED): Rio de Janeiro, 1992.

[4] Kolpin, D. W.; Furlong, E. T.; Meyer, M. T.; Thurman, E. M.; Zaugg, S. D.; Barber, L. B.; Buxton, H. T., Pharmaceuticals, hormones, and other organic wastewater contaminants in U.S. streams, 1999-2000: A national reconnaissance. *Environ. Sci. Technol.* 2002, *36*, (6), 1202-1211.

[5] POSEIDON *Assessment of technologies for the removal of pharmaceuticals and personal care products in sewage and drinking water facilities to improve the indirect potable water reuse. Contract No. EVK1-CT-2000-00047*; http//www.eu-poseidon.com, 2001-2004.

[6] Stackelberg, P. E.; Furlong, E. T.; Meyer, M. T.; Zaugg, S. D.; Henderson, A. K.; Reissman, D. B., Persistence of pharmaceutical compounds and other organic

wastewater contaminants in a conventional drinking-water-treatment plant. *Sci. Total Environ.* 2004, *329*, (1-3), 99-113.
[7] Barceló, D., Emerging pollutants in water analysis. *TrAC Trends Anal. Chem.* 2003, *22*, (10), xiv-xvi.
[8] Klavarioti, M.; Mantzavinos, D.; Kassinos, D., Removal of residual pharmaceuticals from aqueous systems by advanced oxidation processes. *Environ. Int.* 2009, *35*, (2), 402-417.
[9] Ziylan, A.; Ince, N. H., The occurrence and fate of anti-inflammatory and analgesic pharmaceuticals in sewage and fresh water: Treatability by conventional and non-conventional processes. *J. Hazard. Mater.* 2011, *187*, (1-3), 24-36.
[10] Federal Water Pollution Control Amendments 33 U.S.C. In *P.L. 92-500*, 92nd United States Congress, 1972; p 1251.
[11] Water Framework Directive (2000/60/EC). In Parliament, E., Ed. OJL 327, 22 December, 2000; pp 1-73.
[12] Stumm-Zollinger, E.; Fair, G. M., Biodegradation of steroid hormones. *J. Water Pollut. Cont. Fed.* 1965, *37*, 1506-1510.
[13] Hignite, C.; Azarnoff, D. L., Drugs and drug metabolites as environmental contaminants: Chlorophenoxyisobutyrate and salicylic acid in sewage water effluents. *Life Sci.* 1977, *20*, 337-341.
[14] Watts, C. D.; Crathorne, B.; Fielding, M.; Stell, C. P., *Analysis of Organic Micropollutants in Water*. Reidal Publishing Co.: Derdrecht, Germany, 1983.
[15] Tabak, H. H.; Bunch, R. L., Steroid hormones as water pollutants. I. Metabolism of natural and synthetic ovulation-inhibiting hormones by microorganisms of activated sludge and primary settled sewage. *Dev. Ind. Microbiol.* 1970, *11*, 367-376.
[16] Tabak, H. H.; Bloomhuff., R. N.; Bunch, R. L., Steroid hormones as water pollutants. II. Studies on the persistence and stability of natural urinary and synthetic ovulation-inhibiting hormones in untreated and treated wastewaters. *Dev. Ind. Microbiol.* 1981, *22*, 497-519.
[17] Aherne, G. W.; Briggs, R., The relevance of the presence of certain synthetic steroids in the aquatic environment. *J. Pharm. Pharmacol.* 1989, *41*, 735-736.
[18] Aherne, G. W.; J., E.; Marks, V., The role of immunoassay in the analysis of microcontaminants in water samples. *Ecotocol. Environ. Saf.* 1985, *9*, 79-83.
[19] Bevans, H. E.; Goodbred, S. L.; Miesner, J. F.; Watkins, S. A.; Gross, T. S.; Denslow, N. D.; Schoeb, T., Synthetic organic compounds and carp endocrinology and histology in Las Vegas Wash and Las Vegas and Callville Bays Lake Mead, Nevada, 1992 and 1995. *Water—Resources Investigations Report* 1996, 96-4266.
[20] Dresdow, C.; Routledge, E. J.; Brighty, G. C.; Sumpter, J. P.; Waldock, M., Identification of estrogenic chemicals in STW effluent. 1. Chemical fractionation and in vitro biological screening. *Environ. Sci. Technol.* 1998, *32*, (11), 1549-1558.
[21] Jobling, S.; Noylan, M.; Tyler, C. R.; G., B.; Sumpter, J. P., Widespread sexual disruption in wild fish. *Environ. Sci. Technol.* 1998, *32*, 2498-2506.
[22] Kramer, V. J.; Miles-Richardson, S.; Pierens, S. L.; Giesy, J. P., Reproductive impairment and induction of alkaline-labile phosphate, a biomarker of estrogen exposure, in fathead minnows (Pimephales promelas) exposed to waterborne 17 beta-estradiol. *Aquat. Toxicol.* 1998, *40*, (4), 335-360.

[23] Snyder, S. A.; Villeneuve, D. L.; Snyder, E. M.; Giesy, J. P., Identification and quantification of estrogen receptor agonists in wastewater effluents. *Environ. Sci. Technol.* 2001, *35*, (18), 3620-3625.
[24] Purdom, C. E.; Hardiman, P. A.; Bye, V. J.; Eno, N. C.; Tyler, C. R.; Sumpter, J. P., Estrogenic effects of effluents from sewage treatment works. *Chem. Ecol.* 1994, *8*, (4), 275-285.
[25] Daughton, C. G., Pharmaceutical ingredients in drinking water: Overview of occurrence and significance of human exposure. In *Contaminants of Emerging Concern in the Environment: Ecological and Human Health Considerations*, American Chemical Society: 2010; Vol. 1048, pp 9-68.
[26] Stan, H. J.; Heberer, T.; Linkerhägner, M., Vorkommen von Clofibrinsäure im aquatischen System—Führt die therapeutische Anwendung zu einer Belastung von Oberflächen-, Grund- und Trinkwasser? [Occurrence of clofibric acid in the aquatic system—Is their therapeutic use responsible for the loads found in surface, ground- and drinking water?]. *Vom Wasser* 1994, (83), 57-68.
[27] Guidelines for Water Reuse. U.S. Environmental Protection Agency. In *EPA/625/R-04/108* September 2004.
[28] Cunningham, V. L.; Buzby, M.; Hutchinson, T.; Mastrocco, F.; Parke, N.; Roden, N., Effects of human pharmaceuticals on aquatic life: Next steps. *Environ. Sci. Technol.* 2006, *40*, 3456-3462.
[29] Calamari, D., Assessment of persistent and bioaccumulating chemicals in the aquatic environment. *Toxicol.* 2002, *181*, 183-186.
[30] Richardson, M. L.; Bowron, J. M., The fate of pharmaceutical chemicals in the aquatic environment. *J. Pharm. Pharmacol.* 1985, *37*, 1-12.
[31] Petrovic, M.; Eljarrat, E.; López de Alda, M. J.; Barceló, D., Endocrine disrupting compounds and other emerging contaminants in the environment: A survey on new monitoring strategies and occurrence data. *Anal. Bional. Chem.* 2004, *378*, 549-562.
[32] Carlsen, E.; Giwercman, A.; Keiding, N.; Skakkebaek, N. E., Evidence for decreasing quality of semen during past 50 years. *Br. Med. J.* 1992, *305*, 609-613.
[33] Daughton, C. G.; Ternes, T. A., Pharmaceuticals and personal care products in the environment: Agents of subtle change? *Environ. Health Perspect.* 1999, *107*, 907-938.
[34] Ternes, T. A.; Meisenheimer, M.; McDowell, D.; Sacher, F.; Brauch, H.-J. r.; Haist-Gulde, B.; Preuss, G.; Wilme, U.; Zulei-Seibert, N., Removal of pharmaceuticals during drinking water treatment. *Environ. Sci. Technol.* 2002, *36*, (17), 3855-3863.
[35] Mompelat, S.; Le Bot, B.; Thomas, O., Occurrence and fate of pharmaceutical products and by-products, from resource to drinking water. *Environ. Int.* 2009, *35*, (5), 803-814.
[36] Zuccato, E.; Castiglioni, S., Illicit drugs in the environment. *Philos. Trans. R. Soc. A* 2009, *367*, 3965-3978.
[37] Zuccato, E.; Castiglioni, S.; Fanelli, R., Identification of the pharmaceuticals for the human use contaminating the Italian aquatic environment. *J. Hazard. Mater.* 2005, *122*, 205-209.
[38] Monteiro, S. C.; Boxall, A. B. A., Occurrence and fate of human pharmaceuticals in the aquatic environment. In *Reviews Environ. Contam. Toxicol.*, Whitacre, D. M., Ed. Springer: New York, 2010; Vol. 202, pp 53-154.
[39] Daughton, C. G., Illicit drugs: contaminants in the environment and utility in forensic epidemiology. *Rev. Environ. Contam. Toxicol.* 2011, *210*, 59-110.

[40] Gielen, G.; Clinton, P. W.; Van den Heuvel, M. R.; Kimberley, M. O.; Greenfield, L. G., Influence of sewage and pharmaceuticals on soil microbial function. *Environ. Toxicol. Chem.* 2011, *30*, (5), 1086-1095.

[41] Murray, K. E.; Thomas, S. M.; Bodour, A. A., Prioritizing research for trace pollutants and emerging contaminants in the freshwater environment. *Environ. Pollut.* 2011, *158*, (12), 3462-3471.

[42] Halling-Sorensen, B.; Nors Nielsen, S.; Lanzky, P. F.; Ingerslev, F.; Holten LÜtzhoft, H. C.; Jorgensen, S. E., Occurrence, fate and effects of pharmaceutical substance in the environment—A review. *Chemosphere* 1998, *36*, 357-393.

[43] Khetan, S. K.; Collins, T. J., Human pharmaceuticals in the aquatic environment: A challenge to green chemistry. *Chem. Rev.* 2007, *107*, 2319-2364.

[44] Kemper, N., Veterinary antibiotics in the aquatic and terrestrial environment. *Ecol. Indic.* 2008, *8*, 1-13.

[45] Heberer, T., Occurrence, fate, and removal of pharmaceutical residues in the aquatic environment: A review of recent research data. *Toxicol. Lett.* 2002, *131*, 5-17.

[46] Krümmerer, K., Significance of antibiotics in the environment. *J. Antimicrob. Chemother.* 2003, *52*, 5-7.

[47] Hernando, M. D.; Heat, E.; Petrovic, M.; Barceló, D., Trace-level determination of pharmaceutical residues by LC-MS-MS in natural and treated waters. A pilot-survey study. *Anal Bional Chem.* 2006, *385*, 985-991.

[48] Radjenovic, J.; Petrovic, M.; Ventura, F.; Barcelo, D., Rejection of pharmaceuticals in nanofiltration and reverse osmosis membrane drinking water treatment. *Water Res.* 2008, *42*, (14), 3601-3610.

[49] Vanderford, B. J.; Snyder, S. A., Analysis of pharmaceuticals in water by isotope dilution liquid chromatography/tandem mass spectrometry. *Environ. Sci. Technol.* 2006, *40*, 7312-7320.

[50] Zhao, X.; Metcalfe, C. D., Characterizing and compensating for matrix effects using atmospheric pressure chemical ionization liquid chromatography-tandem mass spectrometry: Analysis of neutral pharmaceutics in wastewater. *Analytical Chemistry* 2008, *80*, 2010-2017.

[51] Ternes, T., Pharmaceuticals and metabolites as contaminants of the aquatic environment—an overview. *Abstracts of Papers of ACS* 2000, *219*, U622-U623.

[52] Jones, O. A. H.; Voulvoulis, N.; Lester, J. N., Human pharmaceuticals in wastewater treatment processes. *Crit. Rev. Environ. Sci. Technol.* 2005, *35*, 401-427.

[53] Gomez, M. J.; Bueno, M. J. M.; Lacorte, S.; Fernandez-Alba, A. R.; Aguera, A., Pilot survey monitoring pharmaceuticals and related compounds in a sewage treatment plant located on the Mediterranean coast. *Chemosphere* 2007, *66*, (6), 993-1002.

[54] Zuccato, E.; Castiglioni, S.; Fanelli, R.; Reitano, G.; Bagnati, R.; Chiabrando, C.; Pomati, F.; Rossetti, C.; Calamari, D., Pharmaceuticals in the environment in Italy: Causes, occurrence, effects and control. *Environ. Sci. & Pollut. Res.* 2006, *13* (1), 15-21.

[55] *Pharmaceuticals in the environment. Sources, Fate, Effects and Risks.* K. Kumerer (ed.). Springer 2004.

[56] Löffler, D.; Römbke, J.; Meller, M.; Ternes, T. A., Environmental fate of pharmaceuticals in water/sediment systems. *Environ. Sci. Technol.* 2005, *39*, (14), 5209-5218.

[57] Jones, O. A. H.; Voulvoulis, N.; Lester, J. N., Potential ecological and human health risks associated with the presence of pharmaceutically active compounds in the aquatic environment. *Crit. Rev. Toxicol.* 2004, *34*, (4), 335-350.

[58] Webb, S. F., A data based perspective on the environmental risk assessment of human pharmaceuticals. III. Indirect exposure. . In *Pharmaceuticals in the Environment*, Kümmerer, K., Ed. Springer: Heidelberg, Germany, 2001; p 221.

[59] Schwatz, T.; Kohnen, W.; Jansen, B.; Obst, U., Detection of antibiotic-resistant bacteria and their resistance genes in wastewater, surface water, and drinking water biofilms. *FEMS Microbiol. Ecol.* 2003, *43*, 325-335.

[60] Schaiger, J.; Ferling, H.; Mallow, U.; Wintermayr, H.; Negele, R. D., Toxic effects of the non-steroidal anti-Inflammatory drug diclofenac. Part I: Histopathological alterations and bioaccumulation in rainbow trout. *Aquatic Toxicol.* 2004, *68*, 141-150.

[61] Baquero, F.; Martínez, J. L.; Cantón, R., Antibiotics and antibiotic resistance in water environments. *Curr. Opin. Biotechnol.* 2008, *19*, 260-265.

[62] Guardabassi, L.; Dalsgaard, A.; Olsen, J. E., Phenotypic characterization and antibiotic resistance of Acinetobacter Spp. isolated from aquatic sources. *J. Appl. Microbiol.* 1999, *87*, 659-667.

[63] Muela, A.; Porcino, M.; Arana, I.; Justo, J. I.; Iriberri, J.; Barcina, I., Effect of growth phase and parental cell survival in river water on plasmid transfer between Eschericachia Coli strains. *Appl. Env. Microbiol.* 1994, *60*, 4273-4278.

[64] Carlsson, C.; Johansson, A. K.; Alvan, G.; Bergman, K.; Kühler, T., Are pharmaceuticals potent environmenal pollutants? Part I: Environmental risk assessments of selected active pharmaceutical ingredients. *Sci.Total Environ.* 2006, *364*, 67-87.

[65] Goñi-Uriza, M.; Capdepuy, M.; Arpin, C.; Raymond, N.; Pierre Caumette, C. Q., Impact of an urban effluent on antibiotic resistance of riverine Enterobacteriaceae and Aeromonas Spp. *Appl. Env. Microbiol.* 2000, *66*, 125-132.

[66] di Delupis, G. D.; Macri, A.; Civitareale, A. C.; Migliore, L., Antibiotics of zootechnical use: Effects of actue high and low dose contamination on Daphnia Magna Straus. *Aquat. Toxicol.* 1992, *22*, 53-59.

[67] Pomati, F.; Netting, A. G.; Calamari, D.; Neilan, B. A., Effects of erythromycin, tetrcycline and ibuprofen on the growth of Synechocystis Sp. and Lemna Minor. *Aquatic Toxicol.* 2004, *67*, 387-396.

[68] Westergaard, K.; Müller, A. K.; Christensen, S.; Bloem, J.; Sorensen, S. J., Effects of tylosin as a disturbance on the soil microbial community. *Soil Biol. Biochem.* 2001, *33*, 2061-2071.

[69] Sommer, C.; Bibby, B. M., The influence of veterinary medicines on the decomposition of dung organic matter in soil. *Eur. J. Soil Biol.* 2002, *38*, 155-159.

[70] Contaminant Candidate List 3—CCL In United States Environmental Protection Agency: http://www.epa.gov/safewater/ccl/index.html.

[71] Daughton, C. G. In *Pharmaceuticals in the environment: Overarching issues and overview*, Pharmaceuticals and personal care products in the environment scientific and regulatory issues, Washington, DC, 2001; Daughton, C. G.; Jones, T., Eds. Washington, DC, 2001; pp 2-38.

[72] Tauxe-Wuersch, A.; De Alencastro, L. F.; Grandjean, D.; Tarradellas, J., Occurrence of several acidic drugs in sewage treatment plants in Switzerland and risk assessment. *Water Res.* 2005, *39*, (9), 1761-1772.

[73] Yang, X.; Flowers, R. C.; Weinberg, H. S.; Singer, P. C., Occurrence and removal of pharmaceuticals and personal care products (PPCPs) in an advanced wastewater reclamation plant. *Water Res.* 2011, *45*, (16), 5218-5228.

[74] Ternes, T. A., Occurrence of drugs in German sewage treatment plants and rivers. *Water Res.* 1998, *32*, (11), 3245-3260.

[75] Jones, O. A. H.; Voulvoulis, N.; Lester, J. N., Human pharmaceuticals in the aquatic environment—A review. *Environ. Technol.* 2001, *22*, (12), 1383-1394.

[76] Jones, O. A.; Lester, J. N.; Voulvoulis, N., Pharmaceuticals: a threat to drinking water? *Trends Biotechnol.* 2005, *23*, (4), 163-167.

[77] Heberer, T., Tracking persistent pharmaceutical residues from municipal sewage to drinking water. *J. Hydrol.* 2002, *266*, (3-4), 175-189.

[78] Matamoros, V.; Arias, C.; Brix, H.; Bayona, J. M., Preliminary screening of small-scale domestic wastewater treatment systems for removal of pharmaceutical and personal care products. *Water Res.* 2009, *43*, (1), 55-62.

[79] Onesios, K. M.; Yu, J. T.; Bouwer, E. J., Biodegradation and removal of pharmaceuticals and personal care products in treatment systems: A review. *Biodegrad.* 2009, *20*, (4), 441-466.

[80] Bruchet, A.; Hochereau, C.; Picard, C.; Decottignies, V.; Rodrigues, J. M.; Janex-Habibi, M. L., Analysis of drugs and personal care products in French source and drinking waters: The analytical challenge and examples of application. *Water Sci. Technol.* 2005, *52*, (8), 53-61.

[81] Gibs, J.; Stackelberg, P. E.; Furlong, E. T.; Meyer, M.; Zaugg, S. D.; Lippincott, R. L., Persistence of pharmaceuticals and other organic compounds in chlorinated drinking water as a function of time. *Sci. Total Environ.* 2007, *373*, (1), 240-249.

[82] Benotti, M. J.; Trenholm, R. A.; Vanderford, B. J.; Holady, J. C.; Stanford, B. D.; Snyder, S. A., Pharmaceuticals and endocrine disrupting compounds in US drinking water. *Environ. Sci. Technol.* 2009, *43*, (3), 597-603.

[83] Newcombe, G.; Dixon, D., *Interface Science in Drinking Water Treatment.* Academic Press: 2006.

[84] Adams, C.; Wang, Y.; Loftin, K.; Meyer, M., Removal of antibiotics from surface and distilled water in conventional water treatment processes. *J. Environ. Eng.—ASCE* 2002, *128*, (3), 253-260.

[85] Huber, M. M.; Korhonen, S.; Ternes, T. A.; von Gunten, U., Oxidation of pharmaceuticals during water treatment with chlorine dioxide. *Water Res.* 2005, *39*, (15), 3607-3617.

[86] Ikehata, K.; Naghashkar, N. J.; Ei-Din, M. G., Degradation of aqueous pharmaceuticals by ozonation and advanced oxidation processes: A review. *Ozone: Sci. Eng.* 2006, *28*, (6), 353-414.

[87] Pinkston, K. E.; Sedlak, D. L., Transformation of aromatic ether- and amine-containing pharmaceuticals during chlorine disinfection. *Environ. Sci. Technol.* 2004, *38*, (14), 4019-4025.

[88] P-Three Project. Removal of persistent polar pollutants through improved treatment of wastewater effluent. In *http://www.pthree.de/*, Project Reference: EVK1-CT-2006-00116.
[89] Wang, L. K.; Hung, Y. T.; Shammas, N. K., *Handbook of Environmental Engineering*. Human Press; 1st Ed.: 2007.
[90] Opennländer, T., *Photochemical purification of water and air: advanced oxidation processes (AOPs): Principles, reaction mechenisms, reactor concepts*. Wiley-VCH: 2003.
[91] Ernst, M.; Jekel, M., Advanced treatment combination for groundwater recharge of municipal wastewater by nanofiltration and ozonation. *Water Sci. Technol.* 1999, *40*, 277-284.
[92] Gogate, R.; Pandit, A. B., A review of imperative technologies for wastewater treatment I: oxidation technologies at ambient conditions. *Adv. Environ. Res.* 2004, *8*, 501-551.
[93] Brillas, E.; Sires, I.; Arias, C.; Cabot, P. L.; Centellas, F.; Rodriguez, R. M.; Garrido, J. A., Mineralization of paracetamol in aqueous medium by anodic oxidation with a boron-doped diamond electrode. *Chemosphere* 2005, *58*, (4), 399-406.
[94] Comninellis, C.; Kapalka, A.; Malato, S.; Parsons, S. A.; Poulios, I.; Mantzavinos, D., Advanced oxidation processes for water treatment: Advances and trends for R&D. *J. Chem. Technol. Biotechnol.* 2008, *83*, 769-776.
[95] *Cambridge Crystallografic Data Center. Reciprocal Net site Software, 0.9.0-246.* ; Copyright ©: 2002-2008.
[96] Bosch, M. E.; Sánchez, A. J. R.; Rojas, F. S.; Ojeda, C. B., Determination of paracetamol: Historical evolution. *J. Pharm. Biomed. Anal.* 2006, *42*, (3), 291-321.
[97] Larson, A. M.; Polson, J.; Fontana, R. J.; Davern, T. J.; Lalani, E.; Hynan, L. S.; Reisch, J. S.; Schiodt, F. V.; Ostapowicz, G.; Shakil, A. O.; Lee, W. M.; Acute Liver Failure Study, G., Acetaminophen-induced acute liver failure: Results of a United States multicenter, prospective study. *Hepatology* 2005, *42*, (6), 1364-1372.
[98] Sheen, L.; Dillon, J. F.; Bateman, D. N.; Simpson, K. J.; Macdonald, T. M., Paracetamol toxicity: epidemiology, prevention and costs to the health-care system. *QJM* 2002, *95*, 609-619.
[99] Farmaco, A. I. d., Bolletino di informazione. *Ministero della Salute, Roma* 2005.
[100] Sebastine, I. M.; Wakeman, R. J., Consumption and environmental hazards of pharmaceutical substances in the UK. *Process Saf. Environ. Prot.* 2003, *81*, (B4), 229-235.
[101] Tambosi, J. L.; Yamanaka, L. Y.; Jose, H. J.; Moreira, R.; Schroder, H. F., Recent research data on the removal of pharmaceuticals from sewage treatment plants (STP) *Quim. Nova* 2010, *33*, (2), 411-420.
[102] Mirasol, F., Acetaminophen market sees moderate price hike. *Chem. Mark. Rep.* 1998, *254*, 12.
[103] Ellenhorn, M. J.; Barceloux, D. G., *Medical Toxicology-Diagnosis and Treatment of Human Poisoning*. Elsevier Science: New York, 1988.
[104] Schomburg, D.; Salzmann, M., *Handbook, Part 4*. Springer-Verlag: Berlin, Heidelberg, 1991.

[105] Dalmazio, I.; Alves, T. M. A.; Augusti, R., An appraisal on the degradation of paracetamol by TiO_2/UV system in aqueous medium. Product identification by gas chromatography-mass spectrometry (GC-MS). *J. Braz. Chem. Soc.* 2008, *19*, (1), 81-88.

[106] Andreozzi, R.; Caprio, V.; Marotta, R.; Vogna, D., Paracetamol oxidation from aqueous solutions by means of ozonation and H_2O_2/UV system. *Water Res.* 2003, *37*, (5), 993-1004.

[107] Bonvin, F.; Rutler, R.; Chèvre, N.; Halder, J.; Kohn, T., Spatial and temporal presence of a wastewater-derived micropollutant plume in lake Geneva. *Environ. Sci.Technol.* 2011, *45*, (11), 4702-4709.

[108] Ginebreda, A.; Muñoz, I.; López de Alda, M.; Brix, R.; López-Doval, J.; Barceló, D., Environmental risk assessment of pharmaceuticals in rivers: Relationships between hazard indexes and aquatic macroinvertebrate diversity indexes in the Llobregat River (NE Spain). *Env. Int.* 2010, *36*, 153-162.

[109] Wiegel, S.; Aulinger, A.; Brockmeyer, R.; Harms, H.; Löffler, J.; Reincke, H.; Schmidt, R.; Stachel, B.; von Tümpling, W.; Wanke, A., Pharmaceuticals in the river Elbe and its tributaries. *Chemosphere* 2004, *57*, (2), 107-126.

[110] Bound, J. P.; Voulvoulis, N., Predicted and measured concentrations for selected pharmaceuticals in UK rivers: Implications for risk assessment. *Water Res.* 2006, *40*, (15), 2885-2892.

[111] Naidenko, O.; Leiba, N.; Sharp, R.; Houlihan, J., Bottled water quality investigation: 10 major brands, 38 pollutants. Bottled water contains disinfection byproducts, fertilizer residue, and pain medication. In Environmental Working Group (EWG) ed.; Washington, DC, 2009; pp 33 http://www.ewg.org/reports/bottledwater, http://www.ewg.org/node/27011.

[112] Lin, A. Y.-C.; Panchangam, S. C.; Chen, H.-Y., Implications of human pharmaceutical occurrence in the Sindian river of Taiwan: A strategic study of risk assessment. *J. Environ. Monitor.* 2010, *12*, 261-270.

[113] Brun, G. L.; Bernier, M.; Losier, R.; Doe, K.; Jackman, P.; Lee, H. B., Pharmaceutically active compounds in Atlantic Canadian sewage treatment plant effluents and receiving waters, and potential for environmental effects as measured by acute and chronic aquatic toxicity. *Environ. Toxicol. Chem.* 2006, *25*, (8), 2163-2176.

[114] Chiron, S.; Gomez, E.; Fenet, H., Nitration processes of acetaminophen in nitrifying activated sludge. *Environ. Sci. Technol.* 2010, *44*, (1), 284-289.

[115] Matsuo, H.; Sakamoto, H.; Arizono, K.; Shinohara, R., Behavior of pharmaceuticals in waste water treatment plant in Japan. *Bull. Environ. Contam. Toxicol.* 2011, *87*, 31-35.

[116] Pedrouzo, M.; Borrull, F.; Pocurull, E.; Marcé, R. M., Presence of pharmaceuticals and hormones in waters from sewage treatment plants. *Water Air Soil Pollut.* 2011, *217*, (1-4), 267-281.

[117] Boleda, M. R.; Galceran, M. T.; Ventura, F., Behavior of pharmaceuticals and drugs of abuse in a drinking water treatment plant (DWTP) using combined conventional and ultrafiltration and reverse osmosis (UF/RO) treatments. *Environ. Pollut.* 2011, *159*, (6), 1584-1591.

[118] Rosal, R.; Rodriguez, A.; Perdigon-Melon, J. A.; Petre, A.; Garcia-Calvo, E.; Gomez, M. J.; Aguera, A.; Fernandez-Alba, A. R., Occurrence of emerging pollutants in urban wastewater and their removal through biological treatment followed by ozonation. *Water Res.* 2010, *44*, (2), 578-588.

[119] Han, G. H.; Hur, H. G.; Kim, S. D., Ecotoxicological risk of pharmaceuticals from wastewater treatment plants in Korea: Occurrence and toxicity to Daphnia magna. *Environ. Toxicol. Chem.* 2006, *25*, (1), 265-271.

[120] Wennmalm, Å.; Gunnarsson, B., Pharmaceutical management through environmental product labeling in Sweden. *Environ. Int.* 2009, *35*, (5), 775-777.

[121] Morasch, B.; Bonvin, F.; Reiser, H.; Grandjean, D.; de Alencastro, L. F.; Perazzolo, C.; Chevre, N.; Kohn, T., Occurence and fate of micropollutants in the Vidy Bay of Lake Geneva, Switzerland. Part II: Micropollutant removal between wastewater and raw drinking water. *Environ. Toxicol. Chem.* 2010, *29*, (8), 1658-1668.

[122] Lin, A. Y. C.; Yu, T. H.; Lin, C. F., Pharmaceutical contamination in residential, industrial, and agricultural waste streams: Risk to aqueous environments in Taiwan. *Chemosphere* 2008, *74*, (1), 131-141.

[123] Jones, O. A. H.; Voulvoulis, N.; Lester, J. N., The occurrence and removal of selected pharmaceutical compounds in a sewage treatment works utilising activated sludge treatment. *Environ. Pollut.* 2007, *145*, (3), 738-744.

[124] Boyd, G. R.; Reemtsma, H.; Grimm, D. A.; Mitra, S., Pharmaceuticals and personal care products (PPCPs) in surface and treated waters of Louisiana, USA and Ontario, Canada. *Sci. Total Environ.* 2003, *311*, (1-3), 135-149.

[125] Roberts, P. H.; Thomas, K. V., The occurrence of selected pharmaceuticals in wastewater effluent and surface waters of the lower Tyne catchment. *Sci. Total Environ.* 2006, *356*, (1-3), 143-153.

[126] Gros, M.; Petrovic, M.; Barceló, D., Development of a multi-residue analytical methodology based on liquid chromatography-tandem mass spectrometry (LC-MS/MS) for screening and trace level determination of pharmaceuticals in surface and wastewaters. *Talanta* 2006, *70*, (4), 678-690.

[127] Togola, A.; Budzinski, H., Multi-residue analysis of pharmaceutical compounds in aqueous samples. *J. Chromatogr. A* 2008, *1177*, (1), 150-158.

[128] Kim, S. D.; Cho, J.; Kim, I. S.; Vanderford, B. J.; Snyder, S. A., Occurrence and removal of pharmaceuticals and endocrine disruptors in South Korean surface, drinking, and waste waters. *Water Res.* 2007, *41*, (5), 1013-1021.

[129] Gómez, M. J.; Agüera, A.; Mezcua, M.; Hurtado, J.; Mocholí, F.; Fernández-Alba, A. R., Simultaneous analysis of neutral and acidic pharmaceuticals as well as related compounds by gas chromatography-tandem mass spectrometry in wastewater. *Talanta* 2007, *73*, (2), 314-320.

[130] Gómez, M. J.; Petrovic, M.; Fernandez-Alba, A. R.; Barcelo, D., Determination of pharmaceuticals of various therapeutic classes by solid-phase extraction and liquid chromatography-tandem mass spectrometry analysis in hospital effluent wastewaters. *J. Chromatogr. A* 2006, *1114*, (2), 224-233.

[131] Radjenovic, J.; Petrovic, M.; Barceló, D., Analysis of pharmaceuticals in wastewater and removal using a membrane bioreactor. *Anal. Bioanal. Chem.* 2007, *387*, (4), 1365-1377.

[132] Radjenovic, J.; Petrovic, M.; Barceló, D., Fate and distribution of pharmaceuticals in wastewater and sewage sludge of the conventional activated sludge (CAS) and advanced membrane bioreactor (MBR) treatment. *Water Res.* 2009, *43*, (3), 831-841.

[133] Bernabeu, A.; Vercher, R. F.; Santos-Juanes, L.; Simon, P. J.; Lardin, C.; Martinez, M. A.; Vicente, J. A.; Gonzalez, R.; Llosa, C.; Arques, A.; Amat, A. M., Solar

photocatalysis as a tertiary treatment to remove emerging pollutants from wastewater treatment plant effluents. *Catal. Today* 2011, *161*, (1), 235-240.

[134] Lin, A. Y. C.; Lin, C. F.; Tsai, Y. T.; Lin, H. H. H.; Chen, J.; Wang, X. H.; Yu, T. H., Fate of selected pharmaceuticals and personal care products after secondary wastewater treatment processes in Taiwan. *Water Sci. Technol.* 2010, *62*, (10), 2450-2458.

[135] Glassmeyer, S. T.; Furlong, E. T.; Kolpin, D. W.; Cahill, J. D.; Zaugg, S. D.; Werner, S. L.; Meyer, M. T.; Kryak, D. D., Transport of chemical and microbial compounds from known wastewater discharges: Potential for use as indicators of human fecal contamination. *Environ. Sci. Technol.* 2005, *39*, (14), 5157-5169.

[136] Benotti, M. J.; Brownawell, B. J., Distributions of pharmaceuticals in an urban estuary during both dry- and wet-weather conditions. *Environ. Sci. Technol.* 2007, *41*, (16), 5795-5802.

[137] Yu, J. T.; Bouwer, E. J.; Coelhan, M., Occurrence and biodegradability studies of selected pharmaceuticals and personal care products in sewage effluent. *Agric. Water Manag.* 2006, *86*, (1-2), 72-80.

[138] Focazio, M. J.; Kolpin, D. W.; Barnes, K. K.; Furlong, E. T.; Meyer, M. T.; Zaugg, S. D.; Barber, L. B.; Thurman, M. E., A national reconnaissance for pharmaceuticals and other organic wastewater contaminants in the United States - II Untreated drinking water sources. *Sci. Total Environ.* 2008, *402*, (2-3), 201-216.

[139] Kolpin, D. W.; Skopec, M.; Meyer, M. T.; Furlong, E. T.; Zaugg, S. D., Urban contribution of pharmaceuticals and other organic wastewater contaminants to streams during differing flow conditions. *Sci. Total Environ.* 2004, *328*, (1-3), 119-130.

[140] Stackelberg, P. E.; Gibs, J.; Furlong, E. T.; Meyer, M. T.; Zaugg, S. D.; Lippincott, R. L., Efficiency of conventional drinking-water-treatment processes in removal of pharmaceuticals and other organic compounds. *Sci. Total Environ.* 2007, *377*, (2-3), 255-272.

[141] Alvarez, D. A.; Stackelberg, P. E.; Petty, J. D.; Huckins, J. N.; Furlong, E. T.; Zaugg, S. D.; Meyer, M. T., Comparison of a novel passive sampler to standard water-column sampling for organic contaminants associated with wastewater effluents entering a New Jersey stream. *Chemosphere* 2005, *61*, (5), 610-622.

[142] Zhang, S.; Zhang, Q.; Darisaw, S.; Ehie, O.; Wang, G., Simultaneous quantification of polycyclic aromatic hydrocarbons (PAHs), polychlorinated biphenyls (PCBs), and pharmaceuticals and personal care products (PPCPs) in Mississippi river water, in New Orleans, Louisiana, USA. *Chemosphere* 2007, *66*, (6), 1057-1069.

[143] Barnes, K. K.; Kolpin, D. W.; Furlong, E. T.; Zaugg, S. D.; Meyer, M. T.; Barber, L. B., A national reconnaissance of pharmaceuticals and other organic wastewater contaminants in the United States - I Groundwater. *Sci. Total Environ.* 2008, *402*, (2-3), 192-200.

[144] Frick, E. A.; Henderson, A. K.; Moll, D. M.; Furlong, E. T.; Meyer, M. T. In 2001 GeorgiaWater Resources Conference, Athens, GA, 2001; Hatcher, K. J., Ed. Institute of Ecology, University of Georgia: Athens, GA, 2001; p 282. (cited in Ref 25).

[145] Ostapowicz, G.; Fontana, R. J.; Schiodt, F. V.; Larson, A.; Davern, T. J.; Han, S. H. B.; McCashland, T. M.; Shakil, A. O.; Hay, J. E.; Hynan, L.; Crippin, J. S.; Blei, A. T.; Samuel, G.; Reisch, J.; Lee, W. M.; Grp, U. S. A. L. F. S., Results of a prospective study of acute liver failure at 17 tertiary care centers in the United States. *Ann. Intern. Med.* 2002, *137*, (12), 947-954.

[146] Lee, W. M., Acetaminophen and the US Acute Liver Failure Study Group: Lowering the risks of hepatic failure. *Hepatology* 2004, *40*, (1), 6-9.
[147] Lee, W. M., Acetominophen Toxicity, Changing perceptions on social/medical issue. *Hepatology* 2007, (46), 966-970.
[148] Bound, J. P.; Voulvoulis, N., Pharmaceuticals in the aquatic environment—a comparison of risk assessment strategies. *Chemosphere* 2004, *56*, (11), 1143-1155.
[149] Doc. Ref. EMEA/CHMP/SWP/4447/00) Guideline on the environmental risk assessment of medicinal products for human use. In *European Medicines Agency Pre-Authorisation of Medicines for Human Use* Committee for medicinal products for human use (chmp): 2006.
[150] Initial assessment of eleven pharmaceuticals using EMEA guideline in Norway. *Department of Local Environmental Management* 2006, *TA-2216/20006 ISBN 82-7655-295-1*.
[151] Schowanek, D.; Webb, S., Exposure simulation for pharmaceuticals in European surface waters with GREAT-ER. *Toxicol. Lett.* 2002, *131*, (1-2), 39-50.
[152] Jones, O. A.; Voulvoulis, N.; Lester, J. N., Partiotioning behavior of five pharmaceutical compounds to activated sludge and river sediment. *Arch. Environ. Contam. Toxicol.* 2006, *50*, 297-305.
[153] Löffler, D.; Römbke, J.; Meller, M.; Ternes, T. A., Environmental fate of pharmaceutical compounds to activated sludge and river sediment. *Env. Sci. Technol.* 2005, *25*, 220-225.
[154] Henschel, K. P.; Wenzel, A.; Diedrich, M.; Fliedner, A., Environmental hazard assessment of pharmaceuticals. *Regul. Toxicol. Pharmacol.* 1997, *25*, (3), 220-225.
[155] IUCLID dataset paracetamol. *European Commission—European Chemicals Bureau.* 2000, 76.
[156] Gravel, A.; Vijayan, M. M., Salicylate disrupts interrenal steroidogenesis and brain glucocoricoid receptor expression in rainbow trout. *Toxicol. Sci.* 2006, *93*, 41-49.
[157] Pascoe, D.; Karntanut, W.; Muller, C. T. M., Do pharmaceuticals affect freshwater invertebrates? A study with the Cnidarian Hydra vulgaris. *Chemosphere* 2003, *51*, 521-528.
[158] Technical guidance document in support of commission directive 93/67/EEC on risk assessment for new notified substances and commission regulation (EC) No 1488/94 on risk assessment for existing substances. In *Commission of the European Communities.*, Office for Official Publications of the European Communities: Luxembourg, 1996.
[159] Brain, R. A.; Johnson, D. J.; Richards, S. M.; Hanson, M. L.; Sanderson, H.; Lam, M. W.; Young, C.; Mabury, S. A.; Sibley, P. K.; Solomon, K. R., Microcosm evaluation of the effects of an eight pharmaceutical mixture to the aquatic macrophytes Lemna gibba and Myriophyllum sibiricum. *Aquat. Toxicol.* 2004, *70*, (1), 23-40.
[160] Borgmann, U.; Bennie, D. T.; Ball, A. L.; Palabrica, V., Effect of a mixture of seven pharmaceuticals on Hyalella azteca over multiple generations. *Chemosphere* 2007, *66*, 1278-1283.
[161] Sanderson, H.; Johnson, D. J.; Wilson, C. J.; Brain, R. A.; Solomon, K. R., Probabilistic hazard assessment of environmentally occurring pharmaceuticals toxicity to fish, daphnias and algae by ECOSAR screening. *Toxicol. Lett.* 2003, *144*, 383-395.

[162] Parolini, M.; Binelli, A.; Cogni, D.; Riva, C.; Provini, A., An in vitro biomarker approach for the evaluation of the ecotoxicity of non-steroidal anti-inflammatory drugs (NSAIDs). *Toxicol. Vitro* 2009, *23*, 935-942.

[163] Calleja, M. C.; Persoone, G.; Geladi, P., Comparative acute toxicity of the first 50 multicenter evaluation of in-vitro cytotoxicity chemicals to aquatic non-vertebrates. *Arch. Environ. Contam. Toxicol.* 1994, *26*, 69-78.

[164] EPA, U. S., Search in Ecotoxicology Database System (U. S. EPA MED-Duluth). *http:\\www.epa.gov/medecotx/ecotox home.htm* 1999.

[165] World Health Organization (WHO) guidelines for drinking-water quality. In World Health Organization: Geneva, 2004; p 451.

[166] Miles, A. M.; Singer, P. C.; Ashley, D. L.; Lynberg, M. C.; Mendola, P.; Langlois, P. H.; Nuckols, J. R., Comparison of trihalomethanes in tap water and blood. *Environ. Sci.Technol.* 2002, *36*, (8), 1692-1698.

[167] Bedner, M.; MacCrehan, W. A., Reactions of the amine-containing drugs fluoxetine and metoprolol during chlorination and dechlorination processes used in wastewater treatment. *Chemosphere* 2006, *65*, (11), 2130-2137.

[168] Glassmeyer, S. T.; Shoemaker, J. A., Effects of chlorination on the persistence of pharmaceuticals in the environment. *Bull. Environ. Contam. Toxicol.* 2005, *74*, (1), 24-31.

[169] Bedner, M.; MacCrehan, W. A., Transformation of acetaminophen by chlorination produces the toxicants 1,4-benzoquinone and N-acetyl-p-benzoquinone imine. *Environ. Sci. Technol.* 2006, *40*, (2), 516-522.

[170] Skoumal, M.; Cabot, P. L.; Centellas, F.; Arias, C.; Rodriguez, R. M.; Garrido, J. A.; Brillas, E., Mineralization of paracetamol by ozonation catalyzed with Fe^{2+}, Cu^{2+} and UVA light. *Applied Catal., B* 2006, *66*, (3-4), 228-240.

[171] Pérez, S.; Barceló, D., First evidence for occurrence of hydroxylated human metabolites of diclofenac and aceclofenac in wastewater using QqLIT-MS and QqTOF-MS. *Anal. Chem.* 2008, *80*, (21), 8135-8145.

[172] Poyatos, J. M.; Munio, M. M.; Almecija, M. C.; Torres, J. C.; Hontoria, E.; Osorio, F., Advanced oxidation processes for wastewater treatment: State of the art. *Water Air Soil Pollut.* 2010, *205*, 187-204.

[173] Yang, L.; Yu, L. E.; Ray, M. B., Degradation of paracetamol in aqueous solutions by TiO_2 photocatalysis. *Water Res.* 2008, *42*, (13), 3480-3488.

[174] Yang, L. M.; Yu, L. E.; Ray, M. B., Photocatalytic oxidation of paracetamol: Dominant reactants, intermediates, and reaction mechanisms. *Environ. Sci. Technol.* 2009, *43*, (2), 460-465.

[175] Waterston, K.; Wang, J. W. J.; Bejan, D.; Bunce, N. J., Electrochemical waste water treatment: Electrooxidation of acetaminophen. *J. Appl. Electrochem.* 2006, *36*, (2), 227-232.

[176] Boudreau, J.; Bejan, D.; Bunce, N., Competition between electrochemical advanced oxidation and electrochemical hypochlorination of acetaminophen at boron-doped diamond and ruthenium dioxide based anodes. *Can. J.Chem.* 2010, *88*, 418-425.

[177] Sirés; Arias, C.; Cabot, P. L.; Centellas, F.; Rodríguez, R. M.; Garrido, J. A.; Brillas, E., Paracetamol mineralization by advanced electrochemical oxidation processes for wastewater treatment. *Environ. Chem.* 2004, *1*, (1), 26-28.

[178] Sirés, I.; Garrido, J. A.; Rodriguez, R. M.; Cabot, P. I.; Centellas, F.; Arias, C.; Brillas, E., Electrochemical degradation of paracetamol from water by catalytic action of Fe^{2+}, Cu^{2+}, and UVA light on electrogenerated hydrogen peroxide. *J. Electrochem. Soc.* 2006, *153*, (1), D1-D9.

[179] Almeida, L. C.; Garcia-Segura, S.; Bocchi, N.; Brillas, E., Solar photoelectro-Fenton degradation of paracetamol using a flow plant with a Pt/air-diffusion cell coupled with a compound parabolic collector: Process optimization by response surface methodology. *Appl. Cat. B - Environ.* 2011, *103*, (1-2), 21-30.

[180] Kim, I.; Yamashita, N.; Tanaka, H., Performance of UV and UV/H_2O_2 processes for the removal of pharmaceuticals detected in secondary effluent of a sewage treatment plant in Japan. *J. Hazard. Mat.* 2009, *166*, (2-3), 1134-1140.

[181] Klamerth, N.; Miranda, N.; Malato, S.; Aguera, A.; Fernandez-Alba, A. R.; Maldonado, M. I.; Coronado, J. M., Degradation of emerging contaminants at low concentrations in MWTPs effluents with mild solar photo-Fenton and TiO_2. *Catal. Today* 2009, *144*, (1-2), 124-130.

[182] Trovó, A. G.; Melo, S. A. S.; Nogueira, R. F. P., Photodegradation of the pharmaceuticals amoxicillin, bezafibrate and paracetamol by the photo-Fenton process—Application to sewage treatment plant effluent. *J. Photochem. Photobiol., A* 2008, *198*, (2-3), 215-220.

[183] Durán, A.; Monteagudo, J. M.; Carnicer, A.; Ruiz-Murillo, M., Photo-Fenton mineralization of synthetic municipal wastewater effluent containing acetaminophen in a pilot plant. *Desalination* 2011, *270*, (1-3), 124-129.

[184] Jordá, L. S. J.; Martín, M. M. B.; Gómez, E. O.; Reina, A. C.; Sánchez, I. M. R.; López, J. L. C.; Pérez, J. A. S., Economic evaluation of the photo-Fenton process. Mineralization level and reaction time: The keys for increasing plant efficiency. *J. Hazard. Mat.* 2011, *186*, (2-3), 1924-1929.

[185] Klamerth, N.; Malato, S.; Maldonado, M. I.; Agura, A.; Fernandez-Alba, A. R., Application of photo-Fenton as a tertiary treatment of emerging contaminants in municipal wastewater. *Environ. Sci. Technol.* 2010, *44*, (5), 1792-1798.

[186] Santos-Juanes, L.; Sanchez, J. L. G.; Lopez, J. L. C.; Oller, I.; Malato, S.; Perez, J. A. S., Dissolved oxygen concentration: A key parameter in monitoring the photo-Fenton process. *Appl. Catal., B* 2011, *104*, (3-4), 316-323.

[187] Zhang, X.; Wu, F.; Wu, X. W.; Chen, P. Y.; Deng, N. S., Photodegradation of acetaminophen in TiO_2 suspended solution. *J. Hazard. Mat.* 2008, *157*, (2-3), 300-307.

[188] Miranda-García, N.; Suárez, S.; Sánchez, B.; Coronado, J. M.; Malato, S.; Maldonado, M. I., Photocatalytic degradation of emerging contaminants in municipal wastewater treatment plant effluents using immobilized TiO_2 in a solar pilot plant. *Appl. Catal., B* 2011, *103*, (3-4), 294-301.

[189] Isariebel, Q. P.; Carine, J. L.; Ulises-Javier, J. H.; Anne-Marie, W.; Henri, D., Sonolysis of levodopa and paracetamol in aqueous solutions. *Ultrason. Sonochem.* 2009, *16*, (5), 610-616.

[190] Pereira, V. J.; Weinberg, H. S.; Linden, K. G.; Singer, P. C., UV degradation kinetics and modeling of pharmaceutical compounds in laboratory grade and surface water via direct and indirect photolysis at 254 nm. *Environ. Sci. Technol.* 2007, *41*, (5), 1682-1688.

[191] Centi, G.; Perathoner, S., Use of solid catalysts in promoting water treatment and remediation technologies. In *Catalysis*, Spivey, J. J., Ed. The Royal Society of Chemistry: UK, 2005; Vol. 18, pp 46-68.

[192] Ternes, T. A.; Stüber, J.; Herrmann, N.; McDowell, D.; Ried, A.; Kampmann, M.; Teiser, B., Ozonation: A tool for removal of pharmaceuticals, contrast media and musk fragrances from wastewater? *Water Res.* 2003, *37*, (8), 1976-1982.

[193] Hoigne, J., *Mechanisms, rates and selectivities of oxidations of organic compounds initiated by ozonation of water*. Ann Arbor Science Publ., Ann Arbor: MI, 1982.

[194] Baus, C.; Sona, M.; Brauch, H. J., Ozonation and combined ozone/H_2O_2, UV/ozone and UV/H_2O_2 for treatment of fuel oxygenates MTBE, ETBE, TAME, and DIPE from water—a comparison of removal efficiencies. *Water Sci. Technol.* 2007, *55*, (12), 307-311.

[195] Fenton, H. J., Oxidative properties of the H_2O_2/Fe^{2+} system and its application. *J. Chem. Soc.* 1884, *65*, 889-899.

[196] Haber, F.; Weiss, J., The catalytic decomposition of hydrogen peroxide by iron salts. *J. Proc. Roy. Soc. London A* 1934, *147*, 332-351.

[197] Tekin, H.; Bilkay, O.; Ataberk, S. S.; Balta, T. H.; Ceribasi, I. H.; Sanin, F. D.; Dilek, F. B.; Yetis, U., Use of Fenton oxidation to improve the biodegradability of a pharmaceutical wastewater. *J. Hazard. Mat.* 2006, *136*, (2), 258-265.

[198] Soon, A. N.; Hameed, B. H., Heterogeneous catalytic treatment of synthetic dyes in aqueous media using Fenton and photo-assisted Fenton process. *Desalination* 2011, *269*, (1-3), 1-16.

[199] Martínez, N. S. S.; Fernández, J. F.; Segura, X. F.; Ferrer, A. S., Pre-oxidation of an extremely polluted industrial wastewater by the Fenton's reagent. *J. Hazard. Mat.* 2003, *101*, (3), 315-322.

[200] Guidelines for testing of Chemicals, Simulation Test-Aerobic Sewage Treatment. In Organisation for Economic Cooperation and development (OECD), 303A, 1999.

[201] Fujishima, A.; Honda, K., Electrochemical photolysis of water at a semiconductor electrode. *Nature* 1972, *238*, 37-38.

[202] Ollis, D. F.; Al-Ekabi, H., *Photocatalytic purification and treatment of water and air*. Elsevier: Amsterdam, 1993.

[203] Pelizzetti, E.; Serpone, N., *Photocatalysis: fundamental and applications*. Wiley: New York, 1989.

[204] Legrini, O.; Oliveros, E.; Braun, A. M., Photochemical processes for water treatment. *Chem. Rev.* 1993, *93*, 671-698.

[205] Méndez-Arriaga, F.; Esplugas, S.; Giménez, J., Photocatalytic degradation of non-steroidal anti-inflammatory drugs with TiO_2 and simulated solar irradiation. *Water Res.* 2008, *42*, (3), 585-594.

[206] Choi, H.; Stathatos, E.; Dionysiou, D., Sol-gel preparation of mesoporous photocatalytic TiO2 films and TiO_2/Al_2O_3 composite membranes for environmental applications. *Appl. Catal., B* 2006, *63*, 60-67.

[207] Fernández, A.; Lassaletta, G.; Jimenez, V. M.; Justo, A.; Gonzalez-Elipe, A. R.; Herrmann, J. M., Preparation and characterization of TiO_2 photocatalysts supported on various rigid supports (glass, quartz and stainless steel). Comparative studies of photocatalytic activity in water purification. *Appl. Catal., B* 1995, *7*, 49-63.

[208] Hsien, Y. H.; Chang, C. F.; Chen, Y. H.; Cheng, S., Photodegradation of aromatic pollutants in water over TiO_2 supported on molecular sieves. *Appl. Catal., B* 2001, *31*, 241-249.
[209] Velasco, L. F.; Parra, J. B.; Ania, C. O., Role of activated carbon features on photodegradation of phenol. *Appl. Surf. Sci.* 2010, *256*, 5254- 5258.
[210] Velasco, L. F.; Parra, J. B.; Ania, C. O., Phenol adsorption and photo-oxidation on porous C/Ti composites. *Adsorpt. Sci. Technol.* 2010, *17*, 726-739.
[211] Bussi, J.; Ohanian, M.; Vazquez, M.; Dalchiele, E. A., Photocatalytic removal of Hg from solid wastes of chlor-alkali plant. *J. Environ. Eng.* 2002, *128*, (8), 733-739.
[212] Eggins, B. R.; Palmer, F. L.; Byrne, J. A., Photocatalytic treatment of humic substances in drinking water. *Water Res.* 1997, *31*, 1223-1226.
[213] Mills, A.; LeHunte, S., An overview of semiconductor photocatalysis. *J. Photochem. Photobiol., A* 1997, *108*, 1-35.
[214] Shephard, G. S.; Stockenstrom, S.; de Villiers, D.; Engelbrecht, W. J.; Wessels, G. F. S., Degradation of microcystin toxins in a falling film photocatalytic reactor with immobilized titanium dioxide catalyst. *Water Res.* 2002, *36*, 140-146.
[215] Chen, G., Electrochemical technologies in wastewater treatment. *Sep. Purif. Technol.* 2004, *38*, (1), 11-41.
[216] Sirés, I.; Brillas, E., Remediation of water pollution caused by pharmaceutical residues based on electrochemical separation and degradation technologies: A review. *Environ. Int.* 2011, *doi:10.1016/j.envint.2011.07.012.*
[217] Grimm, J.; Bessarabov, D.; Sanderson, R., Review of electro-assisted methods for water purification. *Desalination* 1998, *115*, (3), 285-294.
[218] Martinez-Huitle, C. A.; Ferro, S., Electrochemical oxidation of organic pollutants for the wastewater treatment: Direct and indirect processes. *Chem. Soc. Rev.* 2006, *35*, (12), 1324-1340.
[219] Comninellis, C.; Pulgarin, C., Electrochemical oxidation of phenol for wastewater treatment using SnO_2, anodes. *J. Appl. Electrochem.* 1993, *23*, 108-112.
[220] Rajeshwar, K.; Ibanez, J. G.; Swain, G. M., Electrochemistry and the environment. *J. Appl. Electrochem.* 1994, *24*, 1077-1091.
[221] Comninellis, C., Electrochemical treatment of waste water containing phenol, Institution of Chemical Engineers Symposium Series, vol. 127. *Electrochem. Eng. Environ.* 1992, *92*, 189-201.
[222] Deshpande, A.; Lokesh, K. S.; Bejankiwar, R. S.; Gowda, T. P. H., Electrochemical oxidation of pharmaceutical effluent using cast iron electrode. *J. Environ. Sci. Eng.* 2005, *47*, 21–24.
[223] Deshpande, A. M.; Satyanarayan, S.; Ramakant, S., Electrochemical pretreatment of wastewater from bulk drug manufacturing industry. *J. Environ. Eng.* 2009, *135*, 716-719.
[224] Naddeo, V.; Belgiorno, V.; Ricco, D.; Kassinos, D., Degradation of diclofenac during sonolysis, ozonation and their simultaneous application. *Ultrason. Sonochem.* 2009, *16*, (6), 790-794.
[225] Hartmann, J.; Bartels, P.; Mau, U.; Witter, M.; Tümpling, W. V.; Hofmann, J.; Nietzschmann, E., Degradation of the drug diclofenac in water by sonolysis in presence of catalysts. *Chemosphere* 2008, *70*, (3), 453-461.

[226] Bandosz, T. J.; Ania, C. O., Surface chemistry of activated carbons and its characterization. In *Activated Carbon Surfaces in Environmental Remediation*, Bandosz, T. J., Ed. Elsevier: New York, 2006; Vol. 7, pp 159-229.

[227] Marsh, H.; Rodríguez-Reinoso, F., *Activated Carbon*. Elsevier: Oxford, 2006; p 536.

[228] Sing, K. S. W., Reporting physisorption data for gas/solid systems, with special reference to the determination of surface area and porosity. *Pure & Appl.Chem.* 1982, *54*, (11), 2201-2218.

[229] Ania, C. O.; Beguin, F., Mechanism of adsorption and electrosorption of bentazone on activated carbon cloth in aqueous solutions. *Water Res.* 2007, *41*, 3372 - 3380.

[230] Ania, C. O.; Beguin, F., Electrochemically assisted adsorption/desorption of bentazone on activated carbon cloth. *Adsorption* 2007, *13*, 579-586.

[231] Afkhami, A.; Conway, B. E., Investigation of removal of Cr(VI), Mo(VI), W(VI), V(IV), and V(V) oxy-ions from industrial wastewaters by adsorption and electrosorption at high-area carbon cloth. *J. Colloid Interface Sci.* 2002, *251*, 248-255.

[232] Ayranci, E.; Hoda, N., Adsorption of bentazone and propanil from aqueous solutions at the high area activated carbon cloth. *Chemosphere* 2004, *57*, 755-762.

[233] Przepiórski, J., Activated carbon filters and their industrial applications. In *Activated Carbon Surfaces in Environmental Remediation*, Bandosz, T. J., Ed. Elsevier: New York, 2006; Vol. 7, pp 421-474.

[234] Karanfil, T., Activated carbon adsorption in drinking water treatment. In *Activated Carbon Surfaces in Environmental Remediation*, Bandosz, T. J., Ed. Elsevier: New York, 2006; Vol. 7, pp 345-374.

[235] Bandosz, T. J. (Ed.), Activated Carbon Surfaces in Environmental Remediation. In *Interface Science and Technology*, Hubbard, A., Ed. Elsevier Ltd: UK, 2006; Vol. 7.

[236] Bottani, E.; Tascón, J., *Adsorption by Carbons*. Elsevier Ltd: Oxford, 2008.

[237] Quesada-Penate, I.; Julcour-Lebigue, C.; Jauregui-Haza, U. J.; Wilhelm, A. M.; Delmas, H., Comparative adsorption of levodopa from aqueous solution on different activated carbons. *Chem. Eng. J.* 2009, *152*, (1), 183-188.

[238] Mestre, A. S.; Pinto, M. L.; Pires, J.; Nogueira, J. M. F.; Carvalho, A. P., Effect of solution pH on the removal of clofibric acid by cork-based activated carbons. *Carbon* 2010, *48*, (4), 972-980.

[239] Mestre, A. S.; Pires, J.; Nogueira, J. M. F.; Carvalho, A. P., Activated carbons for the adsorption of ibuprofen. *Carbon* 2007, *45*, (10), 1979-1988.

[240] Mestre, A. S.; Pires, J.; Nogueira, J. M. F.; Parra, J. B.; Carvalho, A. P.; Ania, C. O., Waste-derived activated carbons for removal of ibuprofen from solution: Role of surface chemistry and pore structure. *Bioresour. Technol.* 2009, *100*, (5), 1720-1726.

[241] Ania, C. O.; Parra, J. B.; Menendez, J. A.; Pis, J. J., Microwave assisted regeneration of activated carbon loaded with pharmaceuticals. *Water Res.* 2007, *41*, 3299-3306

[242] Ania, C. O.; Parra, J. B.; Pis, J. J., Effect of texture and surface chemistry on adsorptive capacities of activated carbons for phenolic compounds removal. *Fuel Process. Technol.* 2002, *77-78*, 337-343.

[243] Ania, C. O.; Parra, J. B.; Pis, J. J., Influence of oxygen containing functional groups on active carbon adsorption of selected organic compounds. *Fuel Process. Technol.* 2002, *79*, 265-271.

[244] Nakamura, T.; Oida, Y.; Matsumoto, K.; Kawasaki, N.; Tanada, S., Inhibitory effect of sorbitol on acetaminophen adsorption by activated carbon. *J. Environ. Sci. Health, Part A* 2002, *37*, (5), 905-912.

[245] Thomas, S. H. L., Paracetamol (acetaminophen) poisoning. *Pharmacol. Ther.* 1993, *60*, (1), 91-120.

[246] Tenenbein, P. K.; Sitar, D. S.; Tenenbein, M., Interaction between N-acetylcysteine and activated charcoal: Implications for the treatment of acetaminophen poisoning. *Pharmacotherapy* 2001, *21*, (11), 1331-1336.

[247] Chamberlain, J. M.; Gorman, R. L.; Oderda, G. M.; Klein-Schwartz, W.; Klein, B. L., Use of activated charcoal in a simulated poisoning with acetaminophen: A new loading dose for N-acetylcysteine? *Ann. Emerg. Med.* 1993, *22*, (9), 1398-1402.

[248] Hoegberg, L. C. G.; Christophersen, A. B.; Christensen, H. R.; Angelo, H. R., Comparison of the adsorption capacities of an activated-charcoal-yogurt mixture versus activated-charcoal-water slurry in vivo and in vitro. *Clin. Toxicol.* 2005, *43*, (4), 269-275.

[249] Hoegberg, L. C. G.; Groenlykke, T. B.; Abildtrup, U.; Angelo, H. R., Combined paracetamol and amitriptyline adsorption to activated charcoal. *Clin. Toxicol.* 2010, *48*, (9), 898-903.

[250] Hoegberg, L. C. G.; Angelo, H. R.; Christophersen, A. B.; Christensen, H. R., The effect of food and ice cream on the adsorption capacity of paracetamol to high surface activated charcoal: In vitro studies. *Pharmacol. Toxicol.* 2003, *93*, (5), 233-237.

[251] Christophersen, A. B.; Levin, D.; Hoegberg, L. C. G.; Angelo, H. R.; Kampmann, J. P., Activated charcoal alone or after gastric lavage: A simulated large paracetamol intoxication. *Br. J. Clin. Pharmacol.* 2002, *53*, (3), 312-317.

[252] Hoegberg, L. C. G.; Angelo, H. R.; Christophersen, A. B.; Christensen, H. R., Effect of ethanol and pH on the adsorption of acetaminophen (paracetamol) to high surface activated charcoal, in vitro studies. *J. Toxicol.-Clin. Toxicol.* 2002, *40*, (1), 59-67.

[253] Rutherfoord, R. S.; Gorman, R. L.; Oderda, G. M.; Klein-Schwartz, W.; Watson, W. A., Simulated acetaminophen overdose: Pharmacokinetics and effectiveness of activated charcoal. *Ann. Emerg. Med.* 1991, *20*, (10), 1064-1068.

[254] Willson, R. A.; Thompson, R. P. H.; Winch, J.; Williams, R., Rapid removal of paracetamol by hemoperfusion through coated charcoal. In-vivo and in-vitro studies in the pig. *The Lancet* 1973, *301*, (7794), 77-79.

[255] Winchester, J. F.; Edwards, R. O.; Tilstone, W. J.; Woodcock, B. G., Activated charcoal hemoperfusion and experimental acetaminophen poisoning. *Toxicol. Appl. Pharmacol.* 1975, *31*, (1), 120-127.

[256] Cabrita, I.; Ruiz, B.; Mestre, A. S.; Fonseca, I. M.; Carvalho, A. P.; Ania, C. O., Removal of an analgesic using activated carbons prepared from urban and industrial residues. *Chem. Eng. J.* 2010, *163*, (3), 249-255.

[257] Mestre, A. S.; Bexiga, A. S.; Proença, M.; Andrade, M.; Pinto, M. L.; Matos, I.; Fonseca, I. M.; Carvalho, A. P., Activated carbons from sisal waste by chemical activation with K_2CO_3: Kinetics of paracetamol and ibuprofen removal from aqueous solution. *Bioresour. Technol.* 2011, *102*, (17), 8253-8260.

[258] Ruiz, B.; Cabrita, I.; Mestre, A. S.; Parra, J. B.; Pires, J.; Carvalho, A. P.; Ania, C. O., Surface heterogeneity effects of activated carbons on the kinetics of paracetamol removal from aqueous solution. *Appl. Surf. Sci.* 2010, *256*, (17), 5171-5175.

[259] Cotoruelo, L. M.; Marques, M. D.; Leiva, A.; Rodriguez-Mirasol, J.; Cordero, T., Adsorption of oxygen-containing aromatics used in petrochemical, pharmaceutical and food industries by means of lignin based active carbons. *Adsorption* 2011, *17*, (3), 539-550.

[260] *Roskill Report, The Economics of Activated Carbon, 6th ed. Roskill Information Services Ltd*; Claphham Road, London, 1998.

[261] Terzyk, A. P., Describing adsorption of paracetamol from aqueous solution on carbons while utilizing the most widespread isotherm models-the impact of surface carbonyl and basic groups. *J. Colloid Interface Sci.* 2002, *247*, (2), 507-510.

[262] Beninati, S.; Semeraro, D.; Mastragostino, M., Adsorption of paracetamol and acetylsalicylic acid onto commercial activated carbons. *Adsorpt. Sci. Technol.* 2008, *26*, (9), 721-734.

[263] Wisniewski, M.; Pacholczyk, A.; Terzyk, A. P.; Rychlicki, G., New phosphorus-containing spherical carbon adsorbents as promising materials in drug adsorption and release. *J. Colloid Interface Sci.* 2011, *354*, (2), 891-894.

[264] Terzyk, A. P., The influence of activated carbon surface chemical composition on the adsorption of acetaminophen (paracetamol) in vitro: Part II. TG, FTIR, and XPS analysis of carbons and the temperature dependence of adsorption kinetics at the neutral pH. *Colloids Surf., A* 2001, *177*, (1), 23-45.

[265] Terzyk, A. P., Adsorption of biologically active compounds from aqueous solutions on to commercial unmodified activated carbons. Part IV. Do the properties of amphoteric carbon surface layers influence the adsorption of paracetamol at acidic pH levels? *Adsorpt. Sci. Technol.* 2003, *21*, (1), 93-123.

[266] Terzyk, A. P., Adsorption of biologically active compounds from aqueous solutions on to commercial unmodified activated carbons. Part III. Theoretical description of paracetamol adsorption data at neutral pH. *Adsorpt. Sci. Technol.* 2002, *20*, (1), 63-81.

[267] Terzyk, A. P., The impact of carbon surface composition on the diffusion and adsorption of paracetamol at different temperatures and at neutral pH. *J. Colloid Interface Sci.* 2000, *230*, (1), 219-222.

[268] Terzyk, A. P., Adsorption of biologically active compounds from aqueous solutions on to commercial unmodified activated carbons. Part II. Temperature dependence of adsorption kinetics of 4-hydroxyacetanilide (paracetamol) at neutral pH. *Adsorpt. Sci. Technol.* 2000, *18*, (5), 477-508.

[269] Terzyk, A. P., Molecular properties and intermolecular forces—factors balancing the effect of carbon surface chemistry in adsorption of organics from dilute aqueous solutions. *J. Colloid Interface Sci.* 2004, *275*, (1), 9-29.

[270] Terzyk, A. P.; Cwiertnia, M. S.; Wisniewski, M.; Gauden, P. A.; Rychlicki, G.; Szymanski, G. S., Impact of the interaction with the positive charge in adsorption of benzene and other organic compounds from aqueous solutions on carbons. *Appl. Surf. Sci.* 2007, *253*, (8), 4006-4009.

[271] Terzyk, A. P.; Rychlicki, G., The influence of activated carbon surface chemical composition on the adsorption of acetaminophen (paracetamol) in vitro: The temperature dependence of adsorption at the neutral pH. *Colloids Surf., A* 2000, *163*, (2-3), 135-150.

[272] Terzyk, A. P.; Rychlicki, G.; Biniak, S.; Lukaszewicz, J. P., New correlations between the composition of the surface layer of carbon and its physicochemical properties

exposed while paracetamol is adsorbed at different temperatures and pH. *J. Colloid Interface Sci.* 2003, *257*, (1), 13-30.

[273] Villaescusa, I.; Fiol, N.; Poch, J.; Bianchi, A.; Bazzicalupi, C., Mechanism of paracetamol removal by vegetable wastes: The contribution of □illaescusa, I.; Fiol, N.; bonding and hydrophobic effect. *Desalination* 2011, *270*, (1-3), 135-142.

[274] Bekçi, Z.; Seki, Y.; Kadir Yurdakoç, M., A study of equilibrium and FTIR, SEM/EDS analysis of trimethoprim adsorption onto K10. *J. Mol. Struct.* 2007, *827*, (1-3), 67-74.

[275] Bekçi, Z.; Seki, Y.; Yurdakoç, M. K., Equilibrium studies for trimethoprim adsorption on montmorillonite KSF. *J. Hazard. Mat.* 2006, *133*, (1-3), 233-242.

[276] Gereli, G.; Seki, Y.; Murat Kusoglu, I.; Yurdakoç, K., Equilibrium and kinetics for the sorption of promethazine hydrochloride onto K10 montmorillonite. *J. Colloid Interface Sci.* 2006, *299*, (1), 155-162.

[277] Bajpai, A. K.; Rajpoot, M.; Mishra, D. D., Studies on the correlation between structure and adsorption of sulfonamide compounds. *Colloids Surf., A* 2000, *168*, (3), 193-205.

[278] Lorphensri, O.; Intravijit, J.; Sabatini, D. A.; Kibbey, T. C. G.; Osathaphan, K.; Saiwan, C., Sorption of acetaminophen, 17 alpha-ethynyl estradiol, nalidixic acid, and norfloxacin to silica, alumina, and a hydrophobic medium. *Water Res.* 2006, *40*, (7), 1481-1491.

[279] Xiao, P.; Dudal, Y.; Corvini, P. F. X.; Shahgaldian, P., Polymeric cyclodextrin-based nanoparticles: synthesis, characterization and sorption properties of three selected pharmaceutically active ingredients. *Polym. Chem.* 2011, *2*, (1), 120-125.

In: Acetaminophen: Properties, Clinical Uses
Editors: Atash Javaherian and Pasha Latifpour
ISBN: 978-1-61942-374-9

Chapter 5

ACETAMINOPHEN OVERDOSE, BIOMARKERS, AND MANAGEMENT

M. Sattari[1] and S. O. Mashayekhi[2,*]
[1]Neurosciences Research Centre, Tabriz University of Medical Sciences, Tabriz, Iran
[2]NPMC, Tabriz University of Medical Sciences, Tabriz, Iran

ABSTRACT

Acetaminophen is manufactured in huge quantities worldwide. Approximately 3.2 thousand million tablets of acetaminophen are consumed by the public every year in the UK (mean of 55 tablets/person).

Acetaminophen poisoning accounts for up to 48% of all poisons admissions to hospital. It is a weak inhibitor of COX-1 and COX-2 in peripheral tissues and possesses no significant anti-inflamatory effects. The oral dose of acetaminophen is 0.5-1g per 4-6 h to a maximum of 4 g in a day. Approximately 95% of acetaminophen is metabolised to glucuronide and sulphate conjugates which are excreted in the urine.

About 5% of acetaminophen is metabolised through the cytochrome P-450 2E1 to produce a highly reactive toxic metabolite, N-acetyl-p-benzoquinonimine (NAPQI). At therapeutic doses, the small amounts of NAPQI produced by acetaminophen metabolism are detoxified by liver stores of hepatic glutathione and is excreted in bile or urine as mercapturic acid conjugate. In overdose, stores of glutathione become depleted. Without the glutathione substrate, NAPQI becomes available to bind to proteins and DNA of hepatocytes causing direct cellular injury.

Generation of reactive oxygen species and nitric oxide, lipid peroxidation, mitochondrial dysfunction, disruption of calcium homeostasis and induction of apoptosis are all mechanisms have suggested that may be involved in acetaminophen-induced hepatotoxicity. Severe liver damage has been defined as an increase in plasma activities of aspartate aminotransferase (AST), alanine aminotransferase (ALT), sorbitol dehydrogenase (SDH), ornithine carbamyltransferase (OCT), lactic dehydrogenase (LDH), hydroxybutyrate dehydrogenase (HBDH), glutathione S-transferases, and F-protein. Increase in prothrombin time, plasma concentrations of creatinine, biliverdin,

* Tel: +98 411 3855905, Fax: +98 411 3344798, E-mail: mashayekhis@yahoo.co.uk

bilirubin, and phosphate, and reduction in blood pH, bicarbonate, and glucose have also been demonstrated as biomarkers of acetaminophen overdose.

We recently showed an increase in plasma concentration of taurine as a probable biomarker of acetaminophen poisoning. Different antidotes such as: cimetidine, cysteamine, methionine, and glycyrrhizin have already used for the treatment of acetaminophen overdose.

However, N-acetylcysteine (NAC) is a clinically approved drug which is used with three treatment regimens: a 20-hour continuous infusion of NAC, a 48-hour regimen of intermittent intravenous infusions and a 72-hour regimen of intermittent oral doses. NAC should be given if the plasma acetaminophen concentration is above a line joining 200mg/L (1.32mmol/L) at four hours after ingestion and 30mg/L (0.20mmol/L) at 15 hours on a semilogarithmic plot.

Few adverse reactions have been reported in 5% of patients who receive NAC particularly in intravenous forms. The most of these reactions are anaphylactoid such as flushing, pruritus, urticaria, angioedema, cough, headache, shortness of breath, wheezing, hypotension, status epilepticus, and cortical blindness.

EPIDEMIOLOGY

Acetaminophen is a widely used analgesic and antipyretic which is available over-the counter and as a prescription drug. Its lack of unwanted gastrointestinal side effects and rapid absorption from the gastrointestinal tract has made it a popular analgesic in the last 30 years. Acetaminophen-induced hepatotoxicity is a common consequence of acetaminophen overdose and may lead to acute liver failure (ALF). Currently acetaminophen is the most common cause of ALF in both United States and United Kingdom, with a trend to increasing incidence in the United States *(Chun et al., 2009)*.

Acetaminophen-related hepatotoxicity is more common in patients with unintentional overdoses, alcohol abuse, and underlying liver disease *(Myers et al., 2008)*. Mortality from acetaminophen overdose is now about 0.4%, although without treatment, severe liver damage occurs in at least half of people with blood acetaminophen levels above the UK standard treatment line *(Buckley et al., 2007)*. Cerebral edema is a major cause of death in acute acetaminophen overdose *(Craig et al., 2010)*.

Acetaminophen poisoning accounts for at least 42% of USA acute liver failure cases seen at tertiary-care centers and one third of the deaths. The percentage of all ALF cases in a study that were due to acetaminophen, doubled in 6 years *(Larson et al., 2005)*. In a study, the proportion of admissions involving acetaminophen increased significantly from 35.9% in 1989 to 44.4% in 2002 in the UK *(Ghandforoush-Sattari et al., 2007)*.

In other studies by *Quigley et al (Quigley et al., 1994)* in Northern Ireland from 1976-1991, *Hawton and Fagg (Hawton et al., 1992)* in Oxford from 1976-1990, by *Bialas et al (Bialas et al., 1996)* in Cardiff from 1987-1993, and *Townsend et al (Townsend et al., 2001)* in Oxford from 1985-1997, many authors observed that the proportion of episodes involving acetaminophen increased over time.

Legislation was introduced in the UK in 1998 to limit over-the-counter sales due to rising rates of deliberate self-poisoning. Despite this legislation, Bateman and colleagues reported an annual hospitalization rate for acetaminophen overdose in Scotland of 124.4 per 100 000 during the following year *(Bateman et al., 2003)*. Another study in Canada showed the incidence of acetaminophen overdose was 46 per 100 000 population (~1/2200) between 1997 and 2002 *(Myers et al., 2007)*.

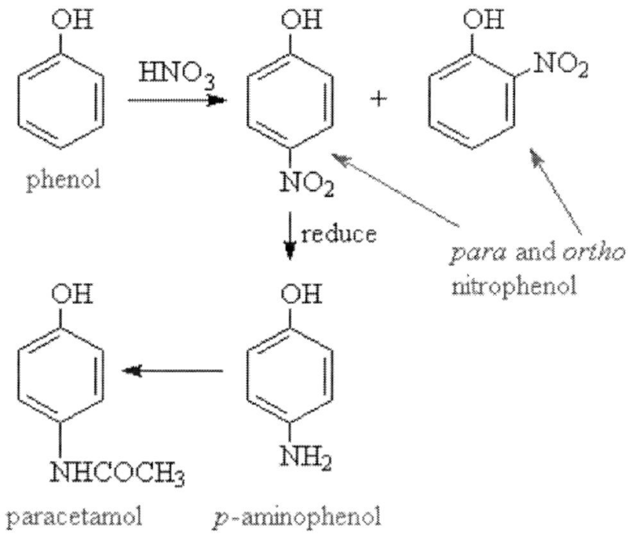

Figure 1. Production of Acetaminophen from Phenol.

Structure

Acetaminophen is manufactured in huge quantities worldwide. The starting material for the commercial manufacture of acetaminophen is phenol, which is nitrated to give a mixture of the *ortho* and *para*-nitrotophenol. The *o*-isomer is removed by steam distillation, and the *p*-nitro group reduced to a *p*-amino group. This is then acetylated to give acetaminophen (Figure 1) *(Atkins, 1987)*.

Pharmacology of Acetaminophen

Acetaminophen is an active metabolite of phenacetin and is responsible for phenacetin's analgesic effect. It is a weak inhibitor of COX-1 and COX-2 in peripheral tissues and possesses no significant anti-inflamatory effects *(Katzung, 2004)*. The oral dose of acetaminophen is 0.5-1g per 4-6 h to a maximum of 4 g in a day *(Laurence DR, 1992)*. Acetaminophen (N-acetyl-p-aminophenol) is rapidly absorbed from the gastrointestinal tract and a dose taken by a fasting subject reaches mean peak plasma concentration in 70 minutes. This peak can be delayed to 160 min by slowing gastric emptying e.g. administration of propantheline *(Rumack et al., 1975)*. Its systemic bioavailability is dose-dependent and ranges from 70 to 90%. Its rate of oral absorption is dependent on the rate of gastric emptying, being delayed by food, propantheline, pethidine, and diamorphine, and enhanced by metoclopramide. Acetaminophen is also well absorbed from the rectum. It distributes rapidly and evenly throughout most tissues and fluids and has a volume of distribution of approximately 0.9 L/kg. Ten to 20% of the drug is bound to red blood cells *(Forrest et al.,*

1982). In acute acetaminophen poisoning, the plasma acetaminophen half-life is the most reliable early guide to prognosis, and is prolonged if acetaminophen-induced liver damage occurs *(Prescott et al., 1971)*. The half-life of acetaminophen in overdose is variable due to saturable conjugation and the effects of hepatotoxicity on metabolism *(Prescott et al., 1973; Slattery et al., 1979)*. The plasma half-life in healthy subjects ranges from 1.9 to 2.5 hours and the total body clearance from 4.5 to 5.5mL/kg/min. Age has little effect on the plasma half-life, but it is reduced in patients taking enzyme inducers (e.g. anticonvulsants). The plasma half-life is usually normal in patients with mild chronic liver disease, but it is prolonged in those with decompensated liver disease *(Forrest et al., 1982)*. Acetaminophen is largely removed from the circulation by hepatic metabolism to glucuronide and sulphate conjugates *(Lau et al., 1994)*, and only about 4% of a therapeutic dose is excreted unchanged in the urine *(Cummings et al., 1967)*.

Toxicity

In Adults, hepatotoxicity may occur after ingestion of a single dose of 10-15g (150-250 mg/kg) of acetaminophen. Doses of 20-25g or greater are potentially fatal *(Goodman et al., 2008)*.

History

The use of acetaminophen for self-poisoning has increased greatly in many countries in recent years. Its use for this purpose has been influenced by cultural factors and local fashions of analgesic use. Acetaminophen poisoning accounts for up to 48% of all poisons admissions to hospital *(Hawton et al., 1992)* and a current estimated 200-300 deaths per year in the UK *(Neeleman et al., 1997; Spooner et al., 1993)*. In contrast, only 9.4% of overdoses were due to analgesics (including acetaminophen, aspirin, and nonsteroidal drugs) and only 80 deaths were reported due to acetaminophen poisoning in the US in 1996 *(Litovitz et al., 1997)*

Mechanisms of Toxicity

Acetaminophen is normally metabolised by the liver to form inactive, non-toxic compounds. Under normal circumstances, approximately 95% of acetaminophen is metabolised to glucuronide and sulphate conjugates which are excreted in the urine *(Johnston et al., 1997)*. About 5% of acetaminophen is metabolised through the cytochrome P-450 2E1 to produce a highly reactive toxic metabolite, N-acetyl-ρ-benzoquinonimine (NAPQI). At therapeutic doses, the small amounts of NAPQI produced by acetaminophen metabolism are detoxified by liver stores of hepatic glutathione and is excreted in bile *(Glazenburg et al., 1983)* or urine as mercapturic acid conjugate *(Waters et al., 2001)* (Figure 2). In overdose, stores of glutathione become depleted. Without the glutathione substrate, NAPQI becomes available to bind to proteins and DNA of hepatocytes causing direct cellular injury *(Boess et al., 1998; Flanagan et al., 1991; Jones, 1998a)*. The damaged hepatocytes release factors that both attract and activate hepatic macrophages, causing cell necrosis by release of proteolytic lysosomal enzymes, and reactive oxygen species *(Weinstein et al., 1988).*

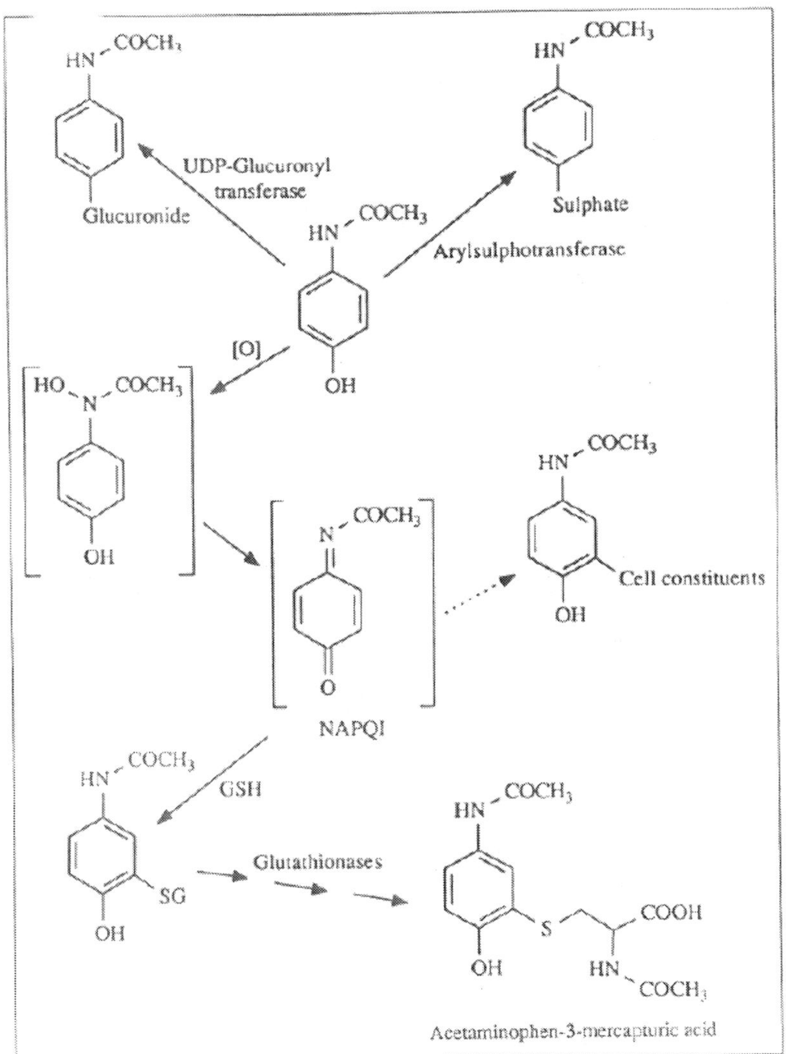

Figure 2. Summary of metabolism of Acetaminophen (Flanagan et al., 1991).

3-(Cysteine-S-yl) acetaminophen-protein adducts have been found in plasma after acetaminophen overdose in humans (Hinson et al., 1990). There is evidence that acetaminophen toxicity can result in an impairment of mitochondrial function, which precedes the loss of plasma membrane integrity (Burcham et al., 1990). Generation of reactive oxygen species (Adamson et al., 1993) and nitric oxide (Gardner et al., 1998), lipid peroxidation (Kamiyama et al., 1993), mitochondrial dysfunction and loss of the ability of the mitochondria to synthesize ATP; and loss of ATP (Donnelly et al., 1994), disruption of calcium homeostasis (Salas et al., 1997) and induction of apoptosis (Ray et al., 1996) are all mechanisms have suggested that may be involved in acetaminophen-induced hepatotoxicity. Studies have shown that activated kupffer cells and their products such as cytokines may also play a role in this liver injury (McClain et al., 1999). Masson et al revealed detrimental effects of Kupffer cells, neutrophils, and NK/NKT cells in the pathophysiology of acetaminophen-induced liver injury (Masson et al., 2008). The limited role of innate immune cells in acetaminophen hepatotoxicity under normal conditions is consistent with the fact that isolated mouse hepatocytes can be killed by acetaminophen with a mechanism similar to the one observed in vivo. This suggests that under specific circumstances innate immune cells may aggravate the toxicity of acetaminophen in certain individuals (Jaeschke et al., 1989).

Adverse Reactions

In a minority of severely poisoned patients (in practice, generally those who present too late for effective treatment with N-acetyleysteine or methionine), acute liver failure supervenes after around 3-6 days later with deepening jaundice, and drowsiness, asterixis, tremor, confusion and delirium progressing to coma. Associated findings include hypoglycemia, metabolic acidosis, hyperventilation, cerebral oedema, renal failure, sepsis, disseminated intravascular coagulation, haemorrhage and terminal cardiac arrythmias *(Ruvalcaba et al., 1966).*

Chronic Overdose

The amount necessary to produce chronic toxicity is not well defined but is less than the amount needed to produce acute effects. Doses of acetaminophen greater than the recommended daily maximum therapeutic dose (4g) but less than the single acutely toxic dose, if taken for days to weeks may produce liver injury. Patients with pre-existing hepatic dysfunction (e.g., chronic abusers of alcohol), concomitant use of other medications, specifically cytochrome P450-inducers (e.g. isoniazid, rifampin, the anticonvulsants, phenobarbital, and phenytoin), and short-term fasting and malnutrition may be at increased risk *(Lane et al., 2002).* Since the kidney also contains the oxidising enzymes, renal failure may occur with high doses of acetaminophen *(Laurence DR, 1992).* A recent study on short courses of acetaminophen did not show any subclinical hepatocellular injury in alcoholics *(Bartels et al., 2008).*

Acute Overdose

Patients ingesting toxic quantities of acetaminophen may show three phases in their course. Anorexia, nausea and vomiting followed by right upper quadrant abdominal pain and hepatic tenderness *(Prescott, 1996)* may be the only symptoms seen initially. Renal damage, which may lead to acute renal failure, occurs in 1-5% of patients up to 14 days after ingestion, sometimes without evidence of hepatic damage *(Prescott et al., 1982).* As acetaminophen is used in many products, there will often be symptoms due to co-ingested agents. In the second phase these symptoms may persist in a less severe form for up to 48 hours. Meanwhile, hepatic enzymes, bilirubin, and prothrombin time rise into the abnormal range as hepatic necrosis ensues. Clinically there is pain in the right hypochondrium, as the liver becomes enlarged and tender. Urinary output may be reduced due to dehydration, renal damage, and the antidiuretic effect of the drug. Rarely, anuria may develop in association with hepatic failure, but the plasma urea may be disproportionately low as the liver damage reduces formation of urea *(Rumack et al., 1975)*.

The third phase follows at three to five days and is marked by hepatic necrosis, with jaundice, coagulation defects, hypoglycaemia, and encephalopathy as well as renal failure and cardiomyopathy. Death is primarily due to hepatic failure and is dependent upon the degree of hepatic necrosis *(Rumack et al., 1975)*. Nephrotoxicity following acetaminophen overdose consists of oliguric renal failure, which develops within 24-48h and is normally accompanied by back pain, renal tenderness, proteinuria and microscopic haematuria. It usually occurs in association with hepatotoxicity, but has been reported rarely in patients who only have had mild liver damage with plasma aminotransferase activity less than 1000 units l^{-1} *(Prescott, 1996)*. *Hengy et al* reported few cases of acute renal failure following acute liver failure without hepatic coma *(Hengy et al., 2009)*. Renal insufficiency occurs in approximately 1–2% of patients with acetaminophen overdose. The pathophysiology of renal toxicity in acetaminophen poisoning has been attributed to cytochrome P-450 mixed function oxidase isoenzymes present in the kidney, although other mechanisms have been elucidated, including the role of prostaglandin synthetase and N-deacetylase enzymes *(Mazer et al., 2008)*. The onset of renal failure typically occurs between day two and day five after the overdose with peak creatinine levels on day seven *(Mazer et al., 2008)*. Since the serum creatinine concentration usually raises minimum 48 hours following acetaminophen ingestion, renal failure might easily be missed if patients are discharged home before this *(Waring et al., 2010)*. The degree of liver injury is dependent on:

1) The total quantity (and presumably the rate) of acetaminophen absorbed
2) The concentration of acetaminophen achieved
3) The metabolic activity of the cytochrome P450 mixed function oxidase (in particular CYP2E1, 1A2, 3A4 subtypes)
4) The rate of elimination and disposition of the toxic and nontoxic acetaminophen metabolites
5) The amount and rate of regeneration of hepatic glutathione *(Jones et al., 1998b)*.

Associated findings included hypoglycaemia, metabolic acidosis, hyperventilation, cerebral oedema, renal failure, sepsis, disseminated intravascular coagulation, haemorrhage, cardiac arrhythmias *(Prescott, 1996)* and pancreatitis *(Caldarola et al., 1986)*. Depression of consciousness with very high plasma acetaminophen concentrations was associated with hypothermia in a 1-year old child *(Lieh-Lai et al., 1984)*. Myocardial damage has been documented in at least five cases of overdose with acetaminophen. ST segment abnormalities, T wave flattening, and pericarditis during life as well as post-mortem findings of subendocardial haemorrhage and myocardial necrosis have been noted *(Pimstone et al., 1968)*. Agranolocytosis has been described in a single patient consuming four tablets with a fall of the white count to $600/mm^3$ *(Lloyd, 1961)*. A case of pruritic maculopapular rash has been described *(Henriques, 1970)*.

Ingestion by an adult of 10-15 g of acetaminophen in a single dose may result in hepatic damage and death from fulminant hepatic failure *(Prescott, 1983)*. Severity of poisoning can be assessed by measuring the blood acetaminophen concentration. If the plasma concentration four hours after the overdose exceeds 300mg/L or 50mg/L after 12 hours hepatic toxicity is likely *(Sherlock et al., 1993).*

Biochemical Abnormalities (Biomarkers)

Biomarkers are defined as an objectively measured change in DNA, protein or metabolite levels that is reflective of a normal biological process, pathological condition or correlates with the pharmacological action of a therapeutic agent *(Antoine et al., 2009; Blazka et al., 1996).* The ideal biomarker of liver damage would have the following characteristics:

- Reflective of the actual hepatic injury/repair status
- Rapidly assayed and can be assayed in any laboratory
- Non-invasive, i.e. present in the blood or urine compartment
- Transferable across in vitro, in vivo and clinical systems to further inform and accelerate drug safety screening
- Able to precede the onset of massive hepatic injury–secreted markers rather than their leakage
- A low baseline variability in control samples and normal population
- Accurately identifiable and quantifiable with a suitable dynamic range to detect upon drug treatment *(Laverty et al., 2010)*

Numerous biomarkers for drug-induced liver injury have been explored, but less than ten are adopted or qualified as valid by the US FDA *(Shi et al., 2010).* Severe liver damage has been defined as an increase in serum aspartate aminotransferase (AST or SGOT) or alanine aminotransferase (ALT or SGPT) activity above 1000 IU/L and renal impairment as a rise in the plasma creatinine concentration from normal to over 300μmol/L (3.4mg/100mL) *(Buckley et al., 1999; Prescott et al., 1979; Routledge et al., 1998).* A less sensitive measure with more prognostic significance such as a prolonged protrombin time (INR* >2.0) may be more appropriate when examining the effectiveness of late treatment *(Buckley et al., 1999; Ros et al., 1994). Whyte et al,* showed a small rise in INR after acetaminophen poisoning without hepatic injury. They postulated that acetaminophen reduces functional concentrations of two vitamin K-dependent clotting factors (VII and IX), by inhibiting gamma carboxylation *(Whyte et al., 2000).*

In patients with acute liver failure due to acetaminophen overdose, a poor prognosis is obtained when PT>100sec (Harrison et al., 1990). In one study, a rise in PT (or INR) on days 3 or 4 was associated with only 7% survival, while survival was 79% in patients with no rise in INR (Trull et al., 2002). In one study, clotting factor VII was shown to provide, a good indication of prognosis of severe liver damage after acetaminophen overdose (Harrison et al., 1990). In coagulation of blood process, factor VII with factors V and X catalyse influence of calcium ions to form prothrombin activator (Guyton, 1984). Dramatic increases in plasma enzyme activity in acetaminophen poisoning was reported for lactic dehydrogenase (>37400 IU/L) and hydroxybutyrate dehydrogenase (>5000 IU/L) (Prescott, 1996).

* = International Normalized Ratio

Acetaminophen-induced hepatic necrosis also causes a dramatic increase in the activity of plasma glutathione S-transferases (GST), a group of cytosolic proteins of low molecular weight present in high concentration in hepatocytes. The increase preceded the rise in aminotransferases and provided a much more sensitive index of hepatocellular integrity *(Beckett et al., 1989; Hayes et al., 1983)*. The plasma concentration of F-protein, another cytosolic protein, is also a sensitive indicator of acetaminophen-induced hepatic injury. It has been suggested that glutathione S-transferase and F-protein have advantage over ALT for detecting minor degrees of acute liver dysfunction, particularly when only centrilobular damage may be involved *(Beckett et al., 1989)*.

Hepatic biliverdin reductase activity is also reduced after an overdose of acetaminophen and serum biliverdin concentrations are greatly increased in patients with fatal liver toxicity (Wardle et al., 1981). An elevated serum bilirubin is an important indicator of drug-induced acute liver failure. However, in acetaminophen overdose, death may occur before bilirubin has increased significantly in those patients with hyperacute liver failure (Trull et al., 2002).

Increased blood hydrogen ion concentrations, reduced blood pH and reduced plasma bicarbonate concentrations (i.e. features of metabolic acidosis) have been frequently observed in patients with severe acetaminophen poisoning and in those who have developed fulminant hepatic failure that is persistent and resistant to correction *(Prescott, 1996)*. The severity of the acidosis is an important prognostic factor *(Gray et al., 1987)*.

Hypoglycaemia is always associated with severe hepatic damage and liver failure and it indicated a very poor prognosis (Prescott, 1996). Blood ammonia concentrations are increased in patients with severe liver damage causing hepatic encephalopathy. In such circumstances the hepatic production of urea is reduced, resulting in low plasma urea concentrations that do not increase with the onset of renal failure (Emby et al., 1977).

Gray et al demonstrated that hyperlactataemia, with or without significant acid-base disturbance, was common following acetaminophen overdose particularly in those who were severely poisoned *(Gray et al., 1987)*.

In a recent study, early high anion gap metabolic acidosis was present in 41% of acetaminophen overdose patients on admission and persisted for 1.5 ± 0.1 days *(Zein et al., 2010)*. It was also shown that the mean plasma taurine concentration in the acetaminophen-poisoned patients (mean 26.4 ± 1.6 mg/l) was significantly different from the control groups (mean 5.6 ± 0.2 mg/l) ($P<0.0001$) *(Ghandforoush-Sattari et al., 2008a)*. Taurine's raised concentration in plasma and urine has already been reported after surgical trauma, X-radiation, muscle necrosis, carbon tetrachloride-induced liver damage *(Waterfield et al., 1991)*, and acataminophen overdose *(Ghandforoush-Sattari et al., 2008a; Harry et al., 1999)*. Changes in taurine concentrations typically occur in stress states, e.g., osmotic changes, anoxia, prolonged illumination of photoreceptors, cell proliferation, brain development *(Huxtable, 1992)*, pneumococcal meningitis *(Guerra-Romero et al., 1993)*, lung cancer *(Kirk et al., 1993)*, myocardial infarction *(Bhatnagar et al., 1990)*, stroke *(Ghandforoush-Sattari et al., 2011)*, speedy exercise *(Ward et al., 1999)*, hepatic encephalopathy *(Butterworth, 1996)*, and heroin addiction *(Ghandforoush-Sattari et al., 2010a)*. Taurine is produced by the liver in response to a toxic insult and subsequent leakage from damaged cells leads to increased concentrations in plasma and urine. The high serum taurine concentration 6 hours or more after acetaminophen overdose could be a useful indicator of liver damage in acetaminophen poisoning *(Ghandforoush-Sattari et al., 2009)*.

A recent study has suggested that a serum phosphate concentration above 1.2mmol/L at 48-96 hours following acetaminophen overdose might be a sensitive and highly specific predictor of patients with liver failure and very little chance of spontaneous survival. Hyperphosphatemia may be caused by renal dysfunction in the absence of hepatic regeneration *(Schmidt et al., 2002)*. Hypokalemia is another non-specific biomarker of acetaminophen overdose. *Zyoud et al* showed serum concentration of K^+ less than 3.5mmol/L in 63.6% of patients with acute acetaminophen overdose *(Zyoud et al., 2010)*.

A recent study indicated that β-catenin activation was an early event and was vital for regeneration after acetaminophen-induced ALF. Interestingly, activation of β-catenin was observed even before biochemical or histological hallmarks of liver injury were evident *(Apte et al., 2009)*. A number of elevated circulating microRNAs in plasma have also been shown as potential biomarkers for drug-induced liver injury in an animal experiment *(Wang et al., 2009)*. Another study showed the elevation of some cytokines such as interleukin 6, interleukin 8, interleukin 10, and monocyte chemoattractant protein 1 in patients with serum alanine aminotransferase >1000 IU/L following acetaminophen overdose *(James et al., 2005)*. Cytokines are interesting candidates for novel biomarkers as they are relatively accessible (by blood sampling) and accurately quantifiable *(Laverty et al., 2010)*. *Demirbas et al* and *Erdinc Cakir et al* demonstrated the preclinical utility of neopterin as a biomarker for the animal model of acetaminophen-induced liver injury *(Cakir et al., 2010; Demirbas et al., 2011)*.

Two previous studies evaluating acetaminophen half-life determinations to predict toxicity found that half-lives less than 2.5 hours and 3 hours respectively make toxicity unlikely *(Dawson et al., 2001; Smilkstein et al., 1994)*. Studies have also shown that half-lives of greater than four hours put the patient at increased risk of hepatotoxicity and demonstrate the longer the half-life, the higher the rate of hepatotoxicity *(Prescott et al., 1971; Schiodt et al., 2002)*. Typically, the use of acetaminophen half-lives to predict toxicity is not recommended due to lack of specificity and multiple confounders such as ongoing gastrointestinal absorption, or co-ingestions *(Sutter et al., 2010)*. James et al, detected protein adducts of acetaminophen in some patient samples 12 days post-ingestion. They suggested that the persistence and specificity of acetaminophen-protein adducts as correlates of toxicity support their use as specific biomarkers of acetaminophen toxicity in patients with acute liver injury *(James et al., 2009)*. These adducts are formed by hepatic metabolism of acetaminophen to *N*-acetyl-*p*-benzoquinone imine, which covalently binds to hepatic proteins as 3-(cystein-*S*-yl)-acetaminophen adducts. Arginase I, sorbitol dehydrogenase, glutamate dehydrogenase, paraxonase, malate dehydrogenase, and purine nucleoside phosphorylase have also been introduced as biomarkers of liver necrosis *(Ozer et al., 2008)*.

Risk Factors

Malnutrition

Fasting may enhance hepatotoxicity and an important mechanism appears to be decreased hepatic stores of glutathione in man (Johnston et al., 1997). Fasting also reduces the glucuronide conjugation of acetaminophen in rats, and toxicity is increased as a result of correspondingly enhanced metabolic activation (Price et al., 1987).

Interactions

Factors that have been reported to enhance risk of hepatotoxicity caused by acetaminophen include enzyme inducing drugs, chronic alcohol misuse and eating disorders, and in each of these, contexts treatment is advisable below the treatment line *(Bridger et al., 1998)*. Treatment line in acetaminophen overdose will be discussed later.

Drugs

Any factor that decreases the rate of absorption or metabolic activation of acetaminophen would reduce the rate of formation of the toxic metabolite and thus reduce the risk of liver damage.

It was suggested that patients who take mixed overdoses of acetaminophen and antimuscarinic drugs are less likely to suffer liver damage because gastric emptying and acetaminophen absorption are delayed *(Prescott, 1996)*. A similar effect might occur with combined overdose with acetaminophen and dextropropoxyphene or codeine and in some reports, associated hypothermia probably provides additional protection by slowing down the metabolic activation of acetaminophen *(Prescott, 1996)*.

Piperonyl butoxide, a known inhibitor of the hepatic microsomal metabolism, has been demonstrated in some investigations on animals to protect against acetaminophen hepatotoxicity *(Mitchell et al., 1973)*. Patients with potentially induced metabolism and hence more rapid production of toxic metabolites have been shown to develop more severe hepatonecrosis than patients who were not induced *(Smith et al., 1986; Wrights et al., 1973)*. Acetaminophen toxicity has been found to be potentiated by anticonvulsant drugs, because of direct induction of cytochrome P450 enzymes *(Bray et al., 1992)*.

A female patient receiving carbamazepine developed severe liver damage after an overdose of acetaminophen. Antidotal therapy was not administered because her plasma acetaminophen concentration was below the treatment line *(Smith et al., 1986)* (Figure 3).

Alcohol

There have been some reports claiming that the hepatotoxicity of acetaminophen is increased in chronic alcoholics, and that such individuals not only carry an increased risk of severe and fatal liver damage after overdose *(Artnak et al., 1998; Johnson et al., 1981; Wrights et al., 1973; Yasunaga et al., 1985)* but that similar serious liver damage may also occur with therapeutic use *(Barker et al., 1977; Himmelstein et al., 1984)*. Alcohol inhibits the hepatic microsomes *(Thummel et al., 1989)* and produces a major reduction in the fractional urinary excretion of the cysteine and mercapturic acid conjugates of acetaminophen in healthy nonalcoholic volunteers *(Banda et al., 1982)* as well as in heavy drinkers *(Prescott, 2000)*.

The interactions between acetaminophen and ethanol are complex and many questions remain to be answered. In animals, chronic administration of ethanol causes microsomal enzyme induction with increased toxic metabolic activation of acetaminophen and enhanced hepatotoxicity.

Conversely, the acute administration of ethanol inhibits the potentially toxic oxidative metabolism of acetaminophen and protects against liver damage. This protective effect disappears when the ethanol is eliminated and the time interval between the intake of ethanol and acetaminophen is critical *(Prescott, 1996)*. In a prospective study, the prevalence of hepatotoxicity was 5.1% in those who ingested ethanol, compared to 15.2% in those who did not *(Waring et al., 2008a)*.

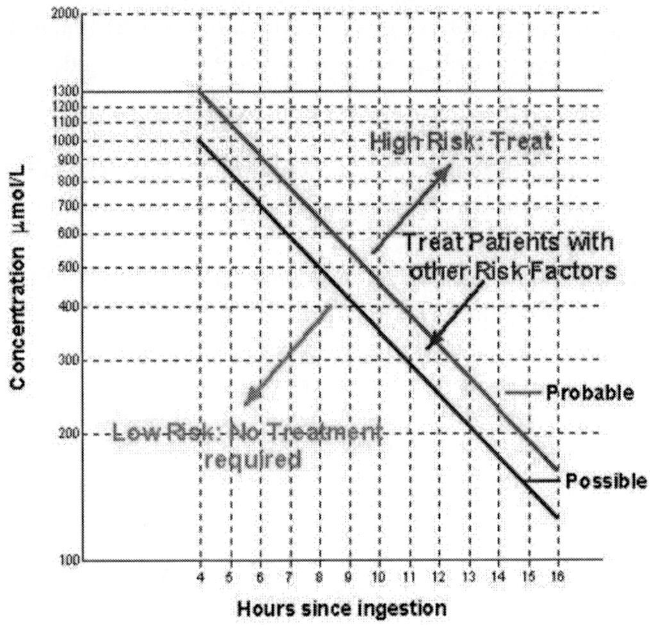

Figure 3. Rumack-Matthew nomogram for single acute acetaminophen poisoning: A semi-logarithmic plot of plasma-acetaminophen concentration against hours after ingestion (Vale, et al 1995).

Patients chronically abusing ethanol are more susceptible to the hepatotoxic effects of acetaminophen. Severe liver failure was reported in three chronic alcoholics after they ingested acetaminophen for therapeutic reasons (McClain et al., 1980). There are several possible mechanisms whereby chronic alcoholism may enhance the toxicity of acetaminophen. First, long-term ethanol ingestion is known to induce a variety of hepatic microsomal drug metabolizing enzymes (Johnston et al., 1997). Second, alcoholics with or without cirrhosis often have inadequate dietary intake of protein. This may adversely affect their hepatic glutathione concentration. Third, alcoholics may also have depressed serum vitamin E and selenium concentrations compared with those of abstinent control subjects. Animal studies have demonstrated that both feeding protein-deficient diets or diets deficient in selenium and vitamin E measurably augmented acetaminophen hepatotoxicity. Vitamin E presumably exerts a protective effect through its role as a general antioxidant and selenium through its catalytic function for the enzyme glutathione peroxidase (McClain et al., 1980).

Lauterberg and Velez indicated that chronic excessive ethanol consumption was associated with decreased circulating concentrations of GSH. Either an increase in the catabolism of plasma GSH or a decreased release of GSH by the liver, possibly because of malnutrition or a direct effect of ethanol, could account for this observation *(Lauterburg et al., 1988)*. Degradation of GSH by the enzyme gamma glutamyl transferase, an enzyme the activity of which is commonly found to be raised in serum of alcoholic patients, is the major route of catabolism of GSH *(Burgunder et al., 1987)*.

Other Factors

It has been suggested that acetaminophen hepatotoxicity might have been enhanced by psittacosis (Davis et al., 1983), human immunodeficiency virus (HIV) infection (Shriner et al., 1992) and co-existing mercury intoxication (Zwiener et al., 1994). Two weeks after halothane anaesthesia for a breast biopsy, a 40-year-old woman was admitted with mildly abnormal liver function tests and acute renal failure. She was said to have taken only 500 mg of acetaminophen on the third and second days before admission and this toxicity was attributed, without evidence, to a synergistic reaction of halothane and acetaminophen (Grinbalt et al., 1980). Nguyen et al have recently described an increased risk of acute liver injury (ALI) due to acetaminophen overdose in patients with hepatitis C virus (HCV). ALI occurred in 16.7% and 7.1% of HCV-positive and HCV-negative patients, respectively (Nguyen et al., 2008). The fractional urinary recovery of the cysteine and mercapturic conjugates of acetaminophen are significantly increased in subjects with Gilbert's disease [*] *(Esteban et al., 1993)* and patients with hepatocellular carcinoma *(Leung et al., 1991)* suggesting that they might have increased susceptibility to hepatotoxicity. *Douglas et al* suggested that not only was acetaminophen elimination impaired in Gilbert's syndrome, but that its distribution kinetics are also abnormal *(Douglas et al., 1978)*.

MANAGEMENT OF ACETAMINOPHEN OVERDOSE

The treatment of a single acute acetaminophen overdose depends on two factors: the interval between overdose and presentation and the plasma concentration of acetaminophen *(Ferner, 1993)*. On admission blood should be taken for emergency estimation of the plasma acetaminophen concentration, remembering that values obtained before four hours after ingestion may not be reliable because of the possibility of continued absorption. The plasma acetaminophen concentration after four hours following overdose is the single most important factor in the decision for or against therapy *(Atwood, 1980)*. However, a recent study showed that dose of acetaminophen ingested did not seem to play a role in prognosis. The most important prognostic factor was coma grade on admission to study. Acetaminophen dosing information is not always obtainable. When it is, it adds little to the clinical assessment. Severity of encephalopathy is a more reliable indicator of prognosis in these critically ill patients *(Gregory et al., 2010)*. Activated charcoal, gastric lavage, and ipecacuanha are able to reduce the absorption of acetaminophen, but the clinical benefit is unclear. Of these, activated charcoal seems to have the best risk-benefit ratio *(Brok et al., 2006)*. Gastric lavage is not indicated unless in potentially life-threatening poisoning and unconscious presentation *(Vale, 1997)*. One non-systematic review of gastric lavage in all forms of poisoning found no evidence that gastric lavage improved outcome in poisoned people *(Vale, 1997)*. Efforts to prevent absorption of the drug with activated charcoal or cholestyramine within four hours after overdose have been attempted *(Dordoni et al., 1973)*. Activated charcoal is unlikely to be beneficial at or beyond 2 h after an overdose of acetaminophen *(Mullins et al., 2009)*. *Spiller et al* suggested that the use of activated charcoal, in addition to the standard NAC

[*] Gilbert's syndrome is an inherited disorder which is characterised by unconjugated hyperbilirubinaemia. Glucuronidation of a number of substrates appears to be impaired in Gilbert's syndrome (Macklon, et al, 1979).

therapy, had improved patient outcome as measured by reduced markers of liver injury, AST and ALT *(Spiller et al., 2006)*. Vomiting induced by syrup of ipeca-guanha has no role in the emergency department management of acetaminophen-poisoned patients *(Zed et al., 1999)*. The role of forced diuresis, haemodialysis and charcoal hemoperfusion in an effort to enhance excretion has been discussed *(Higgins et al., 1996; Matthew, 1973)*, but forced diuresis may be dangerous due to the renal damage and the antidiuretic effect of acetaminophen. Different agents have been used for protection against hepatorenal toxicity of acetaminophen:

Cimetidine

In animals, prior administration of high doses of inhibitors of oxidative metabolism, such as cimetidine, reduces NAPQI formation and thus the frequency and severity of hepatotoxicity. This approach is not appropriate for the treatment of poisoning in humans, for an inhibitor would have to be given before the acetaminophen overdose *(Flanagan et al., 1991)*.

Glutathione (GSH)

GSH for drug use is not widely available and penetrates cell membranes poorly and it is no practical value as a protective agent because huge doses are required *(Williams, 1986)*.

Cysteamine

Cysteamine or (mercaptamine, 2- mercaptoethanolamine), completely prevents severe liver damage when is administered within 10 h in a total dose of 3.2 g intravenously over 20 h. Cysteamine is usually effective in preventing liver toxicity when given within 10 h of ingestion of the acetaminophen but it is ineffective when treatment is delayed beyond 12 h *(Prescott, 1996)*. Unacceptable side effects, including nausea, vomiting, drowsiness, and cardiotoxicity have limited the use of cysteamine *(Byer et al., 1982)*.

Methionine

L-methionine is a precursor of cysteine, and as such, it stimulates glutathione synthesis and was shown to protect animals against acetaminophen-induced liver toxicity *(Neuvonen et al., 1985)*. The N-acetyl-DL-methionine ester of acetaminophen also enhances the hepatic synthesis of glutathione in mice and protects against acetaminophen toxicity *(Skoglund et al., 1988)*. It has been suggested that the problems of liver damage following acetaminophen overdose could be abolished simply by the addition of cysteine or methionine to the tablets *(McLean, 1974; Neuvonen et al., 1985)*. One such formulation was available in the UK (Pameton), although many other formulations are used more widely *(Janes et al., 1992)*. When given within ten hours, oral methionine in a dose of 2.5 g every four hours to a total dose of ten gram is effective in preventing severe liver damage in poisoned patients with plasma acetaminophen concentrations above the standard treatment line *(Crome et al., 1976)*. There are concerns about its efficacy when given late in patients with impending hepatic failure. A further theoretical objection to the use of methionine rather than N-acetylcysteine is that several enzymic reactions are necessary for its conversion to the active form, cysteine. Two of these enzymes contain SH groups that could themselves be inactivated by acetaminophen thus preventing the protective action of methionine. Unlike N-acetylcysteine and other thiols, methionine is unable to prevent direct covalent binding or to reverse post-arylation damage to hepatocytes exposed for a short time to toxic concentrations of acetaminophen *(Tee et al., 1986a; Tredger et al., 1980)*. Vomiting has frequently been described with oral methionine *(Prescott et al., 1979)*.

Glycyrrhizin

Glycyrrhizin, extracted from the roots of licorice (Glycyrrhiza glabra), and its aglycone (glycyrrhetinic acid) have been shown to exert antihepatotoxic activity and protect against carbon tetrachloride and D-galactosamine-induced acute liver injury and chronic cirrhosis. Furthermore, glycyrrhizin has been used in the treatment of chronic hepatitis. It has been reported that glycyrrhizin has significant restorative and protective effects in relation to glutathione S-transferase activity and glutathione content in the liver. Glycyrrhizin and its analogues are also effective in decreasing acetaminophen-induced hepatotoxicity *(Dehpour et al., 1999)*.

Garlic and Related Organosulfurs

Few studies have shown the hepatoprotectivity of garlic and related organosulfurs. The effects of garlic extract on the prevention of reactive oxygen species (ROS) formation and glutathione depletion were demonstrated on freshly isolated rat hepatocytes contacted with acetaminophen suspension *(Anoush et al., 2009b)*. *Gwilt et al* showed that garlic treatment slightly increased sulfate conjugation of acetaminophen on healthy subjects (Gwilt *et al.*, 1994). Garlic oil, as similar to N-acetylcysteine, can eliminate electrophilic intermediates and free radicals through conjugation and reduction reactions. Therefore it protects the liver from toxic doses of a minophen *(Kalantari et al., 2001)*. The protection against acetaminophen-induced hepatotoxicity by fresh garlic homogenates is mainly due to its inhibition of P450-mediated acetaminophen bioactivation *(Wang et al., 1996)*. Components like allyl-mercaptan, diallyl-disulfide, and diallyl-sulfide might have cytoprotective and antioxidant effects *(Anoush et al., 2009a)*.

Taurine

Taurine a sulfur-containing amino acid is a relatively non-toxic substance and a normal constituent of the human diet (Huxtable et al., 1983). Taurine has been shown to protect against membrane damage, maintain membrane organisation, and prevent ion leakage and water influx, thus avoiding cellular swelling (Milei et al., 1992). In the liver ischemia/reperfusion model, taurine prevented hepatocyte injury through its ability to inhibit lipid peroxidation, regulate cellular calcium homeostasis, and stabilise biological membranes (Chen, 1993). Waters et al demonstrated that the administration of a pharmacological dose of taurine (200mg/kg) prevented plasma AST, ALT, and ALP elevation, hepatic DNA fragmentation, and hepatocyte necrosis in an in-vivo rat model. They concluded that administration of taurine has a prophylactic as well as a therapeutic role in preventing acetaminophen-induced hepatotoxicity, possibly through its unique cytoprotective properties such as antioxidant activity, inhibition of nitric oxide, and modulation of calcium homeostasis (Waters et al., 2001). In a study, authors showed that plasma taurine concentration peaked to 86.1±19.0 at 1–2.5 hr of study, plasma elimination half-life ranged from 0.7 to 1.4 hr (mean 1.0±0.3), volume of distribution ranged from 19.8 to 40.7 L (mean 30.0±7.6), ratio of clearance/bioavailability (Cl/F) ranged from 14.0 to 34.4 L/hr (mean 21.1±7.8), and area under curve between 0–8 hr (AUC) ranged from 116.0 to 284.5 mg.hr/L (mean 206.3±63.9) (Ghandforoush-Sattari et al., 2010b).

N-Acetylcysteine (NAC)

Three treatment regimens are thought to be equivalent in efficacy: (1) a 20-hour continuous infusion of NAC, (2) a 48-hour regimen of intermittent intravenous infusions and (3) a 72-hour regimen of intermittent oral doses (James et al., 2002). NAC, a precursor of cysteine, has been in clinical use since the 1960s as a mucolytic agent for the treatment of pulmonary disease and cystic fibrosis *(Prescott et al., 1989; Scheffner, 1983)*, for protection against the toxicity of metals, alkylating agents *(Flanagan, 1987)* and drugs used for cancer chemotherapy *(Botta et al., 1973; Holoye et al., 1983; Myers et al., 1983)*, for treatment of cirrhosis by increasing tissue oxygen use and delivery *(Jones et al., 1994)*, for prevention of damage to human bronchial fibroblast by tobacco smoke condensates *(Aruoma et al., 1989)*, for reversal of acquired tolerance to organic nitrates in cardiovascular disease *(Horowitz et al., 1988)*, and as an effective antidote in acetaminophen poisoning *(Harrison et al., 1991; Keays et al., 1991; Prescott, 1979)*. NAC disrupts disulphide bonds in mucus, making it less viscous, and is reported to offer protection against doxorubicin toxicity and to reduce ifosfamide and cyclophosphamide induced cystitis *(Borgstroem et al., 1986)*. NAC may also have a role in the treatment of toxicity from carbon tetrachloride, chloroform, 1,2-dichloropropane *(Flanagan et al., 1991)* and acrilonitrile inhalation *(Buchter et al., 1984)*. NAC should be given if the plasma acetaminophen concentration is above a line joining 200mg/L (1.32mmol/L) at four hours after ingestion and 30mg/L (0.20mmol/L) at 15 hours on a semilogarithmic plot (Figures 3) *(Flanagan et al., 1991)*. It has been recommended that if the concentration of acetaminophen is below the treatment line, a second acetaminophen concentration should be determined 4-6 hours later. If this concentration is above the treatment line, NAC therapy should be started *(Zed et al., 1999)*. Patients, who are thought to have taken over 7.5 g acetaminophen more than 8 hours previously, however, should be treated immediately without waiting for the plasma acetaminophen result. Also in those patients with high risk of hepatotoxicity caused by acetaminophen include co-ingested enzyme inducing drugs, chronic alcohol misuse and eating disorders treatment is advisable even below the treatment line *(Bridger et al., 1998)*. This nomogram is not always helpful, because an accurate history of the amount and time of acetaminophen ingested often cannot be obtained in cases of suicidal intent or in patients with an altered mental status, the nomogram cannot be applied to many intentional overdose patients or who has ingested an extended-release preparation, who had a repeated supratherapeutic ingestion *(Fontana, 2006; Smith, 2008)*. The nomogram also fails to predict toxicity based on a single serum acetaminophen concentration in patients overdose acetaminophen with an opioid or diphenhydramine *(Dougherty et al., 2011)*. In cases of massive acetaminophen overdose also, standard acetylcysteine dosing may not be adequate and is suggested that elevated serum acetaminophen concentrations at the end of a standard 20-hour acetylcysteine infusion should be discussed with the local poison center *(Wang et al., 2011)*. Although treatment with NAC between 15 and 24 hours is ineffective, it probably does little harm and should be given if the time of ingestion is in doubt. Severe liver damage and renal failure may occur with plasma acetaminophen concentrations below the present treatment line, and in view of the safety of NAC a case has been made for lowering the line to 150 mg/L at 4 hours and 25 mg/L at 15 hours *(Prescott et al., 1979)*.

A plasma acetaminophen measurement before four hours can be misleading due to incomplete absorption. There are several groups such as chronic alcohol abusers who may be at risk of hepatic toxicity from high therapeutic acetaminophen dosage since hepatic GSH may be low initially *(Lauterburg et al., 1988; Seeff et al., 1986)*. For example, for alcoholics, a treatment threshold line of 100mg/mL at 4h is comparable in risk of hepatotoxicity to the 150mg/mL at 4-h line for nonalcoholic patients *(Ali et al., 2008)*. Similarly, HIV-positive individuals may be especially susceptible to acetaminophen-induced hepatotoxicity. The glutathione deficiency occurs in such patients may be due to increased utilisation of this compound because of oxidative stress in HIV patients *(Henry, 1990)*. Other patients, for example those taking anticonvulsants or other enzyme inducers, may form NAPQI more readily and may deplete endogenous GSH more quickly *(Flanagan et al., 1991)*, and this may place them at greater risk.

The above nomogram cannot be used for patients with chronic excess ingestion of acetaminophen or those who have taken slow release formulations for whom there is no substitute for clinical judgement. For example, the maximum plasma concentration of acetaminophen occurs 14 hours after the ingestion of Tylenol Extended Relief (extended-release acetaminophen) *(Bizovi et al., 1996)*. Meanwhile, the use of treatment guidelines, which assess the risk of developing liver failure from blood acetaminophen concentrations corrected for time to NAC treatment, needs careful interpretation due to the unreliability of histories obtained from poisoned patients *(Makin et al., 1995)*.

Pharmacology of NAC

In human volunteers, 20-30% of NAC is cleared by the kidneys (Borgstroem et al., 1986). It can be oxidised to a disulphide, N, N'-diacetylcysteine, and can form mixed disulphides by reacting with other thiols such as cysteine and gluthatione. NAC can be oxidised by reaction with the thiol groups of plasma proteins (Burgunder et al., 1989;

Cotgreave et al., 1987; Olsson et al., 1988). Cysteine and cystine have been identified as the major methabolites of NAC. Inorganic sulphate is the major urinary excreted together with small amounts of taurine and unchanged NAC (Olsson et al., 1988) (Figure 4).

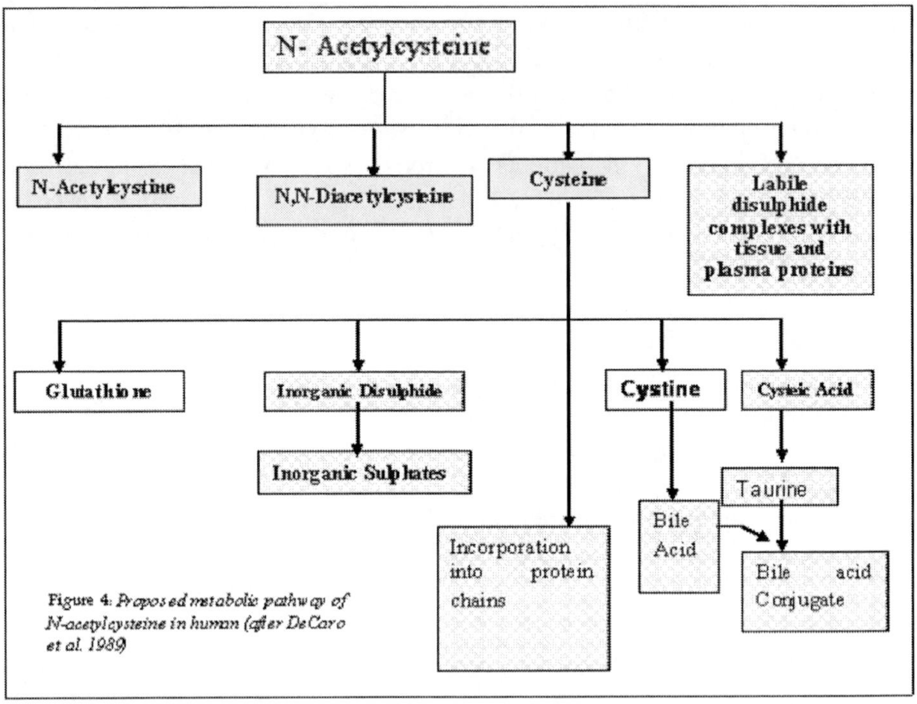

Figure 4. Proposed metabolic pathway of N-acetylcysteine in human (after DeCaro et al. 1989).

NAC is also metabolised to glutathione via cysteine by hepatocytes, which is thought to be an essential mechanism of action when NAC is used in treatment of acetaminophen poisoning (Tee et al., 1986b). Excess cysteine that is not required for protein or glutathione syntesis is catabolised via pyruvate to carbon dioxide and sulphate or to taurine (Weinstein et al., 1988). Only a small amount (3%) of NAC is excreted in faeces (Bonanomi et al., 1980).

Therapeutic Regimens of NAC in Treatment of Acetaminophen Overdose

Oral Regimens

Oral NAC is available in the U.S. as 10% and 20% (weight/volume) solutions and is given orally as a 5% (weight/volume) solution in a soft drink or, if given intragastrically, in water *(Flanagan et al., 1991).* The initial dose of 140mg/kg is followed by 17 maintenance doses (70 mg/kg every 4 hours for 68 hours) *(Smilkstein et al., 1988).* If the patient vomits within 1 hour of a dose, the dose should be repeated. Severe liver damage occurred in 17% of 49 patients treated within 10 hours despite the use of very large doses (130 mg/kg given over three days) *(Prescott et al., 1979).* Absorption is rapid following oral administration of single doses of 100 to 600 mg, but the bioavailability is low *(Prescott et al., 1989).* The low bioavailability of NAC is probably not due to incomplete absorption, but rather to extensive first-pass metabolism *(Olsson et al., 1988)*. This may be because NAC is rapidly oxidised before it reaches the general circulation probably in the gastrointestinal tract. Comparison of intravenous and oral S^{35}-labelled NAC *(Bonanomi et al., 1980)* indicated that the absorption of the radio-label was complete, although NAC in the gut wall of the rat was extensively metabolised to cysteine, glutathione and inorganic sulphite *(Olsson et al., 1988)*.

NAC is only available in the U.S. as an oral product. It is typically mixed in juice or soda to produce a concentration of less than 5% NAC. It is administered with a loading dose 140 mg/kg followed by 70 mg/kg every 4 hours for 17 doses (1300 mg/kg in total) *(Smilkstein et al., 1988)*. The best results have been observed when the NAC has been given within 8 hours of ingestion. However, it appears to be effective and safe when given up to 16 hours post ingestion. Efficacy is not well documented when given beyond 16 hours after ingestion but should be used in cases of confirmed toxic acetaminophen exposure. However, *Smilkstein et al (Smilkstein et al., 1988)* reported that only 41% of their high-risk patients who were treated between 16-24 hours had serious hepatotoxicity in spite of administration of 72-hour oral NAC regimen in comparison to *Prescott et al's (Prescott et al., 1979)* report (89%). *Parker et al* showed the safety of NAC therapy in patients presenting between 16 and 24 hours after acetaminophen intake who had a high risk of liver damage *(Parker et al., 1990)*. *Smilkstein et al* claimed, therefore, that the 72-hour protocol of oral NAC may be superior to the 20-hour intravenous protocol for patients treated 16 hours after the ingestion of acetaminophen *(Smilkstein et al., 1988)*. A prospective study showed that a shortened duration of treatment with oral NAC (20 to 48 hours) might be an effective treatment option in individuals considered to be at no further risk of developing liver toxicity according to the fulfilment of appropriate laboratory criteria before NAC discontinuation *(Betten et al., 2007)*.

The main problem with the oral route is difficulty of administration in severely poisoned patients who are vomiting (Ekins et al., 1987). Vomiting is secondary to both acetaminophen toxicity and NAC side effects, although it can often be controlled with ondansetron (Clark et al., 1996; Reed et al., 1994).

The oral route of administration in encephalopathic and hemodynamically unstable patients may not be safe and bioavailability of NAC is uncertain in these circumstances. In view of the seriousness of acetaminophen hepatotoxicity and the proven efficacy and safety of the intravenous formulation of NAC in Europe, some authors believe it to be imperative that an intravenous formulation of NAC be made available to clinicians in the United States *(Dhawan et al., 1996)*.

Intravenous Regimens

Intravenous NAC BP (20% weight/volume) (Parvolex®), adjusted to pH 7.0, is available in the United Kingdom for intravenous use. It is supplied in 10 mL ampoules (each ampoule contains two gram of NAC). In the treatment of acetaminophen poisoning, an initial dose of 150 mg/kg of body weight of NAC is infused intravenously in 200 mL of 5% dextrose over 15 minutes, followed by 50 mg/kg in 500 mL of 5% dextrose over four hours and 100 mg/kg in one litre of 5% dextrose over the next 16 hours (300 mg/kg of NAC over 20 hours) *(Brent, 1993; Chamberlain et al., 1993; Prescott, 1983)*. *Smilkstein et al* and *Prescott et al (Prescott, 1979; Smilkstein et al., 1991)* mentioned that there was no demonstrated benefit of extended IV treatment with NAC for 48 hours.

Oral NAC has been used for acetaminophen poisoning in the USA *(Carloss et al., 1978; Rumack et al., 1975)*, but severe liver damage has been occurred in 17% of 49 patients treated within 10 hours despite the use of large doses (130 mg/kg given over three days) *(Rumack et al., 1978)*. NAC is apparently more effective when given intravenously than by mouth. In one study most severely poisoned patients have developed early nausea and vomiting, making oral treatment impracticable. In any event, absorption is likely to be delayed or incomplete *(Prescott et al., 1979)* and in one study vomiting apparently occurred in all 416 patients given oral NAC *(Rumack et al., 1978)*. It has been stated that oral NAC is superior to intravenous NAC in presentations later than 15 hours *(Buckley et al., 1999)*.

Intravenous NAC is indicated in patients with plasma acetaminophen concentration above the treatment line if treatment is started within 15 hours of ingestion. Although treatment with NAC between 15 and 24 hours is ineffective, it probably does no harm and should not be withheld if the time of ingestion is in doubt. Severe liver damage and renal failure may occur with plasma acetaminophen concentrations below the present treatment line *(Prescott, 1978)*, and in view of the safety of NAC a case has been made for lowering the line to 150 mg/L at four hours and 25mg/L at 15 hours. A shorter hospital stay, patient and doctor convenience, and the concerns over the reduction in bioavailability of oral NAC by charcoal and vomiting make intravenous NAC preferable for most patients with acetaminophen poisoning *(Brent, 1993; Buckley et al., 1999; Chamberlain et al., 1993)*. A problem with IV-NAC is medication administration errors which occur frequently with IV-NAC in approximately one third of cases compared to oral forms *(Hayes et al., 2008)*.

Previous studies showed no serious adverse reactions judged related to either treatment. Nausea and vomiting were the most common related adverse events and were more common with oral treatment (23% vs 9%). Anaphylactoid reactions were more common with IV administration (6% vs 2%) *(Bebarta et al., 2010; Yip et al., 1998)*. In the US, the Food and Drug administration's approval of intravenous NAC in 2004 represented an advance in the management of acetaminophen poisoning due to a shortened 21-hour course of therapy in uncomplicated cases, ease of administration, and patient adherence even when emesis or depressed mental status are present *(Hayes et al., 2008; Smith et al., 2008)*.

Mechanisms of Action

Glutathione binds to NAPQI to produce a more stable compound that can be further broken down to non-toxic metabolites. NAC protects against liver damage in early acetaminophen poisoning by production of cysteine *(Burgunder et al., 1989)*, which acts as a glutathione precursor. NAC also acts by supplying additional thiol groups which bind directly with the reactive metabolites i.e., it scavenges NAPQI and encourages its reduction to acetaminophen but does not inhibit its production *(Corcoran et al., 1985; Mitchell et al., 1973)*.

Mechanisms of Action in Fulminant Hepatic Failure Associated with Acetaminophen Poisoning

The syndrome of fulminant hepatic failure may include cerebral oedema, infection, circulatory collapse, and renal failure as well as liver failure *(Ellis et al., 1996)*. A case of an infant who developed acute liver failure after administration of acetaminophen for 10 days at a total dose of 720 mg/day (72 mg/kg per day) was reported by *Savino at al.* Intravenous N-acetylcysteine therapy resulted in rapid improvement of the child's clinical condition and laboratory test results *(Savino et al., 2011)*. In 1989, *O'Grady* and colleagues *(O'Grady et al.,*

1989) from King's College Hospital in London, proposed a criteria for fulminant hepatic failure associated with acetaminophen, that is: pH<7.3 at 24h or more following the overdose after correction of hypovolemia or concurrent presence of serum creatinine>300 μmol/L, grade 3 to 4 encephalopathy and prothrombin time more than 100sec. Taking the last two sets of prognostic indicators identified 77% of the deaths from acetaminophen poisoning in their study. Several mechanisms have been suggested for NAC therapy in late acetaminophen poisoning:

1) NAC increases cardiac output in fulminant hepatic failure and thus increases tissue oxygen delivery and increasing peripheral oxygen extraction *(Harrison et al., 1991; Keays et al., 1991)*.
2) Another mechanism proposed includes improved local circulation. Increasing the blood to a critical or failing organ in multiorgan failure state might improve the function of that organ and overall outcome. Improved hepatic microcirculation, as determined by a fibreoptic monitoring system which measures indocyanine green dye clearance, has been reported in patients with fulminant hepatic failure receiving NAC *(Devlin et al., 1997)*.
3) NAC has also been suggested to have chemoprotective properties which may be of value in late poisoning with acetaminophen. Oxygen free radicals are liberated by necrotic hepatic tissue *(Jaeschke et al., 1989)*. NAC has been shown to scavenge such reactive species and may also reduce cytokine concentrations such as interleukin-1 and tumour necrosis factor to prevent migration of neutrophils into the hepatic parenchyma *(Aruoma et al., 1989)*.
4) In isolated hepatocytes, it can also restore the capacity of the intracellular proteolytic system to degrade toxic arylated proteins *(Bruno et al., 1988)*.
5) NAC infusion increases systemic circulating cGMP concentrations in fulminant hepatic failure *(Devlin et al., 1997)*.

In the UK, NAC therapy is routinely given to any patient who presents more than 24 hours after ingestion of more than 150mg/kg of acetaminophen, including those with fulminant hepatic failure but in the US, abnormalities of liver function tests are used to guide NAC therapy when a patient presents beyond 24 hours after a acetaminophen overdose, and total dose ingested is considered less important *(Jones, 1998a)*.

In patients with massive acetaminophen ingestion, erratic absorption may occur, and toxic serum concentrations may persist beyond a standard 21-hour course of intravenous NAC therapy. Acetaminophen concentrations and aminotransferase levels should be evaluated at the completion of the intravenous NAC infusion to ensure complete elimination of acetaminophen and absence of hepatotoxicity and to exclude the need for prolonged treatment *(Smith et al., 2008)*.

Pharmacokinetics of NAC

The results of previous studies of NAC pharmacokinetics in man have varied according to the analytical methods, dose, formulation and route of administration *(Prescott et al., 1989)*. NAC is usually given orally in a 72- hour treatment protocol or intravenously in either a 20- hour or a 48- hour treatment protocol *(Meredith et al., 1995)*. Absorption of NAC occurs rapidly after oral administration of doses of 100-600 mg, although bioavailability is less than 10% *(Burgunder et al., 1989)*.

The volume of distribution ranges from 0.33 to 0.47 L/kg and protein binding is significant, reaching approximately 50% four hours after the dose. Renal clearance has been reported as 0.19 to 0.21 L/kg.hr *(Holdiness, 1991)* and total body plasma clearance 242 mL/min (14.52 L/h) in a person weighing 70 kg. Therefore, 70% of an intravenous dose of NAC is cleared by non-renal routes *(Borgstroem et al., 1986)*.

Twenty to 30% of an intravenous dose is excreted unchanged in the urine and the mean elimination half-life has varied from less than two to more than 6hr in different reports *(Borgstroem et al., 1986; Burgunder et al., 1989; De Caro et al., 1989; Olsson et al., 1988)*.

Adverse Reactions of NAC

There is concern that if clearance of NAC were to be impaired in certain disease states that adverse effects (such as anaphylactoid reactions including systemic vasodilatation and bronchospasm) *(Dawson et al., 1989)* might ensue as they tend to occur when plasma concentrations of the drug are at their highest *(Prescott et al., 1989)*. The effect of liver impairment on NAC clearance has been evaluated in two studies *(Jones et al., 1997; Prescott et al., 1989)*. They showed that the clearance of NAC was reduced in patients with chronic liver disease (4.52±1.87 L/h) compared with controls (6.47±0.78 L/h; $P<0.01$). Most adverse reactions to NAC are believed to be anaphylactoid in nature because the reaction is clinically similar to an anaphylactic reaction in that it is caused by release of histamine but generally not IgE-mediated *(Bailey et al., 1998)*. On the other hand, these effects appear to be concentration-dependent and they are more likely to represent pharmacological effects than "Type B" adverse reactions *(Prescott et al., 1989)*. They may occur in a small percentage (probably less than 5%) of individuals treated with the drug, probably represent a dose-dependent effect, and usually subside rapidly on slowing or discontinuing the infusion *(Dawson et al., 1989; Flanagan et al., 1991)*. The frequency of these reactions have been documented 23% by *Bailey and McGuigan (Bailey et al., 1998)* and 48.5% by *Lynch (Lynch et al., 2004)*.

Although no study has been conducted to evaluate the IgE response to rule out a true anaphylactic reaction to intravenous NAC, the observed reaction is unlikely to be due to true anaphylaxis for two reasons: Firstly, it is very unlikely that the patient has had prior exposure to NAC *(Bailey et al., 1998)*. Secondly, in order to be antigenic, a substance must be of a composition foreign to the organism and must be a complex macromolecule with a molecular weight generally greater than 5000 *(Mota, 1981)*. NAC's molecular weight is only 163 being an acetylated amino acid it is unlikely to be recognised as foreign. Therefore, to induce an allergic response, it would have to act as a hapten by covalently bonding to a carrier protein *(Tenenbein, 1984)*. This reaction takes time in contrast to the rather immediate response observed in patients or healthy volunteers. For these reasons, an allergic aetiology seems unlikely.

High serum acetaminophen concentrations were associated with fewer anaphylactoid reactions in a study, suggesting that these might in some way be protective *(Waring et al., 2008b)*. In another study, severity of adverse effects was correlated with the extent of histamine release. Histamine release appeared independent of tryptase suggesting a non-mast cell source *(Pakravan et al., 2008)*. A relationship has been demonstrated between a low serum acetaminophen at the time of treatment and the development of side effects to NAC *(Schmidt et al., 2001)*. This finding was interpreted by the authors that acetaminophen itself might actually offer some protection against the development of adverse effects to NAC. A similar mechanism was suggested by a study performed in Australia, which showed that side effects were reported only in cases of mild acetaminophen poisoning *(Dawson et al., 1989)*. In a study *(Lynch et al., 2004)* only 7.8% of patients who showed adverse events to NAC had plasma acetaminophen concentrations above the treatment line and plasma acetaminophen concentrations in the remainder (92.8%) were below the treatment line. In a pilot study, the authors performed an investigation on the pharmacokinetics of the intravenous NAC in healthy volunteers. Five healthy male subjects (age between 18-38 years) were recruited to that study. Two subjects were infused NAC intravenously using the accepted UK regimen and three subjects using the Canadian regimen (As the same as UK regimen but the length of the first bag is 45min). Unexpectedly, all five volunteers experienced severe adverse events in association with NAC after 10-20min. The infusion was immediately stopped in all cases and the adverse events were treated with intravenous antihistamine and hydrocortisone *(Ghandforoush-Sattari et al., 2006)*. We speculated that high plasma concentration of acetaminophen in the acetaminophen-poisoned patients might protect patients from the adverse effects of NAC, perhaps by cyclo-oxygenase inhibition as already suggested by others *(Dawson et al., 1989; Schmidt et al., 2001)*. In another study we showed that histamine release occurred in 9 out of 10 healthy subjects, who were receiving IV-NAC according to the UK regimen, at 15min into the study, when plasma NAC was in the highest rate in the body. We concluded that some adverse events occurring during NAC therapy could be attributable to a direct effect of the drug on mast cells and basophils and this effect might be dose dependent. We also suggested that, histamine release might not only mechanism of adverse events associated with NAC and release of some other factors e.g. prostaglandines or tromboxanes could be involved *(Ghandforoush-Sattari et al., 2008b; Ghandforoush-Sattari et al., 2006)*. Since the treatment regimens for NAC are originally derived experimentally, it is still unclear whether reducing the initial bolus dose of intravenous NAC in therapy would produce the same efficacy as the current UK regimen in preventing hepatotoxicity. If it did true, reduction of the loading dose of intravenous NAC might reduce the incidence of adverse reactions with NAC.

Bateman et al suggested that side effects to NAC are caused by a non-allergic release of histamine; this is thought to be a direct and dose dependent pharmacological effect of NAC *(Bateman et al., 1984)*. Therefore a history of drug allergy does not seem to be a risk factor in the development of side effects to NAC *(Schmidt et al., 2001)*.

Anaphylactoid reactions are classified as cutaneous if patients has only "cutaneous" signs such as flushing, pruritus *(Flanagan et al., 1991; Huitema et al., 1998)*, urticaria or angioedema (involvement of deep dermis, subcutaneous or submucosal tissues) *(Dawson et al., 1989)*: or "systemic" if both cutaneous signs and systemic reactions (cough, headache, shortness of breath, wheezing, hypotension, status epilepticus or cortical blindness) are present *(Chan et al., 1994; Dawson et al., 1989; Hershkovitz et al., 1996; Ho et al., 1983; Lorenz et al., 1982)*. It has been believed that asthmatics are at special risk *(Flanagan et al., 1991)*. Systemic side-effects are also more frequent in astmathics but similar in comparison to non-asthmatics *(Schmidt et al., 2001)*. Hypokalaemia and low plasma bicarbonate concentrations have often been noted during the first 72 hours, and there has been a tendency towards low platelet counts, especially in patients with severe liver damage. Serial ECGs have often showed transient generalised T-wave flattening and prominent U waves consistent with hypokalaemia *(Prescott et al., 1979).* The most serious adverse reactions to IV NAC occur during or shortly after the loading dose, are dose related, and generally easily managed. They might be avoided by a slower (30-60 min) infusion of the loading dose. The development of hepatotoxicity should be treated with a prolonged course of IV NAC until liver function is clearly returning towards normal *(Buckley et al., 1999).* Very rarely adverse reactions to excessive dose of NAC have been associated with hypotension and death *(Donovan et al., 1986; Mant et al., 1984).* NAC may also have a direct effect, not necessarily dependent on histamine release *(Sunman et al., 1992).* NAC produces a dose-related vasodilatation of human subcutaneous arterioles in the same concentrations at which it causes anaphylactoid reactions in human being *(Sunman et al., 1992).* This may explain the frequent occurrence of flushing in patients given intravenous NAC. These reactions generally develop between 15 and 60 minutes after the commencement of the infusion (Dawson et al., 1989). In the 20-hour treatment protocol, the time during which half of the total NAC dose is given and when NAC blood concentrations are the highest (Prescott et al., 1989). Moreover, it has been shown that patients, who have had adverse reactions to intravenous NAC, react to high dose intradermally, although not to low dose of NAC. Reactions to intradermal NAC may be prevented by pre-treatment with terfenadine (Bateman et al., 1984). Clinical experience also suggests that antihistamine administration is effective in treating adverse reactions to NAC and preventing their recurrence in man (Bailey et al., 1998).

As with any adverse drug reaction, an anaphylactoid reaction to NAC should prompt a reassessment of the need for NAC therapy. If NAC deemed necessary despite a systemic reaction it is believed that the NAC can be restarted one hour after the administration of an antihistamine *(Bailey et al., 1998).* The 1-hour wait allows the NAC blood concentration to decrease and H_1-receptors to be blocked. The only recurrence of symptoms occurred in a patient in whom NAC was resumed just after diphenhydramine administration (Figure 5). Because the reaction to NAC is apparently dose-related, the use of subsequent doses of diphenhydramine is probably not necessary. Patients have had previous anaphylactoid reactions to NAC should be pre-treated with antihistamine prior to NAC administration *(Bailey et al., 1998).* When NAC is restarted after a life-threatening reaction, administration of ephedrine, cimetidine or both is recommended. Their use has been associated with a decreased incidence of reaction to radio-contrast materials on readministration *(Wittbrodt et al., 1994).* Anaphylactoid reactions to intravenous NAC, either cutaneous or systemic, are rarely life threatening and can be successfully and easily treated with the administration of diphenhydramine. Because of the dose-related nature of the reactions, the administration of diphenhydramine and a delay of 1 hour should be sufficient to allow restarting of intravenous NAC when its use is deemed necessary to prevent acetaminophen-induced hepatotoxicity *(Bailey et al., 1998).* In one reported case *(Nielsen et al., 1996)* an acetaminophen overdosed woman aged 20 who had suffered from severe flushing and urticaria 1h after the administration of IV NAC completely recovered within hours after administration of intravenous glucocorticoids and antihistamines.

Anaphylactoid reactions tend to occur when plasma concentration of NAC is highest (Donovan et al., 1987), i.e. within an hour or two of starting treatment and thus patients with pre-existing liver disease may be more likely to develop anaphylactoid reactions (Jones et al.,

1997). Patients with suspected chronic liver disease, unlike those with acute liver damage due to acetaminophen, may be more likely to develop adverse reactions to NAC as these occur when plasma NAC concentration is highest (Jones et al., 1997).

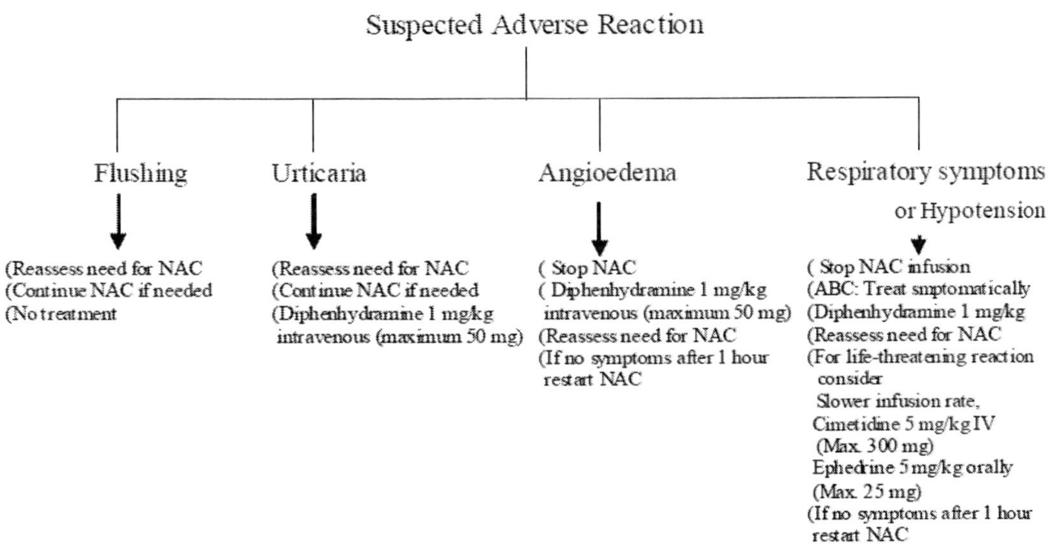

Figure 5. Management guidelines for adverse reactions to NAC (Bailey, et al. 1998).

The dose of intravenous NAC should probably be modified now to avoid these high initial concentrations. Because of the dose-dependent effect of NAC, it should be infused, especially in asthmatics, bolus over a slightly longer period of time, e.g. 30-60min instead of the usual 15min. There is no reason to withhold NAC from any acetaminophen-overdosed patient *(Schmidt et al., 2001).*

To minimise NAC adverse reactions, *Bronstein et al* suggested a 48h IV NAC protocol for the treatment of acetaminophen overdose, in which 140 mg/kg loading dose followed by twelve 70mg/kg maintenance doses at four hours interval*s (Bronstein et al., 1985). Mant et al* suggested substitution of oral methionine instead of NAC, if an anaphylactoid reaction occurs after administration of intravenous NAC *(Mant et al., 1984).*

Biomarkers of NAC Adverse Reactions

Histamine and Methylhistamine

Early diagnosis of anaphylactic-like reactions can be achieved by plasma histamine measurement. The short plasma half-life of histamine (a few minutes) and the difficulties in handling the sample usually preclude this measurement *(Laroche et al., 1991).* The normal means of histamine concentration in healthy volunteers are usually 4-12nM *(Laroche et al., 1991).* Plasma histamine concentrations are maximal at 10-15 min after the anaphylactic-like reaction and return to baseline by 30 min, indicating the completion of mast cell degranulation *(Schwartz et al., 1989).*

Since histamine disappears rapidly from plasma because of its short half-life (3min), and N-methylhistamine is stable and has a longer half-life (30min), determination of its plasma or urine concentration can be a useful biomarker in determination of histamine release *(Takeda et al., 1995)*.

Prostaglandins and Thromboxanes

In vitro studies *(Lages et al., 1989; Panush, 1976; Shalabi, 1992)* have demonstrated that the function of lymphocytes, neutrophils, and thrombocytes is inhibited by toxic, but not by therapeutic concentrations of acetaminophen. It has been suggested that this effect is caused by a reversible inhibition by acetaminophen of cyclo-oxygenase leading to a reduced synthesis of prostaglandins and thromboxanes.

Tryptase

Although a radioimmunologic kit for determination of histamine is routinely available. It has been suggested that the mast cell tryptase could provide an alternative to histamine determination *(Laroche et al., 1991)*. Tryptase is the major known protein component of mast cell secretory granules, existing in both mucosal and connective tissue mast cells. Because small amounts of the enzyme are present in basophils, unlike histamine, tryptase concentrations selectively indicate involvement of mast cell activation.

Tryptase is released in parallel with histamine from activated human mast cells, but its appearance in the circulation is delayed relative to that of histamine, presumably due to a slower rate of diffusion away from its tissue site of release *(Schwartz et al., 1989)*. *Laroche et al* demonstrated that tryptase was a useful marker for severe anaphylactoid reactions, but less so for mild ones.

In some cases, elevated concentrations of tryptase may not be detected during the initial 15-30min. Tryptase concentrations then decline under apparent first order kinetics with a half-life of 2h. Therefore, an appropriate time to obtain samples for tryptase determinations is 1-2h after the precipitating event, but depending on the magnitude of the initial response, elevated concentrations of tryptase may be present in the circulation for several hours *(Laroche et al., 1992)*.

Plasma tryptase concentration in normal healthy human is less than 2 mg/L. Plasma tryptase is very stable and high concentrations of tryptase could be found after storage at -20°C for more than one year.

Blood clotting, haemolysis, freeze-thaw cycle and incubation at room temperature during 48 h have little influence on the measured values. These reasons and the large time interval for sampling make tryptase a very practical biological test for the diagnosis of anaphylactic-like reactions *(Laroche et al., 1991)*.

Liver Transplantation

In a study between 1992 and 2006, from 469 patients with ALF who were admitted to Scottish Liver Transplantation, 104 underwent liver transplantation. Acetaminophen was the most common etiology (68.9%) *(Simpson et al., 2009)*. In patients with acute liver failure and a poor prognosis, early referral to a liver transplant centre is essential.

The King's College criteria (Table 1), a widely used prognostic model in patients with acute liver failure, are used to predict the need for liver transplantation. They are based on the arterial pH, the PT and INR, the severity of encephalopathy, and the serum creatinine concentration *(Schilling et al., 2010)*.

One-year survival after emergency liver transplantation is 70%, but 20% of listed patients die, highlighting the importance of early referral of patients who have ALF with a poor prognosis to a transplant center *(Fontana, 2008)*.

Table 1. King's College criteria for poor prognosis in acute liver failure (O'Grady et al., 1989)

In acetaminophen-induced acute liver failure
Arterial pH < 7.3
Or all of the following:
Grade III or IV encephalopathy
Prothrombin time > 100 seconds
Serum creatinine > 3.4 mg/dL
In acute liver failure from other causes
Prothrombin time > 100 seconds
Or three of the following:
Age < 10 years or > 40 years
Non-A, non-B hepatitis, halothane-induced hepatitis, idiosyncratic drug reactions
More than 7 days of jaundice before the onset of encephalopathy
Prothrombin time > 50 seconds
Serum bilirubin > 18 mg/dL

PREVENTION OF ACETAMINOPHEN OVERDOSE

The clear risk of hepatotoxicity associated with acetaminophen poisoning finally resulted in legislation in the UK in September 1998 to limit pack size of simple (non-opioid) analgesics to 16 tablets in non-pharmacy retail shopping and to 32 from pharmacy outlets *(Hawton et al., 2004; Townsend et al., 2001)*. Mean pack sizes also decreased significantly between 1996-7 and 1998-9 for acetaminophen (35 to 24 tablets per packet). *Hawton* and colleagues showed that legislation restricting pack sizes of analgesics in the UK was beneficial, and suggested that a further reduction in pack sizes could prevent more deaths *(Hawton et al., 2004)*. Several suggestions have been made to reduce the incidence of poisoning in general. Hospital based interventions after admission for self-harm have been postulated in an attempt to reduce repetition *(Eddleston, 2000)*. Improved mental health care, facilities particularly in the community has also been suggested *(Eddleston, 2000)*. In France the content of each pack of acetaminophen is legally limited to 8g. This may be one reason why severe liver damage and deaths after acetaminophen poisoning are 25% less frequent in France than in the UK *(Chan, 2000)*. In one study during 1990-1999 in Scotland, changes in acetaminophen pack-size have been associated with reduced discharge rates *(Bateman et al., 2003)*. However another study on records between 1994-2000 in Scotland observed no reduction in deaths after the introduction of legislation controlling pack-size *(Sheen et al., 2002a)*. These authors suggested that acetaminophen pack-size reduction has not achieved as large as an overdose rate reduction as might have been expected *(Sheen et al., 2002b)*.

Although the effectiveness of using special child-resistant packaging in the prevention of accidental poisonings particularly in the children under the age of 5 has already been well recognised *(Sibert et al., 1977)* but these are sometimes difficult for adults (especially elderly or infirm elderly) to use properly. It has been suggested that liver damage following acetaminophen overdose could be abolished simply by the addition of cysteine or methionine to the tablets *(McLean, 1974; Neuvonen et al., 1985)*. However, this approach has not found favour with legislators. Perhaps further pack-size reduction, as suggested by *Hawton* and colleagues *(Hawton et al., 2004)* may be helpful, although this has to be balanced against the inconvenience that might be caused to the vast majority of the population who only wish to take acetaminophen at therapeutic doses. Education of the public and medical profession might be helpful in increasing awareness of the potential toxic effects of acetaminophen overdose *(Mills et al., 2008)*.

REFERENCES

Adamson GM, Harman AW (1993). Oxidative stress in cultured hepatocytes exposed to acetaminophen. *Biochem. Pharmacol.* 45(11): 2289-2294.

Ali FM, Boyer EW, Bird SB (2008). Estimated risk of hepatotoxicity after an acute acetaminophen overdose in alcoholics. *Alcohol* 42(3): 213-218.

Anoush M, Eghbal MA, Fathiazad F, Hamzei H, Saeedi Kouzehkonani N (2009a). The Protective Effect of Garlic Extract against Acetaminophen-Induced Loss of Mitochondrial Membrane Potential in Freshly Isolated Rat Hepatocytes. *Iranian Journal of Pharmaceutical Sciences* 5(3): 141-150.

Anoush M, Eghbal MA, Fathiazad F, Hamzeiy H, Kouzehkonani NS (2009b). The protective effects of garlic extract against acetaminophen-induced oxidative stress and glutathione depletion. *Pak. J. Biol. Sci.* 12(10): 765-771.

Antoine DJ, Williams DP, Kipar A, Jenkins RE, Regan SL, Sathish JG, *et al.* (2009). High-mobility group box-1 protein and keratin-18, circulating serum proteins informative of acetaminophen-induced necrosis and apoptosis in vivo. *Toxicol. Sci.* 112(2): 521-531.

Apte U, Singh S, Zeng G, Cieply B, Virji MA, Wu T, *et al.* (2009). Beta-catenin activation promotes liver regeneration after acetaminophen-induced injury. *Am. J. Pathol.* 175(3): 1056-1065.

Artnak KE, Wilkinson SS (1998). Fulminant hepatic failure in acute acetaminophen overdose. *Dimens Crit. Care Nurs.* 17(3): 135-144.

Aruoma OI, Halliwell B, Hoey BM, Butler J (1989). The antioxidant action of N-acetylcysteine: its reaction with hydrogen peroxide, hydroxyl radical, superoxide, and hypochlorous acid. *Free Radic. Biol. Med.* 6(6): 593-597.

Atkins P (1987). *Molecules*. edn. W.H. Freeman and Co: New York.

Atwood SJ (1980). The laboratory in the diagnosis and management of acetaminophen and salicylate intoxications. *Pediatr. Clin. North Am.* 27(4): 871-879.

Bailey B, McGuigan MA (1998). Management of anaphylactoid reactions to intravenous N-acetylcysteine. *Ann. Emerg. Med.* 31(6): 710-715.

Banda PW, Quart BD (1982). The effect of mild alcohol consumption on the metabolism of acetaminophen in man. *Res. Commun. Chem. Pathol. Pharmacol.* 38(1): 57-70.

Barker JD, Jr., de Carle DJ, Anuras S (1977). Chronic excessive acetaminophen use and liver damage. *Ann. Intern. Med.* 87(3): 299-301.

Bartels S, Sivilotti M, Crosby D, Richard J (2008). Are recommended doses of acetaminophen hepatotoxic for recently abstinent alcoholics? A randomized trial. *Clin. Toxicol. (Phila)* 46(3): 243-249.

Bateman DN, Bain M, Gorman D, Murphy D (2003). Changes in paracetamol, antidepressants and opioid poisoning in Scotland during the 1990s. *QJM* 96(2): 125-132.

Bateman DN, Woodhouse KW, Rawlins MD (1984). Adverse reactions to N-acetylcysteine. *Hum. Toxicol.* 3(5): 393-398.

Bebarta VS, Kao L, Froberg B, Clark RF, Lavonas E, Qi M, *et al.* (2010). A multicenter comparison of the safety of oral versus intravenous acetylcysteine for treatment of acetaminophen overdose. *Clin. Toxicol. (Phila)* 48(5): 424-430.

Beckett GJ, Foster GR, Hussey AJ, Oliveira DB, Donovan JW, Prescott LF, *et al.* (1989). Plasma glutathione S-transferase and F protein are more sensitive than alanine aminotransferase as markers of paracetamol (acetaminophen)-induced liver damage. *Clin. Chem.* 35(11): 2186-2189.

Betten DP, Cantrell FL, Thomas SC, Williams SR, Clark RF (2007). A prospective evaluation of shortened course oral N-acetylcysteine for the treatment of acute acetaminophen poisoning. *Ann. Emerg. Med.* 50(3): 272-279.

Bhatnagar SK, Welty JD, al Yusuf AR (1990). Significance of blood taurine levels in patients with first time acute ischaemic cardiac pain. *Int. J. Cardiol.* 27(3): 361-366.

Bialas MC, Reid PG, Beck P, Lazarus JH, Smith PM, Scorer RC, *et al.* (1996). Changing patterns of self-poisoning in a UK health district. *Qjm* 89(12): 893-901.

Bizovi KE, Aks SE, Paloucek F, Gross R, Keys N, Rivas J (1996). Late increase in acetaminophen concentration after overdose of Tylenol Extended Relief. *Ann. Emerg. Med.* 28(5): 549-551.

Blazka ME, Elwell MR, Holladay SD, Wilson RE, Luster MI (1996). Histopathology of acetaminophen-induced liver changes: role of interleukin 1 alpha and tumor necrosis factor alpha. *Toxicol. Pathol.* 24(2): 181-189.

Boess F, Bopst M, Althaus R, Polsky S, Cohen SD, Eugster HP, *et al.* (1998). Acetaminophen hepatotoxicity in tumor necrosis factor/lymphotoxin-alpha gene knockout mice. *Hepatology* 27(4): 1021-1029.

Bonanomi L, Gazzaniga A (1980). Toxicological, pharmacokinetic and metabolic studies on acetylcysteine. *Eur. J. Respir. Dis. Suppl.* 111: 45-51.

Borgstroem L, Kagedal B, Paulsen O (1986). Pharmacokinetics of NAC in man. *Eur. J. Pharmacol.* 31: 217-222.

Botta JA, Jr., Nelson LW, Weikel JH, Jr. (1973). Acetylcysteine in the prevention of cyclophosphamide-induced cystitis in rats. *J. Natl. Cancer Inst.* 51(3): 1051-1058.

Bray GP, Harrison PM, O'Grady JG, Tredger JM, Williams R (1992). Long-term anticonvulsant therapy worsens outcome in paracetamol-induced fulminant hepatic failure. *Hum. Exp. Toxicol.* 11(4): 265-270.

Brent J (1993). Are activated charcoal-N-acetylcysteine interactions of clinical significance? *Ann. Emerg. Med.* 22(12): 1860-1862.

Bridger S, Henderson K, Glucksman E, Ellis A, Henry J, Williams R (1998). Death from low dose paracetamol poisoning. *BMJ* 316: 1724-1725.

Brok J, Buckley N, Gluud C (2006). Interventions for paracetamol (acetaminophen) overdose. *Cochrane Database Syst. Rev.*(2): CD003328.

Bronstein A, Linden C, Hall A, Kulig K, Rimack B, Donovan W, *et al.* (1985). Interavenous N- acetylcysteine for acute acetaminophen poisoning. *Vet Hum. Toxicol.* 27: 316.

Bruno MK, Cohen SD, Khairallah EA (1988). Antidotal effectiveness of N-acetylcysteine in reversing acetaminophen-induced hepatotoxicity. Enhancement of the proteolysis of arylated proteins. *Biochem. Pharmacol.* 37(22): 4319-4325.

Buchter A, Peter H, Bolt HM (1984). [N-Acetylcysteine as an antidote in accidental acrylonitrile poisoning]. *Int. Arch. Occup. Environ. Health* 53(4): 311-319.

Buckley N, Eddleston M (2007). Paracetamol (acetaminophen) poisoning. *Clin. Evid. (Online)* 2007.

Buckley NA, Whyte IM, O'Connell DL, Dawson AH (1999). Oral or intravenous N-acetylcysteine: which is the treatment of choice for acetaminophen (paracetamol) poisoning? *J. Toxicol. Clin. Toxicol.* 37(6): 759-767.

Burcham PC, Harman AW (1990). Mitochondrial dysfunction in paracetamol hepatotoxicity: in vitro studies in isolated mouse hepatocytes. *Toxicol. Lett.* 50(1): 37-48.

Burgunder JM, Lauterburg BH (1987). Decreased production of glutathione in patients with cirrhosis. *Eur. J. Clin. Invest.* 17(5): 408-414.

Burgunder JM, Varriale A, Lauterburg BH (1989). Effect of N-acetylcysteine on plasma cysteine and glutathione following paracetamol administration. *Eur. J. Clin. Pharmacol.* 36(2): 127-131.

Butterworth RF (1996). Taurine in hepatic encephalopathy. *Adv. Exp. Med. Biol.* 403: 601-606.

Byer AJ, Traylor TR, Semmer JR (1982). Acetaminophen overdose in the third trimester of pregnancy. *Jama* 247(22): 3114-3115.

Cakir E, Akgul OE, Aydin I, Cayci T, Kurt YG, Onguru O, *et al.* (2010). The association between neopterin and acetaminophen-induced nephrotoxicity. *Ren. Fail* 32(6): 740-746.

Caldarola V, Hassett JM, Hall AH, Bronstein AB, Kulig KW, Rumack BH (1986). Hemorrhagic pancreatitis associated with acetaminophen overdose. *Am. J. Gastroenterol.* 81(7): 579-582.

Carloss H, Forrester J, Austin F, Fuson T (1978). Acute acetaminophen intoxication. *South Med. J.* 71(8): 906-908.

Chamberlain JM, Gorman RL, Oderda GM, Klein-Schwartz W, Klein BL (1993). Use of activated charcoal in a simulated poisoning with acetaminophen: a new loading dose for N-acetylcysteine? *Ann. Emerg. Med.* 22(9): 1398-1402.

Chan TY (2000). Improvements in the packaging of drugs and chemicals may reduce the likelihood of severe intentional poisonings in adults. *Hum. Exp. Toxicol.* 19(7): 387-391.

Chan TY, Critchley JA (1994). Adverse reactions to intravenous N-acetylcysteine in Chinese patients with paracetamol (acetaminophen) poisoning. *Hum. Exp. Toxicol.* 13(8): 542-544.

Chen YX (1993). [Protective action of taurine on ischemia-reperfusion liver injury in rats and its mechanism]. *Zhonghua Yi Xue Za Zhi* 73(5): 276-279, 318-279.

Chun LJ, Tong MJ, Busuttil RW, Hiatt JR (2009). Acetaminophen hepatotoxicity and acute liver failure. *J. Clin. Gastroenterol.* 43(4): 342-349.

Clark RF, Chen R, Williams SR, Johnson CL, Harchelroad F (1996). The use of ondansetron in the treatment of nausea and vomiting associated with acetaminophen poisoning. *J. Toxicol. Clin. Toxicol.* 34(2): 163-167.

Corcoran GB, Racz WJ, Smith CV, Mitchell JR (1985). Effects of N-acetylcysteine on acetaminophen covalent binding and hepatic necrosis in mice. *J. Pharmacol. Exp. Ther.* 232(3): 864-872.

Cotgreave IA, Berggren M, Jones TW, Dawson J, Moldeus P (1987). Gastrointestinal metabolism of N-acetylcysteine in the rat, including an assay for sulfite in biological systems. *Biopharm. Drug Dispos.* 8(4): 377-386.

Craig DG, Lee A, Hayes PC, Simpson KJ (2010). Review article: the current management of acute liver failure. *Aliment Pharmacol. Ther.* 31(3): 345-358.

Crome P, Vale JA, Volans GN, Widdop B, Goulding R (1976). Oral methionine in the treatment of severe paracetamol (Acetaminophen) overdose. *Lancet* 2(7990): 829-830.

Cummings AJ, King ML, Martin BK (1967). A kinetic study of drug elimination: the excretion of paracetamol and its metabolites in man. *Br. J. Pharmacol.* 29(2): 150-157.

Davis AM, Helms CM, Mitros FA, Wong YW, LaBrecque DR (1983). Severe hepatic damage after acetaminophen use in psittacosis. *Am. J. Med.* 74(2): 349-352.

Dawson AH, Henry DA, McEwen J (1989). Adverse reactions to N-acetylcysteine during treatment for paracetamol poisoning. *Med. J. Aust.* 150(6): 329-331.

Dawson AH, Whyte IM (2001). Therapeutic drug monitoring in drug overdose. *Br. J. Clin. Pharmacol.* 52 Suppl 1: 97S-102S.

De Caro L, Ghizzi A, Costa R, Longo A, Ventresca GP, Lodola E (1989). Pharmacokinetics and bioavailability of oral acetylcysteine in healthy volunteers. *Arzneimittelforschung* 39(3): 382-386.

Dehpour A, Zahedi H, Amini S, Akhgari M, Abdollahi M (1999). Effects of glicyrhizza derivatives against acetaminophen -induced hepatotoxicity. *Irn. J. Med. Sci.* 24(1and2): 26-31.

Demirbas S, Cakir E, Akgul EO, Seyrek M, Cayci T, Kurt YG, *et al.* (2011). Elevated serum neopterin levels in acetaminophen-induced liver injury. *Environ. Toxicol. Pharmacol.* 31(1): 165-170.

Devlin J, Ellis AE, McPeake J, Heaton N, Wendon JA, Williams R (1997). N-acetylcysteine improves indocyanine green extraction and oxygen transport during hepatic dysfunction. *Crit. Care Med.* 25(2): 236-242.

Dhawan A, Sorrell MF (1996). Acetaminophen overdose: need to consider intravenous preparation of N-acetylcysteine in the United States. *Am. J. Gastroenterol.* 91(7): 1476.

Donnelly PJ, Walker RM, Racz WJ (1994). Inhibition of mitochondrial respiration in vivo is an early event in acetaminophen-induced hepatotoxicity. *Arch. Toxicol.* 68(2): 110-118.

Donovan J, Jarvie D, Prescott L, Proutfoot A (1987). Adverse reactions of N-acetylcysteine and their relation to plasma levels. *Vet. Hum. Toxicol.* 29: 470 (Abstract).

Donovan J, Proudfoot A, Prescott L (1986). Adverse effects of N-acetylcysteine (Abstract). *Vet. Hum. Toxicology* 28: 487.

Dordoni B, Willson RA, Thompson RP, Williams R (1973). Reduction of absorption of paracetamol by activated charcoal and cholestyramine: a possible therapeutic measure. *Br. Med. J.* 3(5871): 86-87.

Dougherty PP, Klein-Schwartz W (2011). Unexpected Late Rise in Plasma Acetaminophen Concentrations with Change in Risk Stratification in Acute Acetaminophen Overdoses. *J. Emerg. Med.*

Douglas AP, Savage RL, Rawlins MD (1978). Paracetamol (acetaminophen) kinetics in patients with Gilber's syndrome. *Eur. J. Clin. Pharmacol.* 13(3): 209-212.

Eddleston M (2000). Patterns and problems of deliberate self-poisoning in the developing world. *Qjm* 93(11): 715-731.

Ekins BR, Ford DC, Thompson MI, Bridges RR, Rollins DE, Jenkins RD (1987). The effect of activated charcoal on N-acetylcysteine absorption in normal subjects. *Am. J. Emerg. Med.* 5(6): 483-487.

Ellis A, Wendon J (1996). Circulatory, respiratory, cerebral, and renal derangements in acute liver failure: pathophysiology and management. *Semin. Liver Dis.* 16(4): 379-388.

Emby DJ, Fraser BN (1977). Hepatotoxicity of paracetamol enhanced by ingestion of alcohol: report of two cases. *S Afr. Med. J.* 51(7): 208-209.

Esteban A, Perez-Mateo M (1993). Gilbert's disease: a risk factor for paracetamol overdosage? *J. Hepatol.* 18(2): 257-258.

Ferner R (1993). Paracetamol poisoning- an update. *Prescriber's Journal* 33(2): 45-50.

Flanagan RJ (1987). The role of acetylcysteine in clinical toxicology. *Med. Toxicol.* 2(2): 93-104.

Flanagan RJ, Meredith TJ (1991). Use of N-acetylcysteine in clinical toxicology. *Am. J. Med.* 91(3C): 131S-139S.

Fontana RJ (2008). Acute liver failure including acetaminophen overdose. *Med. Clin. North Am.* 92(4): 761-794, viii.

Fontana RJ (2006). "Unintentional" acetaminophen overdose on the rise: who is responsible? Dr Robert J Fontana is interviewed by Paul C Adams. *Can. J. Gastroenterol.* 20(5): 319-324.

Forrest JA, Clements JA, Prescott LF (1982). Clinical pharmacokinetics of paracetamol. *Clin. Pharmacokinet.* 7(2): 93-107.

Gardner CR, Heck DE, Yang CS, Thomas PE, Zhang XJ, DeGeorge GL, *et al.* (1998). Role of nitric oxide in acetaminophen-induced hepatotoxicity in the rat. *Hepatology* 27(3): 748-754.

Ghandforoush-Sattari M, Mashayekhi S (2008a). Evaluation of taurine as a biomarker of liver damage in paracetamol poisoning. *Eur. J. Pharmacol.* 581(1-2): 171-176.

Ghandforoush-Sattari M, Mashayekhi S, Nemati M, Routledge PA (2009). A Rapid Determination of Taurine in Human Plasma by LC. *Chromatographia* 69(11-12): 1427-1430.

Ghandforoush-Sattari M, Mashayekhi S, Nemati M, Seydi A, Azadi H (2010a). Changes in plasma taurine concentration during a period of heroin detoxification. *Toxicological and Environmental Chemistry* 92(8): 1505–1512.

Ghandforoush-Sattari M, Mashayekhi S, Thompson J, Routledge P (2007). Admissions to the Cardiff Poisons Unit involving paracetamol poisoning (1989-2002). *Toxicology Letters* 172: S229-S229.

Ghandforoush-Sattari M, Mashayekhi SO (2008b). A rapid determination of histamine and 3-methylhistamine in human plasma by high performance liquid chromatography. *Toxicological and Environmental Chemistry* 90(4): 787 – 793.

Ghandforoush-Sattari M, Mashayekhi SO, Krishna CV, Thompson JP, Routledge PA (2010b). Pharmacokinetics of Oral Taurine in Healthy Volunteers. *J. Amino Acids* 2010(2010): 1-5.

Ghandforoush-Sattari M, Mashayekhi SO, Nemati M, Ayromlou H (2011). Changes in plasma concentration of taurine in stroke. *Neurosci. Lett.* 496(3): 172-175.

Ghandforoush-Sattari M, Thompson JP, Krishna CV, Routledge PA (2006). Effects of Pre-treatment with Naproxen on the Tolerability of N-acetylcysteine (NAC) in Healthy Volunteers. In: *6th International Congress of Turkish Society of Toxicology*. Antalya, Turkey.

Glazenburg EJ, Jekel-Halsema IM, Scholtens E, Baars AJ, Mulder GJ (1983). Effects of variation in the dietary supply of cysteine and methionine on liver concentration of glutathione and "active sulfate" (PAPS) and serum levels of sulfate, cystine, methionine and taurine: relation to the metabolism of acetaminophen. *J. Nutr.* 113(7): 1363-1373.

Goodman LS, Gilman A, Brunton LL (2008). *Goodman and Gilman's manual of pharmacology and therapeutics*. edn. McGraw-Hill Medical: New York.

Gray TA, Buckley BM, Vale JA (1987). Hyperlactataemia and metabolic acidosis following paracetamol overdose. *Q. J. Med.* 65(246): 811-821.

Gregory B, Larson AM, Reisch J, Lee WM (2010). Acetaminophen dose does not predict outcome in acetaminophen-induced acute liver failure. *J. Investig. Med.* 58(5): 707-710.

Grinbalt J, Lewitus Z, Rosenfeld J (1980). Renal tubular necrosis and liver damage: A possible consequence of low dose of acetaminophen and halotane anaesthesia. *Drug Intelligence and Clinical Pharmacy* 14: 431-435.

Guerra-Romero L, Tureen JH, Fournier MA, Makrides V, Tauber MG (1993). Amino acids in cerebrospinal and brain interstitial fluid in experimental pneumococcal meningitis. *Pediatr. Res.* 33(5): 510-513.

Guyton AC (1984). *Physiology of the Human Body*. 6th. edn. Saunders College Publishing.

Gwilt PR, Lear CL, Tempero MA, Birt DD, Grandjean AC, Ruddon RW, *et al.* (1994). The effect of garlic extract on human metabolism of acetaminophen. *Cancer Epidemiol Biomarkers Prev.* 3(2): 155-160.

Harrison PM, O'Grady JG, Keays RT, Alexander GJ, Williams R (1990). Serial prothrombin time as prognostic indicator in paracetamol induced fulminant hepatic failure. *Bmj* 301(6758): 964-966.

Harrison PM, Wendon JA, Gimson AE, Alexander GJ, Williams R (1991). Improvement by acetylcysteine of hemodynamics and oxygen transport in fulminant hepatic failure. *N. Engl. J. Med.* 324(26): 1852-1857.

Harry F, Hale A, Buss D, Hutchings A, Routledge P (1999). Serum taurine levels in healthy subjects and in paracetamol poisoned patients. *Human and Experimental Toxicology* 18: 531.

Hawton K, Fagg J (1992). Trends in deliberate self poisoning and self injury in Oxford, 1976-90. *Bmj* 304(6839): 1409-1411.

Hawton K, Simkin S, Deeks J, Cooper J, Johnston A, Waters K, *et al.* (2004). UK legislation on analgesic packs: before and after study of long term effect on poisonings. *Bmj* 329(7474): 1076.

Hayes BD, Klein-Schwartz W, Doyon S (2008). Frequency of medication errors with intravenous acetylcysteine for acetaminophen overdose. *Ann. Pharmacother.* 42(6): 766-770.

Hayes JD, Gilligan D, Chapman BJ, Beckett GJ (1983). Purification of human hepatic glutathione S-transferases and the development of a radioimmunoassay for their measurement in plasma. *Clin. Chim. Acta* 134(1-2): 107-121.

Hengy B, Hayi-Slayman D, Page M, Christin F, Baillon JJ, Ber CE, *et al.* (2009). [Acute renal failure after acetaminophen poisoning: report of three cases]. *Can. J. Anaesth.* 56(10): 770-774.

Henriques CC (1970). Acetaminophen sensitivity and fixed dermatitis. *Jama* 214(13): 2336.

Henry J (1990). Glotathione and HIV infection. *Lancet* 335: 235-236.

Hershkovitz E, Shorer Z, Levitas A, Tal A (1996). Status epilepticus following intravenous N-acetylcysteine therapy. *Isr. J. Med. Sci.* 32(11): 1102-1104.

Higgins RM, Goldsmith DJ, MacDiarmid-Gordon A, Taberner D, Venning MC, Ackrill P (1996). Treating paracetamol overdose by charcoal haemoperfusion and long-hours high-flux dialysis. *Qjm* 89(4): 297-306.

Himmelstein DU, Woolhandler SJ, Adler RD (1984). Elevated SGOT/SGPT ratio in alcoholic patients with acetaminophen hepatotoxicity. *Am. J. Gastroenterol.* 79(9): 718-720.

Hinson JA, Roberts DW, Benson RW, Dalhoff K, Loft S, Poulsen HE (1990). Mechanism of paracetamol toxicity. *Lancet* 335(8691): 732.

Ho SW, Beilin LJ (1983). Asthma associated with N-acetylcysteine infusion and paracetamol poisoning: report of two cases. *Br. Med. J. (Clin Res Ed)* 287(6396): 876-877.

Holdiness MR (1991). Clinical pharmacokinetics of N-acetylcysteine. *Clin. Pharmacokinet* 20(2): 123-134.

Holoye PY, Duelge J, Hansen RM, Ritch PS, Anderson T (1983). Prophylaxis of ifosfamide toxicity with oral acetylcysteine. *Semin. Oncol.* 10(1 Suppl 1): 66-71.

Horowitz JD, Henry CA, Syrjanen ML, Louis WJ, Fish RD, Smith TW, *et al.* (1988). Combined use of nitroglycerin and N-acetylcysteine in the management of unstable angina pectoris. *Circulation* 77(4): 787-794.

Huitema AD, Soesan M, Meenhorst PL, Koks CH, Beijnen JH (1998). A dose-dependent delayed hypersensitivity reaction to acetaminophen after repeated acetaminophen intoxications. *Hum. Exp. Toxicol.* 17(7): 406-408.

Huxtable R, Sebring L (1983). Cardiovascular actions of taurine. In: *Sulfur amino acids Biochemical aspects*, Kuriyama K, Huxtable R, Iwata H (eds), pp 5-37. New York: Alan R. Liss, Inc.

Huxtable RJ (1992). Physiological actions of taurine. *Physiol. Rev.* 72(1): 101-163.

Jaeschke H, Mitchell JR (1989). Mitochondria and xanthine oxidase both generate reactive oxygen species in isolated perfused rat liver after hypoxic injury. *Biochem. Biophys. Res. Commun.* 160(1): 140-147.

James LP, Letzig L, Simpson PM, Capparelli E, Roberts DW, Hinson JA, *et al.* (2009). Pharmacokinetics of acetaminophen-protein adducts in adults with acetaminophen overdose and acute liver failure. *Drug. Metab. Dispos.* 37(8): 1779-1784.

James LP, Simpson PM, Farrar HC, Kearns GL, Wasserman GS, Blumer JL, *et al.* (2005). Cytokines and toxicity in acetaminophen overdose. *J. Clin. Pharmacol.* 45(10): 1165-1171.

James LP, Wells E, Beard RH, Farrar HC (2002). Predictors of outcome after acetaminophen poisoning in children and adolescents. *J. Pediatr.* 140(5): 522-526.

Janes J, Routledge PA (1992). Recent developments in the management of paracetamol (acetaminophen) poisoning. *Drug Saf*.7(3): 170-177.

Johnson MW, Friedman PA, Mitch WE (1981). Alcoholism, nonprescription drug and hepatotoxicity. The risk from unknown acetaminophen ingestion. *Am. J. Gastroenterol.* 76(6): 530-533.

Johnston SC, Pelletier LL, Jr. (1997). Enhanced hepatotoxicity of acetaminophen in the alcoholic patient. Two case reports and a review of the literature. *Medicine (Baltimore)* 76(3): 185-191.

Jones AL (1998a). Mechanism of action and value of N-acetylcysteine in the treatment of early and late acetaminophen poisoning: a critical review. *J. Toxicol. Clin. Toxicol.* 36(4): 277-285.

Jones AL, Bangash IH, Bouchier IA, Hayes PC (1994). Portal and systemic haemodynamic action of N-acetylcysteine in patients with stable cirrhosis. *Gut* 35(9): 1290-1293.

Jones AL, Jarvie DR, Simpson D, Hayes PC, Prescott LF (1997). Pharmacokinetics of N-acetylcysteine are altered in patients with chronic liver disease. *Aliment Pharmacol. Ther.* 11(4): 787-791.

Jones DP, Carlson JL, Samiec PS, Sternberg P, Jr., Mody VC, Jr., Reed RL, *et al.* (1998b). Glutathione measurement in human plasma. Evaluation of sample collection, storage and derivatization conditions for analysis of dansyl derivatives by HPLC. *Clin. Chim. Acta* 275(2): 175-184.

Kalantari H, Salehi M (2001). The protective effect of garlic oil on hepatotoxicity induced by acetaminophen in mice and comparison with N-acetylcysteine. *Saudi Med. J.* 22(12): 1080-1084.

Kamiyama T, Sato C, Liu J, Tajiri K, Miyakawa H, Marumo F (1993). Role of lipid peroxidation in acetaminophen-induced hepatotoxicity: comparison with carbon tetrachloride. *Toxicol. Lett.* 66(1): 7-12.

Katzung B (2004). *Basic and Clinical Pharmacology*. 9th edn. McGraw-Hill Companies Inc.

Keays R, Harrison PM, Wendon JA, Forbes A, Gove C, Alexander GJ, *et al.* (1991). Intravenous acetylcysteine in paracetamol induced fulminant hepatic failure: a prospective controlled trial. *Bmj* 303(6809): 1026-1029.

Kirk K, Kirk J (1993). Volume-regulatory taurine release from a human lung cancer cell line. Evidence for amino acid transport via a volume-activated chloride channel. *FEBS Lett.* 336(1): 153-158.

Lages B, Weiss HJ (1989). Inhibition of human platelet function in vitro and ex vivo by acetaminophen. *Thromb. Res.* 53(6): 603-613.

Lane JE, Belson MG, Brown DK, Scheetz A (2002). Chronic acetaminophen toxicity: a case report and review of the literature. *J. Emerg. Med.* 23(3): 253-256.

Laroche D, Duboise F, Lefrancois C, Gerard J, Bricard H (1992). Plasma tryptase concentration is related to the severity grade of the anaphylactoid reaction. *Anesthesiology* 77(3A): A1109.

Laroche D, Vergnaud MC, Sillard B, Soufarapis H, Bricard H (1991). Biochemical markers of anaphylactoid reactions to drugs. Comparison of plasma histamine and tryptase. *Anesthesiology* 75(6): 945-949.

Larson AM, Polson J, Fontana RJ, Davern TJ, Lalani E, Hynan LS, *et al.* (2005). Acetaminophen-induced acute liver failure: results of a United States multicenter, prospective study. *Hepatology* 42(6): 1364-1372.

Lau GS, Critchley JA (1994). The estimation of paracetamol and its major metabolites in both plasma and urine by a single high-performance liquid chromatography assay. *J. Pharm. Biomed. Anal.* 12(12): 1563-1572.

Laurence DR BP (1992). *Clinical Pharmacology*. Seventh edn. Churchill Livingstone: Edinburgh.

Lauterburg BH, Velez ME (1988). Glutathione deficiency in alcoholics: risk factor for paracetamol hepatotoxicity. *Gut* 29(9): 1153-1157.

Laverty HG, Antoine DJ, Benson C, Chaponda M, Williams D, Kevin Park B (2010). The potential of cytokines as safety biomarkers for drug-induced liver injury. *Eur. J. Clin. Pharmacol.* 66(10): 961-976.

Leung NW, Critchley JA (1991). Increased oxidative metabolism of paracetamol in patients with hepatocellular carcinoma. *Cancer Lett.* 57(1): 45-48.

Lieh-Lai MW, Sarnaik AP, Newton JF, Miceli JN, Fleischmann LE, Hook JB*, et al.* (1984). Metabolism and pharmacokinetics of acetaminophen in a severely poisoned young child. *J. Pediatr.* 105(1): 125-128.

Litovitz TL, Smilkstein M, Felberg L, Klein-Schwartz W, Berlin R, Morgan JL (1997). 1996 annual report of the American Association of Poison Control Centers Toxic Exposure Surveillance System. *Am. J. Emerg. Med.* 15(5): 447-500.

Lloyd TW (1961). Agranulocytosis associated with paracetamol. *Lancet* 1: 114-115.

Lorenz W, Doenicke A, Schoning B, Ohmann C, Grote B, Neugebauer E (1982). Definition and classification of the histamine-release response to drugs in anaesthesia and surgery: studies in the conscious human subject. *Klin. Wochenschr.* 60(17): 896-913.

Lynch RM, Robertson R (2004). Anaphylactoid reactions to intravenous N-acetylcysteine: a prospective case controlled study. *Accid. Emerg. Nurs.* 12(1): 10-15.

Makin AJ, Wendon J, Williams R (1995). A 7-year experience of severe acetaminophen-induced hepatotoxicity (1987-1993). *Gastroenterology* 109(6): 1907-1916.

Mant TG, Tempowski JH, Volans GN, Talbot JC (1984). Adverse reactions to acetylcysteine and effects of overdose. *Br. Med. J. (Clin. Res. Ed)* 289(6439): 217-219.

Masson MJ, Carpenter LD, Graf ML, Pohl LR (2008). Pathogenic role of natural killer T and natural killer cells in acetaminophen-induced liver injury in mice is dependent on the presence of dimethyl sulfoxide. *Hepatology* 48(3): 889-897.

Matthew H (1973). Acute acetaminophen poisoning. *Clin. Toxicol.* 6(1): 9-11.

Mazer M, Perrone J (2008). Acetaminophen-induced nephrotoxicity: pathophysiology, clinical manifestations, and management. *J. Med. Toxicol.* 4(1): 2-6.

McClain CJ, Kromhout JP, Peterson FJ, Holtzman JL (1980). Potentiation of acetaminophen hepatotoxicity by alcohol. *Jama* 244(3): 251-253.

McClain CJ, Price S, Barve S, Devalarja R, Shedlofsky S (1999). Acetaminophen hepatotoxicity: An update. *Curr. Gastroenterol. Rep.* 1(1): 42-49.

McLean AE (1974). Letter: Prevention of paracetamol poisoning. *Lancet* 1(7860): 729.

Meredith T, Jacobsen D, Haines J (1995). *Antidotes for poisoning by paracetamol*. edn. Cambridge University Press: Geneva.

Milei J, Ferreira R, Llesuy S, Forcada P, Covarrubias J, Boveris A (1992). Reduction of reperfusion injury with preoperative rapid intravenous infusion of taurine during myocardial revascularization. *Am. Heart J.* 123(2): 339-345.

Mills MO, Lee MG (2008). Acetaminophen overdose in Jamaica. *West Indian Med. J.* 57(2): 132-134.

Mitchell JR, Jollow DJ, Potter WZ, Davis DC, Gillette JR, Brodie BB (1973). Acetaminophen-induced hepatic necrosis. I. Role of drug metabolism. *J. Pharmacol. Exp. Ther.* 187(1): 185-194.

Mota I (1981). *Antigens: Fundamentals of immunology*. edn. Springer-Verlag: New York.

Mullins M, Froelke BR, Rivera MR (2009). Effect of delayed activated charcoal on acetaminophen concentration after simulated overdose of oxycodone and acetaminophen. *Clin. Toxicol. (Phila)* 47(2): 112-115.

Myers C, Bonow R, Palmeri S, Jenkins J, Corden B, Locker G, *et al.* (1983). A randomized controlled trial assessing the prevention of doxorubicin cardiomyopathy by N-acetylcysteine. *Semin. Oncol.* 10(1 Suppl 1): 53-55.

Myers RP, Li B, Fong A, Shaheen AA, Quan H (2007). Hospitalizations for acetaminophen overdose: a Canadian population-based study from 1995 to 2004. *BMC Public Health* 7: 143.

Myers RP, Shaheen AA, Li B, Dean S, Quan H (2008). Impact of liver disease, alcohol abuse, and unintentional ingestions on the outcomes of acetaminophen overdose. *Clin. Gastroenterol. Hepatol.* 6(8): 918-925; quiz 837.

Neeleman J, Wessely S (1997). Drugs taken in fatal and non-fatal self-poisoning: a study in south London. *Acta Psychiatr. Scand.* 95(4): 283-287.

Neuvonen PJ, Tokola O, Toivonen ML, Simell O (1985). Methionine in paracetamol tablets, a tool to reduce paracetamol toxicity. *Int. J. Clin. Pharmacol. Ther. Toxicol.* 23(9): 497-500.

Nguyen GC, Sam J, Thuluvath PJ (2008). Hepatitis C is a predictor of acute liver injury among hospitalizations for acetaminophen overdose in the United States: a nationwide analysis. *Hepatology* 48(4): 1336-1341.

Nielsen PT, Pfeiffer P (1996). Adverse reactions to N-acetylcysteine in Inuit to paracetamol (acetaminophen) overdose. *Arctic Med. Res.* 55(4): 204-205.

O'Grady JG, Alexander GJ, Hayllar KM, Williams R (1989). Early indicators of prognosis in fulminant hepatic failure. *Gastroenterology* 97(2): 439-445.

Olsson B, Johansson M, Gabrielsson J, Bolme P (1988). Pharmacokinetics and bioavailability of reduced and oxidized N-acetylcysteine. *Eur. J. Clin. Pharmacol.* 34(1): 77-82.

Ozer J, Ratner M, Shaw M, Bailey W, Schomaker S (2008). The current state of serum biomarkers of hepatotoxicity. *Toxicology* 245(3): 194-205.

Pakravan N, Waring WS, Sharma S, Ludlam C, Megson I, Bateman DN (2008). Risk factors and mechanisms of anaphylactoid reactions to acetylcysteine in acetaminophen overdose. *Clin. Toxicol. (Phila)* 46(8): 697-702.

Panush RS (1976). Effects of certain antirheumatic drugs on normal human peripheral blood lymphocytes. Inhibition of mitogen- and antigen-stimulated incorporation of tritiated thymidine. *Arthritis Rheum.* 19(5): 907-917.

Parker D, White JP, Paton D, Routledge PA (1990). Safety of late acetylcysteine treatment in paracetamol poisoning. *Hum. Exp. Toxicol.* 9(1): 25-27.

Pimstone BL, Uys CJ (1968). Liver necrosis and myocardiopathy following paracetamol overdosage. *S Afr. Med. J.* 42(11): 259-262.

Prescott L (1996). *Paracetamol (Acetaminophen):A critical bibliographic review*. edn. Taylor and Francis: London.

Prescott L (1979). Prevention of hepatic necrosis following paracetamol overdosage. *Health Bulletin* 36: 204-212.

Prescott LF (1978). The chief scientist reports ... prevention of hepatic necrosis following paracetamol overdosage. *Health Bull. (Edinb)* 36(4): 204-212.

Prescott LF (1983). Paracetamol overdosage. Pharmacological considerations and clinical management. *Drugs* 25(3): 290-314.

Prescott LF (2000). Paracetamol, alcohol and the liver. *Br. J. Clin. Pharmacol.* 49(4): 291-301.

Prescott LF, Donovan JW, Jarvie DR, Proudfoot AT (1989). The disposition and kinetics of intravenous N-acetylcysteine in patients with paracetamol overdosage. *Eur. J. Clin. Pharmacol.* 37(5): 501-506.

Prescott LF, Illingworth RN, Critchley JA, Stewart MJ, Adam RD, Proudfoot AT (1979). Intravenous N-acetylcystine: the treatment of choice for paracetamol poisoning. *Br. Med. J.* 2(6198): 1097-1100.

Prescott LF, Proudfoot AT, Cregeen RJ (1982). Paracetamol-induced acute renal failure in the absence of fulminant liver damage. *Br. Med. J. (Clin Res Ed)* 284(6313): 421-422.

Prescott LF, Roscoe P, Wright N, Brown SS (1971). Plasma-paracetamol half-life and hepatic necrosis in patients with paracetamol overdosage. *Lancet* 1(7698): 519-522.

Prescott LF, Wright N (1973). The effects of hepatic and renal damage on paracetamol metabolism and excretion following overdosage. A pharmacokinetic study. *Br. J. Pharmacol.* 49(4): 602-613.

Price VF, Miller MG, Jollow DJ (1987). Mechanisms of fasting-induced potentiation of acetaminophen hepatotoxicity in the rat. *Biochem. Pharmacol.* 36(4): 427-433.

Quigley N, Galloway R, Kelly C (1994). Changes in the pattern of deliberate self-poisoning presenting at Craigavon Area Hospital: 1976, 1986 and 1991. *Ulster Med. J.* 63(2): 155-161.

Ray SD, Mumaw VR, Raje RR, Fariss MW (1996). Protection of acetaminophen-induced hepatocellular apoptosis and necrosis by cholesteryl hemisuccinate pretreatment. *J. Pharmacol. Exp. Ther.* 279(3): 1470-1483.

Reed MD, Marx CM (1994). Ondansetron for treating nausea and vomiting in the poisoned patient. *Ann. Pharmacother.* 28(3): 331-333.

Ros SP, Conrad HA (1994). Baseline liver function tests following acetaminophen ingestion. What is the utility? *Clin. Pediatr. (Phila)* 33(9): 569-570.

Routledge P, Vale JA, Bateman DN, Johnston GD, Jones A, Judd A, *et al.* (1998). Paracetamol (acetaminophen) poisoning. No need to change current guidelines to accident departments. *Bmj* 317(7173): 1609-1610.

Rumack BH, Matthew H (1975). Acetaminophen poisoning and toxicity. *Pediatrics* 55(6): 871-876.

Rumack BH, Peterson RG (1978). Acetaminophen overdose: incidence, diagnosis, and management in 416 patients. *Pediatrics* 62(5 Pt 2 Suppl): 898-903.

Ruvalcaba RH, Limbeck GA, Kelley VC (1966). Acetaminophen and hypoglycemia. *Am. J. Dis. Child* 112(6): 558-560.

Salas VM, Corcoran GB (1997). Calcium-dependent DNA damage and adenosine 3',5'-cyclic monophosphate-independent glycogen phosphorylase activation in an in vitro model of acetaminophen-induced liver injury. *Hepatology* 25(6): 1432-1438.

Savino F, Lupica MM, Tarasco V, Locatelli E, Garazzino S, Tovo PA (2011). Fulminant hepatitis after 10 days of acetaminophen treatment at recommended dosage in an infant. *Pediatrics* 127(2): e494-497.

Scheffner A (1983). The reduction in vitro in viscosity of mucoprotein solutions by a new mucolytic agent NAC. *Ann. NY Acad. Sci.* 106: 298-310.

Schilling A, Corey R, Leonard M, Eghtesad B (2010). Acetaminophen: old drug, new warnings. *Cleve Clin. J. Med.* 77(1): 19-27.

Schiodt FV, Ott P, Christensen E, Bondesen S (2002). The value of plasma acetaminophen half-life in antidote-treated acetaminophen overdosage. *Clin. Pharmacol. Ther.* 71(4): 221-225.

Schmidt LE, Dalhoff K (2001). Risk factors in the development of adverse reactions to N-acetylcysteine in patients with paracetamol poisoning. *Br. J. Clin. Pharmacol.* 51(1): 87-91.

Schmidt LE, Dalhoff K (2002). Serum phosphate is an early predictor of outcome in severe acetaminophen-induced hepatotoxicity. *Hepatology* 36(3): 659-665.

Schwartz LB, Yunginger JW, Miller J, Bokhari R, Dull D (1989). Time course of appearance and disappearance of human mast cell tryptase in the circulation after anaphylaxis. *J. Clin. Invest.* 83(5): 1551-1555.

Seeff LB, Cuccherini BA, Zimmerman HJ, Adler E, Benjamin SB (1986). Acetaminophen hepatotoxicity in alcoholics. A therapeutic misadventure. *Ann. Intern. Med.* 104(3): 399-404.

Shalabi EA (1992). Acetaminophen inhibits the human polymorphonuclear leukocyte function in vitro. *Immunopharmacology* 24(1): 37-45.

Sheen CL, Dillon JF, Bateman DN, Simpson KJ, MacDonald TM (2002a). Paracetamol-related deaths in Scotland, 1994-2000. *Br. J. Clin. Pharmacol.* 54(4): 430-432.

Sheen CL, Dillon JF, Bateman DN, Simpson KJ, MacDonald TM (2002b). Paracetamol pack size restriction: the impact on paracetamol poisoning and the over-the-counter supply of paracetamol, aspirin and ibuprofen. *Pharmacoepidemiol. Drug Saf.* 11(4): 329-331.

Sherlock S, Dooley J (1993). *Diseases of the Liver and Biliary System.* 9th edn. Blackwell Scientific Publication.

Shi Q, Hong H, Senior J, Tong W (2010). Biomarkers for drug-induced liver injury. *Expert Rev. Gastroenterol. Hepatol.* 4(2): 225-234.

Shriner K, Goetz MB (1992). Severe hepatotoxicity in a patient receiving both acetaminophen and zidovudine. *Am. J. Med.* 93(1): 94-96.

Sibert JR, Craft AW, Jackson RH (1977). Child-resistant packaging and accidental child poisoning. *Lancet* 2(8032): 289-290.

Simpson KJ, Bates CM, Henderson NC, Wigmore SJ, Garden OJ, Lee A, *et al.* (2009). The utilization of liver transplantation in the management of acute liver failure: comparison between acetaminophen and non-acetaminophen etiologies. *Liver Transpl.* 15(6): 600-609.

Skoglund LA, Ingebrigtsen K, Nafstad I, Aalen O (1988). In vivo studies on toxic effects of concurrent administration of paracetamol and its N-acetyl-DL-methionine ester (SUR 2647 combination). *Gen. Pharmacol.* 19(2): 213-217.

Slattery JT, Levy G (1979). Acetaminophen kinetics in acutely poisoned patients. *Clin. Pharmacol. Ther.* 25(2): 184-195.

Smilkstein MJ, Bronstein AC, Linden C, Augenstein WL, Kulig KW, Rumack BH (1991). Acetaminophen overdose: a 48-hour intravenous N-acetylcysteine treatment protocol. *Ann. Emerg. Med.* 20(10): 1058-1063.

Smilkstein MJ, Douglas DR, Daya MR (1994). Acetaminophen poisoning and liver function. *N. Engl. J. Med.* 331(19): 1310-1311; author reply 1311-1312.

Smilkstein MJ, Knapp GL, Kulig KW, Rumack BH (1988). Efficacy of oral N-acetylcysteine in the treatment of acetaminophen overdose. Analysis of the national multicenter study (1976 to 1985). *N. Engl. J. Med.* 319(24): 1557-1562.

Smith JA, Hine ID, Beck P, Routledge PA (1986). Paracetamol toxicity: is enzyme induction important? *Hum. Toxicol.* 5(6): 383-385.

Smith L (2008). ACEP Policy on N-acetylcysteine for Acetaminophen
Overdose. *Am. Fam. Physician.* 77(10): 1464.

Smith SW, Howland MA, Hoffman RS, Nelson LS (2008). Acetaminophen overdose with altered acetaminophen pharmacokinetics and hepatotoxicity associated with premature cessation of intravenous N-acetylcysteine therapy. *Ann. Pharmacother.* 42(9): 1333-1339.

Spiller HA, Winter ML, Klein-Schwartz W, Bangh SA (2006). Efficacy of activated charcoal administered more than four hours after acetaminophen overdose. *J. Emerg. Med.* 30(1): 1-5.

Spooner J, Harvey J (1993). Paracetamol overdosage facts, not misconceptions. *Pharm. J.* 250: 706-707.

Sunman W, Hughes AD, Sever PS (1992). Anaphylactoid response to intravenous acetylcysteine. *Lancet* 339(8803): 1231-1232.

Sutter ME, Daily MF, Owen KP, Daubert GP, Albertson TE (2010). Multiple organ transplantation after suicide by acetaminophen and gunshot wound. *West J. Emerg. Med.* 11(5): 506-509.

Takeda J, Ueda E, Takahashi J, Fukushima K (1995). Plasma N-methylhistamine concentration as an indicator of histamine release by intravenous d-tubocurarine in humans: preliminary study in five patients by radioimmunoassay kits. *Anesth. Analg.* 80(5): 1015-1017.

Tee LB, Boobis AR, Huggett AC, Davies DS (1986a). Reversal of acetaminophen toxicity in isolated hamster hepatocytes by dithiothreitol. *Toxicol. Appl. Pharmacol.* 83(2): 294-314.

Tee LG, Boobis AR, Davies DS (1986b). N-acetylcysteine for paracetamol overdose. *Lancet* 1(8476): 331-332.

Tenenbein M (1984). Hypersensitivity-like reactions to N-acetylcysteine. *Vet. Hum. Toxicol.* 26 Suppl 2: 3-5.

Thummel KE, Slattery JT, Nelson SD, Lee CA, Pearson PG (1989). Effect of ethanol on hepatotoxicity of acetaminophen in mice and on reactive metabolite formation by mouse and human liver microsomes. *Toxicol. Appl. Pharmacol.* 100(3): 391-397.

Townsend E, Hawton K, Harriss L, Bale E, Bond A (2001). Substances used in deliberate self-poisoning 1985-1997: trends and associations with age, gender, repetition and suicide intent. *Soc. Psychiatry Psychiatr. Epidemiol.* 36(5): 228-234.

Tredger JM, Smith HM, Davis M, Williams R (1980). Effects of sulphur-containing compounds on paracetamol activation and covalent binding in a mouse hepatic microsomal system. *Toxicol. Lett.* 5(5): 339-344.

Trull A, Demers L, Holt D, Johnston A, Tredger J, Price C (2002). *Biomarkers of Disease: An evidence-based approach.* edn, vol. Cambridge University Press.

Vale JA (1997). Position statement: gastric lavage. American Academy of Clinical Toxicology; European Association of Poisons Centres and Clinical Toxicologists. *J. Toxicol. Clin. Toxicol.* 35(7): 711-719.

Wang EJ, Li Y, Lin M, Chen L, Stein AP, Reuhl KR, *et al.* (1996). Protective effects of garlic and related organosulfur compounds on acetaminophen-induced hepatotoxicity in mice. *Toxicol. Appl. Pharmacol.* 136(1): 146-154.

Wang GS, Monte A, Bagdure D, Heard K (2011). Hepatic failure despite early acetylcysteine following large acetaminophen-diphenhydramine overdose. *Pediatrics* 127(4): e1077-1080.

Wang K, Zhang S, Marzolf B, Troisch P, Brightman A, Hu Z, *et al.* (2009). Circulating microRNAs, potential biomarkers for drug-induced liver injury. *Proc. Natl. Acad. Sci. U S A* 106(11): 4402-4407.

Ward RJ, Francaux M, Cuisinier C, Sturbois X, De Witte P (1999). Changes in plasma taurine levels after different endurance events. *Amino Acids* 16(1): 71-77.

Wardle EN, Williams R (1981). Raised serum biliverdin in hepatic necrosis. *Biochem. Med.* 26(1): 8-11.

Waring WS, Jamie H, Leggett GE (2010). Delayed onset of acute renal failure after significant paracetamol overdose: A case series. *Hum. Exp. Toxicol.* 29(1): 63-68.

Waring WS, Stephen AF, Malkowska AM, Robinson OD (2008a). Acute ethanol coingestion confers a lower risk of hepatotoxicity after deliberate acetaminophen overdose. *Acad. Emerg. Med.* 15(1): 54-58.

Waring WS, Stephen AF, Robinson OD, Dow MA, Pettie JM (2008b). Lower incidence of anaphylactoid reactions to N-acetylcysteine in patients with high acetaminophen concentrations after overdose. *Clin. Toxicol. (Phila)* 46(6): 496-500.

Waterfield CJ, Turton JA, Scales MD, Timbrell JA (1991). Taurine, a possible urinary marker of liver damage: a study of taurine excretion in carbon tetrachloride-treated rats. *Arch. Toxicol.* 65(7): 548-555.

Waters E, Wang JH, Redmond HP, Wu QD, Kay E, Bouchier-Hayes D (2001). Role of taurine in preventing acetaminophen-induced hepatic injury in the rat. *Am. J. Physiol. Gastrointest. Liver Physiol.* 280(6): G1274-1279.

Weinstein CL, Haschemeyer RH, Griffith OW (1988). In vivo studies of cysteine metabolism. Use of D-cysteinesulfinate, a novel cysteinesulfinate decarboxylase inhibitor, to probe taurine and pyruvate synthesis. *J. Biol. Chem.* 263(32): 16568-16579.

Whyte IM, Buckley NA, Reith DM, Goodhew I, Seldon M, Dawson AH (2000). Acetaminophen causes an increased International Normalized Ratio by reducing functional factor VII. *Ther. Drug Monit.* 22(6): 742-748.

Williams R (1986). *Liver Failure.* edn. Churchill Livingstone Press.

Wittbrodt ET, Spinler SA (1994). Prevention of anaphylactoid reactions in high-risk patients receiving radiographic contrast media. *Ann. Pharmacother.* 28(2): 236-241.

Wrights N, Prescott LF (1973). Potentiation by previous drug therapy of hepatotoxicity following paracetamol overdosage. *Scott. Med. J.* 18(2): 56-58.

Yasunaga M, Matsuda S, Murata M (1985). Two cases of acute liver injury caused by ingesting small dose of acetaminophen. *Acta Hepatologica Japonica* 26: 493-499.

Yip L, Dart RC, Hurlbut KM (1998). Intravenous administration of oral N-acetylcysteine. *Crit. Care Med.* 26(1): 40-43.

Zed PJ, Krenzelok EP (1999). Treatment of acetaminophen overdose. *Am. J. Health Syst. Pharm.* 56(11): 1081-1091; quiz 1091-1083.

Zein JG, Wallace DJ, Kinasewitz G, Toubia N, Kakoulas C (2010). Early anion gap metabolic acidosis in acetaminophen overdose. *Am. J. Emerg. Med.* 28(7): 798-802.

Zwiener RJ, Kurt TL, Ghali F, Day LC, Timmons CF (1994). Potentiation of acetaminophen hepatotoxicity in a child with mercury poisoning. *J. Pediatr. Gastroenterol. Nutr.* 19(2): 242-245.

Zyoud SH, Awang R, Syed Sulaiman SA, Al-jabi SW (2010). High prevalence of hypokalemia after acute acetaminophen overdose: impact of psychiatric illness. *Hum. Exp. Toxicol.* 29(9): 773-778.

In: Acetaminophen: Properties, Clinical Uses
Editors: Atash Javaherian and Pasha Latifpour
ISBN: 978-1-61942-374-9

Chapter 6

ACETAMINOPHEN HEPATOTOXICITY AND POTENTIAL INTERACTIONS WITH DIETARY SUPPLEMENTS*

W. F. Salminen, X. Yang, Q. Shi and A. A. Ali
Food and Drug Administration, Jefferson, Arkansas, US

ABSTRACT

Acetaminophen (APAP) is the leading cause of drug-induced acute liver failure in the United States. At normal therapeutic doses, APAP is a safe drug when used by itself. Problems arise when multiple products containing APAP are used and the therapeutic dose is exceeded.

A recent US FDA Advisory Committee concluded that other factors such as ethnicity, genetics, and nutrition may also play a role in a person's susceptibility to APAP-induced liver injury. One nutrition factor that is likely to play a role is dietary supplements.

Dietary supplement use continues to rise and many consumers consider these products as inherently safe by themselves or in combination with other products, including drugs, since they are "natural".

However, the safety of most dietary supplements by themselves has not been adequately tested and even less data are available on potential drug – dietary supplement interactions. APAP is metabolized by the liver to a reactive metabolite, NAPQI, that causes a wide array of cellular effects such as depletion of cytoprotective molecules, covalent binding to cellular macromolecules, oxidative stress, and impaired mitochondrial function.

Dietary supplements that increase the metabolism of APAP are likely to increase the hepatotoxicity of APAP; whereas, those that decrease APAP metabolism are likely to provide protection. Dietary supplements that affect endpoints downstream of APAP metabolism could also either reduce or increase APAP hepatotoxicity depending on the magnitude and direction of the effect. This chapter reviews the key areas of potential interaction between APAP and dietary supplements and reviews the available data on specific dietary supplements.

---

* *Disclaimer*: This article is not an official guidance or policy statement of the US Food and Drug Administration (FDA). No official support or endorsement by the US FDA is intended or should be inferred.

INTRODUCTION

Acetaminophen (APAP) is a widely used over-the-counter analgesic and antipyretic in the United States. When used at recommended therapeutic doses, APAP is rarely associated with liver injury. Unfortunately, APAP can cause fatal acute liver failure when therapeutic doses are exceeded. This can occur when people purposely take an overdose or accidentally when people consume multiple products containing APAP. Due to this concern, a recent FDA Advisory Panel recommended lowering the maximum therapeutic dose of APAP[1] and this was followed by a Federal Register notice lowering the maximum APAP dose in prescription products[2]. The Committee also concluded that in addition to people unknowingly consuming multiple products containing APAP, some individuals may be especially sensitive to liver injury from APAP and that more research is needed to understand whether ethnicity, genetics, nutrition, or other factors might have a role in making some individuals more sensitive.

One factor that is likely to increase a person's sensitivity to APAP is the consumption of dietary supplements (DS). Some DS have various toxicological effects or alter the toxicity of concomitantly administered drugs[3-7]. Unfortunately, most drug-DS interactions are unknown or, at best, poorly characterized. A general misconception about DS is that they are safe since they are "natural." Potential adverse effects caused by DS are highlighted in a recent prospective clinical study of DILI, which identified that 9% of the cases were caused solely by DS and 18% of the cases by multiple agents, including DS[8].

The United States regulations covering the marketing of DS further magnifies the potential issue since, in contrast to drugs, DS do not require FDA approval of their safety[1] prior to marketing[9]. Instead, under the Dietary Supplement Health and Education Act of 1994 (DSHEA), the DS manufacturer is responsible for ensuring that a DS is safe before it is marketed. Unfortunately, when compared to drugs, limited safety data are typically generated for a given DS and they provide limited insight into the safety of the DS in humans. The FDA can take action against an unsafe DS after it has been marketed but at that point people will have been unnecessarily exposed to the unsafe product. DS sales have seen very strong growth in the US with many popular products exhibiting consistent double digit yearly growth[10-12]. The trend is expected to continue as US consumers continue to focus on what they consider safer "natural" alternative medicines. In correlation with the increased DS sales is an increase in individual consumption of DS with 42.1% of the US population using at least one DS in the past month during a 1988 – 1994 survey compared with 53.1% during 2001 – 2004[13]. As individual consumption of DS increases, the probability of experiencing adverse drug-DS interactions increases; therefore, it is important to identify any drug-DS interactions so that consumers can be informed of the risks.

A good example of the types of warnings that could help inform consumers is the warnings provided for the interaction of warfarin with various DS. Warfarin is an anticoagulant that has a very small therapeutic window. The US FDA drug label for warfarin (US FDA NDA 9-218/S-105) lists multiple DS that should be avoided when taking warfarin due to drug-DS interactions (e.g., garlic, Ginkgo biloba, ginseng, St. John's wort, coenzyme

---

[1] If a dietary supplement contains a "new dietary ingredient", then the "new dietary ingredient" requires FDA approval of safety prior to marketing. A "new dietary ingredient" is a dietary ingredient (e.g., vitamin, mineral, herb/botanical, amino acid) that was not sold in the US in a dietary supplement before October 15, 1994.

Q10). This information helps the physician and patient understand the risks some DS pose during warfarin therapy. Unfortunately, only a handful of drug-DS interactions have been clearly identified and more research is needed to understand the safety of DS in combination with drugs.

ACETAMINOPHEN HEPATOTOXICITY AND POTENTIAL POINTS OF INTERACTION WITH DIETARY SUPPLEMENTS

Due to the concern over APAP-induced liver injury, a tremendous amount of research has been conducted to understand the mechanisms behind the pathogenesis. The least controversial and most critical step is the metabolism of APAP. At therapeutic doses, APAP is predominantly metabolized by the Phase II metabolic pathways of glucuronidation and sulfation (Figure 1). A small portion of APAP is metabolized by the Phase I cytochrome P450 (CYP) metabolic pathway to the reactive metabolite N-acetyl-*p*-benzoquinone imine (NAPQI), which is subsequently detoxified by conjugation with glutathione (GSH)[14-15].

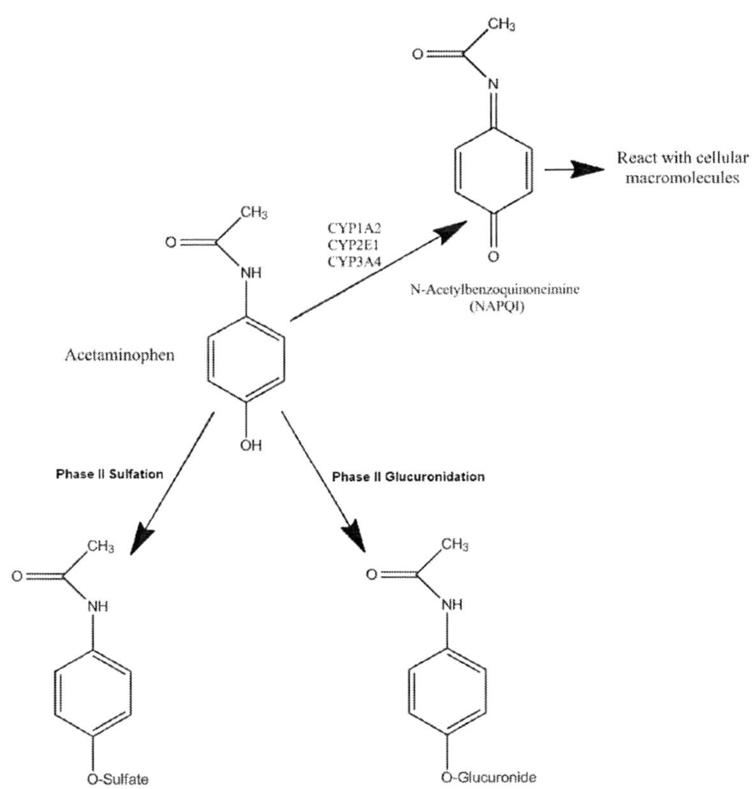

Figure 1. Hepatic metabolism of acetaminophen to the reactive metabolite NAPQI. At therapeutic doses, APAP is metabolized predominantly by the Phase II glucuronidation and sulfation pathways. A small percentage is metabolized by the Phase I CYP enzymes 1A2, 2E1, and 3A4. In overdose, the glucuronidation and sulfation pathways become saturated and a larger fraction of APAP is metabolized by the Phase I pathways to the reactive metabolite NAPQI. NAPQI is detoxified by conjugation with glutathione; however, hepatic glutathione levels are limited and once depleted below a certain threshold, NAPQI can covalently react with cellular macromolecules.

In overdose, the glucuronidation and sulfation pathways are overwhelmed and a larger portion of APAP is metabolized through the Phase I pathway. GSH levels are limited and once depleted below a critical level, NAPQI is free to react with cellular macromolecules. DS that alter the Phase I or Phase II metabolism of APAP could either increase or decrease the toxicity of APAP. If a DS decreases Phase II glucuronidation or sulfation, more APAP will be metabolized via the Phase I pathway and hepatotoxicity is likely to increase. If a DS decreases Phase I metabolism, such as through inhibition of one of the key CYPs responsible for APAP metabolism (i.e., CYP 1A2, 2E1, or 3A4), hepatotoxicity is likely to decrease[5]. Another potential mechanism that may play a role in decreasing APAP hepatotoxicity is if a DS directly scavenges NAPQI, similar to the role of GSH. Lastly, if a DS itself decreases GSH levels, it will likely increase APAP hepatotoxicity; whereas, ones that increase GSH levels or other parts of the GSH system (e.g., glutathione-S-transferase enzymes) will decrease APAP hepatotoxicity.

After formation of significant quantities of NAPQI, the subsequent pathways leading to cellular injury have been extensively investigated but their contribution to the actual pathogenesis are more tentative[15-16]. Based on the weight of evidence, APAP binds various proteins, disrupts their function, leading to altered cellular function. However, there are likely to be other direct or indirect effects of NAPQI leading to cell death, such as alteration of cellular redox status or disruption of signaling pathways. Despite the wide array of cellular pathways that have been shown to play a role in APAP-induced hepatotoxicity, it is clear that disruption of mitochondrial function is one of the key outcomes[17-19]. After covalent binding and GSH depletion occur, APAP induces the mitochondrial permeability transition (MPT), which allows the leakage of mitochondrial constituents into the cytosol. Following activation of the MPT, mitochondria swell, lose membrane potential, and exhibit decreased oxidative phosphorylation with subsequent ATP depletion and necrotic cell death. DS may increase or decrease APAP hepatotoxicity if they alter one or more of these many toxicity pathways by themselves. For example, a DS that decreases mitochondrial function (e.g., uncoupling of oxidative phosphorylation by a compound such as usnic acid) is likely to increase APAP-induced mitochondrial effects and subsequent hepatotoxicity.

Another consideration when assessing APAP-DS interactions is the temporal relationship between the APAP and DS doses. A DS may be consumed as a single dose or chronically as repeated doses. The DS may be consumed before, concurrently with, or after the APAP dose. The temporal differences may lead to differential interactions between APAP and the DS. For example, we have found that when green tea extract is administered prior to the APAP dose in mice, either 2 h or once daily for 3 days before the APAP dose, green tea provides protection against APAP hepatotoxicity. This protection is most likely due to decreased APAP metabolism via green tea-induced CYP inhibition. In contrast, if green tea is administered 6 h after the APAP dose, a significant increase in hepatotoxicity is observed. The mechanism of the potentiation is probably due to glutathione depletion by green tea extract and prolonged maintenance of an oxidizing environment in the liver. Administering a glutathione depleting chemical after the initial APAP insult probably prevents the liver from recovering and propagates the injury. The inhibition of CYP metabolism by green tea at this later timepoint would not be a factor since metabolism and covalent binding of APAP are essentially complete within the first couple of hours after the APAP dose[20].

Since most DS, especially herbal preparations, are a complex mixture of many compounds, it is difficult to predict how a given DS will interact with the many pathways leading to APAP hepatotoxicity. It is possible that one compound will alter a pathway that increases APAP hepatotoxicity but another compound alters a pathway that decreases APAP hepatotoxicity and the ultimate balance depends on the importance of each pathway. Also, if one pathway is a prerequisite for initiation of a subsequent pathway, this will also dictate the role each DS component plays. This highlights the difficulty with predicting toxicity of not only the DS itself, but how it will interact with APAP.

Complicating matters further is that for a given DS, there are often many different types of preparations. The plant, which may be the leaves, stems, roots, seeds, flowers, or a combination of these, may be processed (e.g., dried and ground) into a DS. Alternatively, an extract of the plant may be used in the DS. Different extraction solvents (e.g., hot water or ethanolic) produce different chemical constituent profiles. Even if the same extraction solvent is used, chemical constituent profiles are unlikely to be the same between manufacturers since they use different extraction protocols (e.g., temperature or duration of extraction might be different). Another factor complicating DS assessment is the fact that plants are often sourced from different locations and grown under varying conditions (e.g., time of year, soil condition, hydration status). Even if a DS is sourced from the same location, it has been shown that growing condition variations lead to high batch to batch variability of the botanical chemical constituents[10]. All of the above factors contribute to the difficulty of predicting how a given DS will interact with APAP. One approach to reducing the uncertainty imposed by these factors is to test the single chemical entity representing the active ingredient in the DS. Unfortunately, for most DS, especially herbals, multiple potential active ingredients are present. Even if the active ingredient(s) is known, other chemical constituents may exhibit toxicological effects even if they do not contribute to the efficacy of the supplement. Since people are exposed to all of the various chemical constituents when they consume a botanical-derived DS and not just the active ingredient(s), it is important to test the DS that people are exposed to unless data clearly show that a specific chemical constituent is responsible for the toxicity. Testing individual components can be informative, but it may not provide a complete picture of the potential interactions that may occur with the other components in the DS and APAP.

Dietary Supplement Interactions with APAP

The following sections review the data that are available on the interaction of APAP with various DS. The focus is on those DS that have been shown to have clear interactions with APAP based on preclinical studies or clinical case reports. Some DS are highlighted, even if data on the interaction with APAP are not available, simply because they have been associated with liver injury. For each supplement, a brief introduction about its common use is provided; however, it is important to remember that many of these efficacy claims are only theoretical and not based on robust clinical trials. Another point to keep in mind is that the dose makes the poison. APAP is a perfect example of this. At low therapeutic doses, APAP is a very safe drug. When the dose is increased and the threshold of toxicity is exceeded, APAP can cause severe liver injury. Other compounds, such as DS, follow this same paradigm. Therefore, just because a DS might be inherently unsafe, if it is consumed at a sufficiently low dose, it will not cause harm. The concern with combining APAP with potentially harmful

DS is that the threshold for APAP hepatotoxicity may be lowered and a previously safe dose of APAP now becomes hepatotoxic (Figure 2).

Black Cohosh

Black cohosh (*Cimicifuga racemosa*) is a wildflower native to eastern North America. The roots of the plant are the commonly used part. Black cohosh is commonly taken for the relief of symptoms associated with menopause including hot flashes, depression, mood swings, headaches, sleep disorders, heart palpitations, vaginal dryness, and night sweats. The main active constituents are thought to be triterpene glycosides.

Black cohosh has been associated with cases of liver injury; however, the association is far from conclusive [21-24]. No data are available on the interaction of black cohosh with APAP. One study found that various metabolites produced by incubating black cohosh with rat microsomes (the major metabolic enzymes of the liver) could react with glutathione[25]. However, glutathione-based metabolites were not detected in the urine from women taking black cohosh. These results indicate that one or more black cohosh metabolites might react with and deplete glutathione in the liver and could potentiate APAP hepatotoxicity; however, this is mostly theoretical.

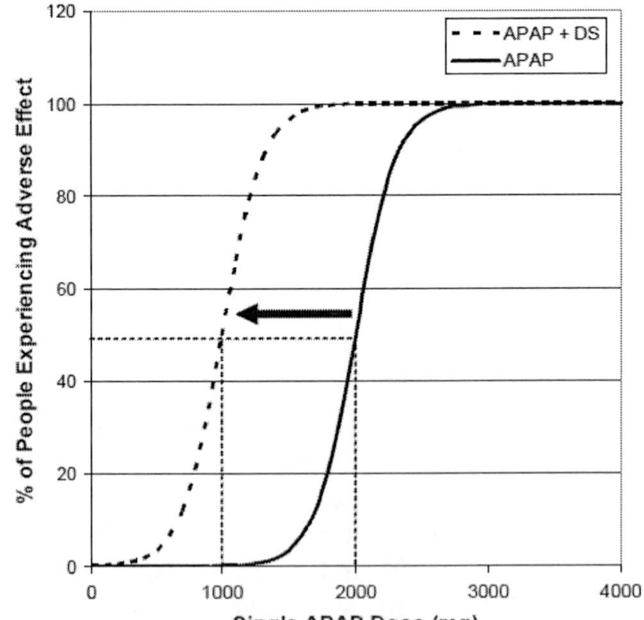

Figure 2. Shifting of the APAP dose response curve by a dietary supplement. A dietary supplement administered before, during, or after the APAP dose may increase the toxicity of APAP and shift the APAP dose response curve to the left. The indicated doses and responses are for demonstration purposes only and should not be taken as true indicators of the APAP dose response in people.

Chaparral

Chaparral (*Larrea tridentata*), also known as creosote bush and greasewood, is an evergreen desert shrub that is used for a variety of ailments such as the common cold, bone and muscle pain, "blood purifying", liver tonic, skin disorders, among others. Chaparral has been associated with clinical cases of hepatotoxicity[4, 26-30]. Due to the potential for chaparral to injure the liver, or at least lower its threshold for other hepatotoxicant insults, APAP should be used with caution in combination with chaparral.

Dong Quai

Dong Quai (*Angelica sinensis*), also known as Dong Gui and female ginseng, is widely used in Chinese traditional medicine to treat gynecological ailments, fatigue, mild anemia and high blood pressure.

Studies

A polysaccharides-enriched fraction from the root of *Angelica sinensis* was orally administered to mice at 25, 50 or 75 mg/kg 6 h and 1 h before the APAP dose (700 mg/kg orally)[31]. The two high doses reduced liver toxicity induced by APAP based on serum alanine-aminotransferase (ALT) activity, hepatic glutathione levels, and liver histopathology.

Assessment

Based on data from a single animal study, it appears that dong quai may have protective effects against APAP-induced hepatotoxicity; however, these limited results should be extrapolated to human use with caution.

Echinacea

Echinacea is a flower native to North America. Echinacea extracts are used for treating and preventing colds, flu and other infections, liver cancer, colon cancer, and stimulating the immune system. There are three different species (*purpurea, angustifolia,* and *pallida*), which contain various concentrations of active compounds in different parts of each plant.

Certain species contain pyrrolizidine alkaloids, which can cause liver toxicity by depleting glutathione[3]. Since glutathione is essential in detoxifying NAPQI produced from APAP metabolism, any concomitant treatment that decrease glutathione levels has the potential to increase APAP hepatotoxicity. Therefore, Echinacea should be used with caution when combined with APAP.

Garlic

Garlic (*Allium sativum)* is a widely used food ingredient. It is commonly used for cardiovascular disease prevention (e.g., reducing serum cholesterol and triglycerides, inhibiting platelet aggregation, antiatherosclerotic, and lowering blood pressure), preventing infections as a broad-spectrum antibiotic, and a chemopreventive and anticancer agent. Garlic contains many sulfur-containing compounds that are believed to be the active ingredients, such as alliin, allicin, S-allylcysteine, S-methylcysteine, and many others.

Studies

Fresh garlic homogenate (5 g/kg orally) administered to mice 2 h before or immediately after APAP (200 mg/kg orally) prevented hepatotoxicity based on serum ALT and lactate dehydrogenase activity and histopathology[32]. A lower dose of garlic (0.5 g/kg) provided partial protection. Garlic inhibited APAP-induced glutathione depletion and the formation of APAP-oxidized metabolites. Several garlic-derived organosulfur compounds and structurally-related compounds were further tested in their ability to reduce APAP hepatotoxicity. It was found that an S-allyl structure was a common feature for most sulfides to inhibit CYP 2E1 activity and provide protection against APAP.

Garlic oil (100, 200, or 500 mg/kg via intraperitoneal injection) administered to mice immediately before an oral dose of APAP (500 mg/kg followed 1 h later by another 500 mg/kg dose orally) provided various degrees of protection against APAP-induced hepatotoxicity based on serum ALT and aspartate-aminotransferase (AST) activity and liver histopathology[33]. When administered 1 h after the APAP dose, garlic oil provided less protection.

In primary rat hepatocytes, garlic extract reduced APAP-induced glutathione depletion and reactive oxygen formation when exposed to the cells 30 minutes before, at the same time, or 30 minutes after APAP addition[34].

In a clinical study, 16 male nonsmoker subjects ingested daily doses of garlic extract (approximately equivalent to 6 to 7 cloves of garlic) for 3 months[35]. A 1 g oral dose of acetaminophen was given to each subject before the start of garlic treatment, at the end of each month, and 1 month after termination of garlic administration. Plasma and urine analysis found no discernible effect on oxidative metabolism of APAP. However, there was a slight increase in sulfate conjugation of APAP.

Various individual components of garlic have been tested for their hepatoprotective effects against APAP-induced injury. One component of garlic, diallyl sulfide, is an inhibitor of CYP 2E1, which is one of the main CYPs responsible for metabolizing APAP to the reactive NAPQI. Various studies have shown that diallyl sulfide, or its metabolites (e.g., diallyl sulfone), can reduce APAP-induced hepatotoxicity in mice and rats when administered prior to, at the same time, or shortly after the APAP dose [36-39]. Ajoene is a garlic-derived sulfur-containing compound. Ajoene reduced indices of APAP-induced hepatocellular injury, such as glutathione depletion and serum glutamic-pyruvic transaminase activity, when administered orally 2 and 24 h prior to the APAP dose (300 mg/kg orally) in mice[40]. *S*-allylmercaptocysteine is a water-soluble organosulfer compound found in ethanol extracts of garlic. When administered to mice at 100 mg/kg orally 2 and 24 h before a single APAP dose (500 mg/kg orally), *S*-allylmercaptocysteine reduced APAP hepatotoxicity based on plasma ALT and glutathione levels[41]. In a follow-up study, a single dose of *S*-allylmercaptocysteine (200 mg/kg orally) administered to mice 0.5 h after APAP administration (500 mg/kg orally) reduced APAP hepatotoxicity based on plasma ALT, liver histopathology, and mortality[42]. As with other garlic-derived sulfur compounds, CYP 2E1 activity was suppressed in both studies.

Assessment

Overall, these results clearly show that at high doses, garlic and one or more of its individual components has the capacity to inhibit CYP metabolism of APAP and decrease its hepatotoxicity, at least in animal and *in vitro* models. Since the protection is mediated by inhibition of CYP activity, garlic needs to be administered prior to, at the same time, or immediately after the APAP dose in order to have a significant affect on the metabolism. Therefore, garlic is unlikely to provide therapeutic benefit in APAP overdose situations where the patient is treated hours after the initial ingestion.

Ginkgo Biloba

Ginkgo biloba is believed to be the world's oldest living tree species. Various parts of the ginkgo tree have been used in traditional Chinese medicine; however, modern ginkgo extracts are typically produced from the leaves.

Ginkgo is commonly taken for improving memory and mental sharpness, alleviating symptoms of Alzheimer's disease, relieving depression, and as an antioxidant. The main active constituents are ginkgo flavone glycosides and terpene lactones.

Studies

In an *in vivo* study using mice, animals were administered a single intraperitoneal injection of 900 mg/kg APAP followed by a single dose of 50 mg/kg *Ginkgo* extract[43]. The actual time elapsed between the APAP and *Ginkgo* doses was not clearly stated in the report. The *Ginkgo* extract reduced APAP hepatotoxicity based on serum ALT and AST levels and liver histopathology. The *Ginkgo* treatment also attenuated APAP-induced glutathione depletion and other indicators of adverse liver effects. In an *in vitro* study using primary rat hepatocytes, *Ginkgo biloba* extract potentiated APAP cytotoxicity[44]. The *Ginkgo* extract was incubated with the hepatocytes for 48 h prior to APAP exposure. The potentiation was found to be a result of increased APAP metabolism by CYP 3A enzymes, which were induced by the *Ginkgo* pre-treatment. Assessment of the different constituents of the extract identified ginkgolide A as being responsible for the induction of CYP 3A.

Assessment

These conflicting results might be explained by the timing of the different exposures. *Ginkgo* was administered to animals after the APAP dose, presumably within several minutes, whereas, cells were incubated with the extract for several days prior to the APAP exposure. When administered right after the APAP dose, the *Ginkgo's* antioxidant properties might have scavenged NAPQI, similar to glutathione, or could have decreased the resulting APAP-induced oxidant damage.

However, when administered for several days prior to APAP exposure *in vitro*, *Ginkgo* had sufficient time to induce CYP 3A and in turn result in increased NAPQI formation once APAP was added to the cultures. The difference in the results could also be due to the different test systems and/or differences in the extracts that were tested. Regardless, these results warrant caution when using *Ginkgo* with acetaminophen, especially if the *Ginkgo* is consumed chronically.

Ginseng

Ginseng (*Panax ginseng*) is also known as "true" ginseng. Other forms of ginseng that are commonly included in this group are Siberian ginseng (*Eleutherococcus senticosus*) and American ginseng (*Panax quinquefolium*). Typical indications include beneficial effects on the central nervous system, protection from stress, antifatigue, enhancement of sexual function, and acceleration of metabolism.

Studies

Total saponins of *Panax japonicus* and *Panax notoginseng* (both contain a variety of ginsenosides) were administered to mice once daily for three days at 50 mg/kg via subcutaneous injection[45]. Between 1 and 12 h after the last dose, APAP (500 mg/kg via intraperitoneal injection) was administered as a single dose. Both saponin preparations reduced APAP hepatotoxicity based on serum ALT and liver histopathology.

Assessment

Based on data from a single animal study, it appears that ginseng may have protective effects against APAP-induced hepatotoxicity; however, these results should be extrapolated to human use with caution.

Green Tea

Green tea (*Camellia sinensis*) is the second most consumed beverage in the world behind water. Green tea is prepared by picking, lightly steaming the leaves, and allowing them to dry. Black tea is made by allowing the leaves to ferment before drying.

The active compounds in green tea are a family of polyphenols (catechins) with antioxidant activity. Tannins, large polyphenol molecules, form the bulk of the active compounds in green tea, with catechins making up nearly 90% of that.

Several catechins predominate such as epicatechin, epigallocatechin, epicatechin gallate, and epigallocatechin gallate. Typical uses of green tea are as an anticancer agent, general antioxidant, reducing cholesterol and triglycerides, enhancing immune function, and weight loss.

Studies

Several clinical case reports have indicated that high doses of green tea may induce liver toxicity[46-48]. In addition, various animal studies have shown that green tea and its components can induce liver toxicity. Liver necrosis was observed in mice and rats administered green tea extract once daily for 14 weeks at up to 1000 mg/kg (orally)[49]. A single dose of (-)-epigallocatechin-3-gallate (an active component of green tea) at 1500 mg/kg (orally) increased plasma ALT activity, induced liver necrosis, and reduced survival[50].

In our laboratory, we have observed increased serum ALT and AST and liver histopathology changes, including liver necrosis, after single doses of green tea extract (1500 and 2000 mg/kg orally). Normal consumption of green tea beverages are unlikely to provide a dose sufficient to reach hepatotoxic levels; however, some of the concentrated extracts might either produce toxicity by themselves or compromise the defenses of the liver and make it more susceptible to other hepatotoxic agents.

A nutrient mixture containing green tea extract was administered to mice via feed (0.5% of weight) for two weeks[51]. APAP (600 mg/kg via intraperitoneal injection) was then administered (the time between the last nutrient mixture exposure and APAP dose was not specified).The nutrient mixture reduced APAP hepatotoxicity based on serum ALT, AST, and alkaline phosphatase activities and liver histopathology. Green tea polyphenols were administered to mice via the diet at 1% (by weight) for five days[52]. The mice were than administered a single dose of APAP (750 mg/kg via intraperitoneal injection); however, the time between the last green tea administration and the APAP dose was not indicated. Green tea polyphenols attenuated APAP hepatotoxicity based on serum ALT activity, glutathione and S-adenosylmethionine depletion, and liver histopathology. In a follow-up study, green tea polyphenols were administered to mice via the diet at 0.25% (by weight)[53]. Green tea polyphenols were found to normalize cyclooxygenase 2 and B-cell lymphoma-2 activation.

In our laboratory, we have found that the temporal relationship between green tea extract exposure and the APAP dose is critical for determining if green tea provides protection or enhances APAP hepatotoxicity. When administered 3 h prior to the APAP dose (150 or 300 mg/kg orally) or once daily for 3 days followed by an APAP dose 24 h later, green tea (500 or 1000 mg/kg orally) provided protection against APAP hepatotoxicity in mice based on serum ALT and AST activity and liver histopathology. In contrast, when green tea extract was administered 6 h after the APAP dose, green tea significantly enhanced APAP hepatotoxicity. Work is ongoing to elucidate the mechanisms behind the differential effects.

Assessment

Since green tea itself is hepatotoxic, caution should be exercised when taking concentrated green tea extracts with APAP. Although some reports have suggested using green tea extract as a therapy for APAP overdose, our data show that the timing of the green tea dose relative to APAP is critical in determining the type of interaction (i.e., synergistic vs. antagonistic). Since we have shown that administering green tea extract after the APAP dose enhances hepatotoxicity, it is unlikely that green tea extract would be beneficial after someone has overdosed on APAP and it is likely to make the hepatotoxicity worse.

Kava

Kava (*Piper methysticum*) is a plant traditionally used by Pacific islanders as a ceremonial intoxicant to help people relax and socialize. More recent claims of commercial preparations are alleviating anxiety, promoting relaxation, aiding sleep, balancing mood, relieving depression, easing symptoms of menopause, and a headache remedy. The active ingredients are kavalactones which act as mild central nervous system depressants.

Kava has been associated with clinical cases of liver injury [4, 54-56].Due to this concern, in 2002, the US Food and Drug Administration (FDA) issued a consumer advisory of the potential risk of liver injury associated with the use of kava[57].

Studies

In our laboratory, we have shown that non-cytotoxic concentrations of kava potentiated APAP cytotoxicity in primary rat hepatocytes[58]. Cells were exposed to the kava and APAP at the same time. The synergistic interaction was due to a combination of kava inducing glutathione depletion and increasing APAP-induced mitochondrial dysfunction.

In whole animal studies, we have observed that kava also potentiates APAP hepatotoxicity in mice based on increased serum ALT and AST levels and liver histopathology.

In contrast to green tea, this synergistic interaction occurred when kava (2000 mg/kg orally) was administered before (once daily for 3 days) or 6 h after the APAP (150 or 300 mg/kg orally) dose.

Assessment

Since kava itself has been associated with clinical cases of hepatotoxicity, it should not be used in combination with APAP. The *in vitro* and *in vivo* data showing that kava can potentiate APAP-induced hepatotoxicity further support this conclusion.

Licorice

Licorice (*Glycyrrhiza uralensis* and *Glycyrrhiza glabra*) is one of the most widely used herbs in Asian medicine. This herb should not be confused with some "licorice" confectionary products that are often flavored with anise. Licorice is used for chronic fatigue, constipation, cough, hepatoprotection against toxicity, herpes, inflammation, ulcers, among many others. Glycyrrhizin is one of the key constituents of licorice.

Studies

Glycyrrhizin (25 mg/kg orally) was administered to mice once daily for 7 days[59]. The animals were than administered APAP (500 mg/kg via intraperitoneal injection); however, the time between the last DS dose and APAP was not specified. APAP-induced hepatotoxicity was decreased by glycyrrhizin based on hepatic glutathione levels and mortality. In a novel *in vitro* model system using gel-entrapped primary rat hepatocytes, licorice extract and glycyrrhizic acid reduced APAP-induced cytotoxicity[60]. In this study, glycyrrhizic acid and APAP were exposed to the cells at the same time. In another *in vitro* study, fractioned extracts of *Glycyrrhiza glabra* decreased APAP-induced cytotoxicity in primary rat hepatocytes[61].

In a rat metabolism study, administration of a *Glycyrrhiza glabra* extract (1 g/kg orally) for 6 days significantly increased the cumulative biliary and urinary excretions of the APAP-glucuronide conjugate after APAP (150 mg/kg via intravenous injection) administration[62]. The level of thioether and sulfate conjugates was not affected. Further analysis found that both the extract and glycyrrhizin (23 mg/kg orally) increased the specific activity of UDP-glucuronosyltransferase (UGT) 1A and increased the concentration of UDP-glucuronic acid.

Assessment

Licorice and one of the main constituents, glycyrrhizic acid, appear to have protective effects against APAP. This protective effect may be through increased glucuronidation.

However, the data are not substantial enough to advocate using licorice as a therapeutic for preventing APAP hepatotoxicity.

Methionine, S-Adenosylmethionine (SAMe)

Methionine is a thiol-containing essential amino acid. It can be enzymatically converted into SAMe, which in turn can be converted into cysteine. Both methionine and SAMe have been approved as prescription drugs in some countries.

In the U.S., only methionine, but not SAMe, is approved by the FDA as a prescription drug. However, SAMe is widely consumed as a food supplement in the U.S.

Studies

Orally administered methionine (50~300 mg/kg) has long been recognized to be protective against APAP hepatotoxicity in rats [63]. Intramuscular injected methionine (7.5 mg/kg) and SAMe (10~20 mg/kg) showed similar protective effects in rats [64].

In mice, which are more sensitive to APAP hepatotoxicity, methionine and SAMe decreased APAP-induced liver injury, even when administered after apparent injury occurred. The protective effects were similar to [65] or even more potent than the standard antidote N-acetyl cysteine [66, 67]. These beneficial effects were also observed in the hamster [68]. The proposed mechanisms for methionine and SAMe in reducing APAP hepatotoxicity include (1) they act as precursors of intracellular glutathione [68, 69], (2) they decrease the covalent binding of APAP to microsomal proteins [64], (3) they prevent mitochondrial dysfunction induced by APAP [70], and/or (4) they reduce the lipid peroxidation after APAP challenge [71].

Assessment

Methionine and SAMe appear to be protective against APAP hepatotoxicity in animal models, but the mechanism(s) awaits further investigation. Previous mechanistic studies are incomplete and a definitive pathway for protection has not been elucidated. Robust clinical trial data are needed to translate these promising animal study results into clinical use.

Mushrooms

Most commercially-available mushrooms pose very little risk to the consumer whether consumed alone or with APAP. However, some wild mushrooms are extremely hepatotoxic. Of the 5000 species of mushrooms, fewer than 100 are poisonous to humans and less than 10 of these are deadly[29]. Extreme caution should be exercised when consuming wild mushrooms by themselves or in combination with APAP.

N-Acetyl Cysteine and Glutathione

N-acetyl cysteine (NAC) is available as a dietary supplement and is used for a variety of different indications such as an antioxidant, supporting the immune system, and a liver protectant. NAC, available as Acetadote (FDA Drug Label NDA 21-539/S-004), is an FDA-approved treatment for APAP overdose.

It is administered via intravenous injection and has the greatest efficacy when administered within 8 – 10 h after an overdose. Efficacy declines when administered after this timeframe; however, it does not appear to worsen APAP-induced hepatotoxicity during this time. NAC most likely protects the liver by maintaining or restoring glutathione levels or by acting as an alternate substrate for conjugation with and thus detoxification of NAPQI. NAC is not without adverse effects since it can cause serious anaphylactoid reactions in a significant number of patients.

Treatment of APAP overdose with NAC should be done by medical professionals using the FDA-approved drug and route of administration instead of an orally-administered form of NAC.

Glutathione within hepatocytes plays a critical role in detoxifying NAPQI. Glutathione is available as a dietary supplement and is used for a variety of different indications such as an antioxidant and aiding cellular function.

Theoretically, administering glutathione would increase glutathione levels and help detoxify APAP; however, any orally-administered glutathione that is absorbed into the blood stream in intact form is not taken up by cells[72]. Instead, glutathione has to be broken down into its individual amino acids and those are taken up by the cells of the liver[73]. Therefore, orally-administered glutathione is not recommended for preventing or reducing APAP-induced hepatotoxicity since NAC is a better alternative.

Niacin (Vitamin B_3)

Niacin, also known as vitamin B_3 and nicotinic acid, is a commonly used water-soluble vitamin. Niacin is hepatotoxic at high doses [74, 75]; therefore, APAP should be used with caution in combination with high dose niacin supplementation.

Skullcap

Skullcap (*Scutellaria lateriflora*) is a native North American perennial herb. It is used as an anti-inflammatory, antispasmodic, astringent, and sedative. Skullcap has been associated with clinical cases of liver injury[4, 76]; therefore, concomitant use with APAP is not recommended.

Usnic Acid

Usnic acid is found is several lichen species, such as *Usnea*. Usnic acid is used as an anti-infective, analgesic, anti-inflammatory, and weight loss aid. Usnic acid has been associated with clinical cases of liver injury[54, 77-79]. Based on research conducted at the US FDA National Center for Toxicological Research, usnic acid appears to be an uncoupler of oxidative phosphorylation and in turn damages mitochondria. Since toxic doses of APAP lead to mitochondrial damage and this is believed to be one of the mechanisms leading to hepatocellular injury, APAP should not be used in combination with usnic acid.

Vitamin A

Vitamin A is a commonly used fat soluble vitamin. Vitamin A is hepatotoxic at high doses [75, 80]; therefore, APAP should be used with caution in combination with high dose vitamin A supplementation. In addition, a variety of animal studies have shown that retinol, a form of vitamin A, potentiates APAP toxicity[81-84].

Vitamin C

Vitamin C is a well-know anti-oxidant. This makes it a reasonable candidate to prevent APAP hepatotoxicity, because oxidative stress is a key mechanism for injury. Indeed, early studies showed that vitamin C was able to decrease APAP hepatotoxicity in a mouse model [85]. However, this effect is critically dependent on the salt forms of vitamin C. Specifically, neither the free acid of vitamin C nor its sodium form is effective [85], but both ascorbyl palmitate [85-87] and ascorbyl stearate [88, 89] are able to reduce APAP hepatotoxicity. The protective effect of vitamin C esters is likely due to (1) they can reduce the toxic metabolite of APAP back to its parent form [88] or (2) they can promote the regeneration of the hepatic glutathione [89]. Confirmatory studies are needed to strengthen these preliminary findings.

Other DS and Combination Products

A variety of studies have assessed the interaction of different DS with APAP. Most of these studies have observed a protective effect; however, the data are limited for each DS and more studies are needed before any conclusions can be made about the role each DS may play in reducing APAP hepatotoxicity. Table 1 summarizes the studies for these different DS.

Conclusions

From the review of the available literature and theoretical considerations of the mechanisms of APAP hepatotoxicity, it remains a difficult task of predicting how a DS will interact with APAP. Further complicating matters is that DS are typically complex mixtures and even for a single type of DS, the spectrum of compounds are likely to change between preparations/batches. Since each compound may have differential affects on APAP hepatotoxicity, variations in composition may result in differential interactions with APAP. Fortunately, when used at recommended therapeutic doses, APAP is a safe drug. Problems arise when people take multiple products containing APAP and the threshold of toxicity is

Table 1. Summary of interactions between APAP and other dietary supplements

Compound	Effect	Dietary Supplement Dose	APAP dose	Model	Responses	References
Alpha-lipoic acid	Protect	Pretreatment (1h before APAP), 100 mg/kg (single), 25 mg/kg (7-day), oral	Oral, Single (2.5 g/kg) and 7-day (750 mg/kg)	Rats	Inhibited NO overproduction and maintained the intracellular antioxidant (GSH) status in liver and kidney.	[90]
	Potentiate	Pretreatment (daily for 15 weeks), 150 mg/kg, diet	Oral, Single (90.5mg/kg)	Cats	Potentiated APAP induced liver toxicity based on oxidant damage and hepatic glutathione levels.	[91]
Alpha-tocopherol	Protect	Pretreatment (12h before APAP), 20 mg/kg, IP	IP, Single (400 mg/kg)	Mice	Reduced APAP induced liver toxicity based on ALT.	[92]
	Protect	Pre- or co-incubation, 50 μM	N/A	Rat hepatocytes	Prevented DNA damage, no effect on cytoxicity.	[93]
Ayurvedic medicine: HD-03[a]	Protect	Pretreatment (daily for 14-days), 750 mg/kg, oral	IP, Single (2 g/kg)	Rats	Reduced APAP induced liver toxicity based on ALT, AST, and hepatic glutathione levels.	[94]
Ayurvedic medicine: polyherbal formulations[b]	Protect	Posttreatment (daily for 7 days), 5.2 ml/kg, oral	Oral, Single (500 mg/kg)	Mice	Reduced APAP induced liver toxicity based on ALT, AST, and liver histopathology.	[95]
Boerhaavia diffusa	Protect	Pretreatment (daily for 7-days), 100 -400 mg/kg, oral	Oral, Single (1.5 g/kg)	Rats	Reduced APAP induced liver toxicity based on ALT, AST and lipid peroxidation.	[96]
C. vitellinum	Protect	Co-incubation, 1 mg/ml, 24h	N/A	Rat liver slices	Prevented APAP-induced ATP depletion and histopathological changes	[97]
Carnosine	Protect	Pretreatment (daily for 4 weeks), 2 g/L,drinking water	IP, Single (350 mg/kg)	Mice	Reduced APAP induced liver toxicity based on ALT, AST, hepatic glutathione levels, and lipid peroxidation. Inhibited CYP2E1.	[98]
CI-1, protein purify from Cajanus indicus	Protect	Posttreatment (daily for 7 days), 100 g/ml, IP	IP, Single (300-500 mg/kg)	Mice	Reduced APAP induced liver toxicity based on decreased mitochondrial damage analyzed by electron micrograph.	[99]
Coenzyme Q10	Protect	Pretreatment (12h before APAP), 5 mg/kg, IP	IP, Single (400 mg/kg)	Mice	Reduced APAP induced liver toxicity based on plasma ALT.	[92]
Curcumin	Protect	Posttreatment (daily for 7 days), 50 and 100 mg/kg, oral	Oral, Single (100mg/kg)	Mice	Reduced APAP induced liver toxicity based on ALT, AST, lipid peroxidation, and liver histopathology.	[100]

Compound	Effect	Dietary Supplement Dose	APAP dose	Model	Responses	References
Cuscuta chinensis (nanoparticle formulation)	Protect	Pretreatment (daily for 7 days), 25-50 mg/kg,oral	IP, Single (835 mg/kg)	Rats	Reduced APAP induced liver toxicity based on ALT, AST, liver histopathology, and lipid peroxidation.	[101]
Ellagic acid	Protect	Posttreatment (daily for 7 days), 50,100 mg/kg, oral	Oral, Single (100 mg/kg)	Mice	Reduced APAP induced liver toxicity based on ALT, AST, lipid peroxidation, and liver histopathology.	[100]
Fulvotoment osides	Protect	Pretreatment (daily for 3-days), 150 mg/kg, oral	IP, Single (500 mg/kg)	Mice	Reduced APAP induced liver toxicity based on ALT,and liver histopathology.	[45]
Gentiana manshurica Kitagawa (GM)	Protect	Pretreatment (2h before APAP), 200 mg/kg,oral	IP, Single (300 mg/kg)	Mice	Reduced APAP induced liver toxicity based on ALT, AST, hepatic glutathione levels, and liver histopathology.	[102]
Gomisin A	Protect	Pretreatment (1h before APAP), 50 mg/kg, ip	Oral, Single (750 mg/kg)	Rats	Reduced APAP induced liver toxicity based on ALT, AST, and hepatic glutathione levels.	[103]
Histidine	Protect	Pretreatment (daily for 4 weeks), 2 g/L,drinking water	IP, Single (350 mg/kg)	Mice	Reduced APAP induced liver toxicity based on ALT, AST, hepatic glutathione levels, and lipid peroxidation. Inhibited CYP2E1.	[98]
L-carnitine	Protect	Pretreatment (daily for 5 days), 500 mg/kg,IP	IP, Single (500 mg/kg)	Mice	Reduced APAP induced liver toxicity based on ALT, AST, hepatic glutathione levels, and liver histopathology.	[104]
Melatonin	Protect	Pretreatment (30 minutes), 10 mg/kg, IP	IP, Single (900 mg/kg)	Mice	Reduced APAP induced toxicity based on liver and kidney serum biomarkers.	[105]
Moutan Cortex	Protect	Pretreatment (daily for 14 days), 200-400 mg/kg,oral	IP, Single (400 mg/kg)	Mice	Attenuated GSH depletion and DNA damage, inhibited CYP2E1 activity.	[106]
Nutrient mixture (NM)[c]	Protect	Pretreatment (2 weeks), diet	IP, Single (600 mg/kg)	Mice	Reduced APAP induced toxicity based on liver and kidney serum biomarkers.	[51]
O. lamiifolium	Protect	Co-incubation, 1 mg/ml, 24h	N/A	Rat liver slices	Prevented APAP-induced ATP depletion and histopathological changes	[97]
Oleanolic acid	Protect	Pretreatment (daily for 3-days), 100 mg/kg, oral	IP, Single (500 mg/kg)	Mice	Reduced APAP induced liver toxicity based on ALT and liver histopathology.	[45]

Table 1. (Continued)

Compound	Effect	Dietary Supplement Dose	APAP dose	Model	Responses	References
Oxymatrine	Protect	Pretreatment (daily for 3-days), 150 mg/kg, oral	IP, Single (500 mg/kg)	Mice	Reduced APAP induced liver toxicity based on ALT and liver histopathology.	[45]
P. japonicus[d]	Protect	Pretreatment (daily for 3-days), 50 mg/kg, oral	IP, Single (500 mg/kg)	Mice	Reduced APAP induced liver toxicity based on ALT and liver histopathology.	[45]
P. notoginseng[e]	Protect	Pretreatment (daily for 3-days), 50 mg/kg, oral	IP, Single (500 mg/kg)	Mice	Reduced APAP induced liver toxicity based on ALT and liver histopathology.	[45]
Phytochemical-nutraceutical mixture (PNM)	Protect	Pretreatment (daily for 4 weeks) 5.7mg per mouse, diet	IP, Single (400 mg/kg)	Mice	Reduced animal mortality, ALT, decrease genomic DNA fragmentation.	[107]
Picroliv	Protect	Posttreatment (daily for 7 days), 50 and 100 mg/kg, oral	Oral, Single (100 mg/kg)	Mice	Reduced APAP induced liver toxicity based on ALT, AST, lipid peroxidation, and liver histopathology.	[100]
Premna tomentosa (L. Verbenaceae)	Protect	Pretreatment (daily for 15 days), 750 mg/kg, oral	IP, Single (640 mg/kg)	Rats	Reduced APAP induced liver toxicity based on decreased lipid oxidation.	[108]
Proanthocyanidins (Grape Seeds)	Protect	Pretreatment (daily 3-days or 7-days), 100 mg/kg, oral	IP, Single (400 mg/kg)	Mice	Reduced animal mortality and liver damage based on serum ALT, DNA damage and histopathology. Inhibit CYP2E1 in mice.	[109]
Probiotic Enterococcus lactis	Protect	Pretreatment (daily for 7-days), 107 -109 units, oral	Oral, 14-day, 1 g/kg	Rats	Restored GSH and other antioxidants, inhibited apoptosis, prevent DNA damage.	[110]
Probiotic Enterococcus lactis [e]	Protect	Pre-, Co-, Post-incubation, 20 µg LAB_{SN} /5 µg silymarin	N/A	Rat hepatocytes	Pre/Co-treatment restored GSH, inhibited apoptosis, prevented mitochondrial and DNA damage, and reduced cytotoxicity.	[111]
Silibin	Protect	Pre or co-incubation, 25 µM	N/A	Rat hepatocytes	Prevented DNA damage, no effect on cytoxicity.	[93]
Silymarin	Protect	Posttreatment (daily for 7 days), 50 and 100 mg/kg, oral	Oral, Single (100 mg/kg)	Mice	Reduced APAP induced liver toxicity based on ALT, AST, lipid peroxidation, hepatic glutathione levels and liver histopathology.	[100]
Syringic acid	Protect	Pretreatment (daily for 6-days), 25-100 mg/kg, oral	IP, Single (750 mg/kg)	Rats	Reduced ALT, AST, ALP, GGT, lipid peroxidation and histopathological damage. Restored antioxidants, including GSH.	[112]

Compound	Effect	Dietary Supplement Dose	APAP dose	Model	Responses	References
Ulva reticulata	Protect	Pretreatment (daily for 15 days), 150 mg/kg, IP	IP, Single (800 mg/kg)	Rats	Reduced ALT, AST, ALP, GGT, lipid peroxidation and histopathological damage. Restored antioxidants, including GSH.	[113]
Vitamin C	Protect	Pretreatment (daily for 7-days), 500 mg/kg, oral	Oral, 14-day, 1 g/kg	Rats	Restored GSH and other antioxidants, inhibited apoptosis, prevented DNA damage.	[110]
Vitamin E	Protect	Pretreatment (30 minutes), 30m g/kg, IP	IP, Single (900 mg/kg)	Mice	Reduced APAP induced toxicity based on liver and kidney serum biomarkers.	[105]
Vitamin E and cysteine	Protect	Pretreatment (daily for 15 weeks),2,200 U/kg (vitamin E), 9.5 g/kg (cysteine), diet	Oral, Single (90.5 mg/kg)	Cats	Reduced APAP induced liver toxicity based on oxidant damage and hepatic glutathione levels.	[91]

Note: a polyherbal formulation_HD-03: Solanum nigrum L.(Solanaceae; whole plant, 30%), Cichorium intybus L. (Compositae; seeds, 20%), Picrorrhiza kurroa Benth. (Scrophulariaceae; roots, 20%), Tephrosia purpurea L. (Papilionaceae; whole plant, 20%) and Andrographis paniculata Nees. (Acanthaceae;Leaves, 10%). b Liv 52, Livergen, Livokin, Octogen, Stimuliv, and Tefroliv; c Nutrient mixture contains: vitamin C (as ascorbic acid and as Mg, Ca, and palmitate ascorbate) 700 mg; L-lysine 1000 mg; L-proline 750 mg; L-arginine 500 mg; N-acetyl cysteine 200 mg; standardized green tea extract (80% polyphenol) 1000 mg; selenium 30 μg;copper 2 mg; manganese 1 mg; d Total saponins of P. japonicus contains ginsengnosides and oleanolate saponin; e Total saponins of P. notoginseng contains ginsengnosides and notogensenosides; e Probiotic Enterococcus lactis IITRHR1 (ElSN) and Lactobacillus acidophilus MTCC447 (LaSN)

exceeded. Problems may also arise if a DS lowers the threshold of toxicity (shifts the toxicity curve to the left- see Figure 2) and a previously safe therapeutic dose now becomes hepatotoxic. A DS may also protect against APAP hepatotoxicity; however, given the availability of the clinically-effective antidote NAC, the role of DS in preventing APAP appears less critical. Also, unless a DS has undergone clinical trails to assess its efficacy in preventing or lessening APAP hepatotoxicity, it is best to use proven therapies and adhere to APAP dosing instructions to prevent APAP hepatotoxicity.

REFERENCES

[1] US-FDA. Joint Meeting of the Drug Safety and Risk Management Advisory Committee with the Anesthetic and Life Support Drugs Advisory Committee and the Nonprescription Drugs Advisory Committee (June 29-30, 2009). Meeting background information, presentations, and minutes/voting results. 2009 [cited; Available from: http://www.fda.gov/AdvisoryCommittees/Calendar/ucm143083.htm.

[2] US-FDA, Prescription drug products containing acetaminophen; actions to reduce liver injury from unintentional overdose. Vol. 76. 2011: Federal Register. 2691-2697.

[3] Abebe, W., Herbal medication: potential for adverse interactions with analgesic drugs. *J. Clin. Pharm. Ther*, 2002. 27(6): p. 391-401.

[4] Estes, J.D., et al., High prevalence of potentially hepatotoxic herbal supplement use in patients with fulminant hepatic failure. *Arch. Surg*, 2003. 138(8): p. 852-8.

[5] Zhou, S.F., et al., Metabolic activation of herbal and dietary constituents and its clinical and toxicological implications: an update. *Curr. Drug Metab*, 2007. 8(6): p. 526-53.

[6] Dara, L., J. Hewett, and J.K. Lim, Hydroxycut hepatotoxicity: a case series and review of liver toxicity from herbal weight loss supplements. *World J. Gastroenterol*, 2008. 14(45): p. 6999-7004.

[7] Guo, L., et al., Analysis of gene expression changes of drug metabolizing enzymes in the livers of F344 rats following oral treatment with kava extract. *Food Chem. Toxicol*, 2009. 47(2): p. 433-42.

[8] Chalasani, N., et al., Causes, clinical features, and outcomes from a prospective study of drug-induced liver injury in the United States. *Gastroenterology*, 2008. 135(6): p. 1924-34, 1934 e1-4.

[9] US-FDA. Overview of Dietary Supplements. 2009 10/14/2009 [cited 2009 11/16/2009].

[10] Talbott, S. and R. Wildman, A guide to understanding dietary supplements: magic bullets or modern snake oil? 1 ed. 2003, Binghamton, NY: The Haworth Press, Inc.

[11] Dennehy, C.E., The use of herbs and dietary supplements in gynecology: an evidence-based review. *J. Midwifery Womens Health*, 2006. 51(6): p. 402-9.

[12] Thurston, C. Dietary Supplements: The Latest Trends and Issues. [Web Page Article] 2009 [cited 2009 11/24/2009]; Article on Dietary Supplement Consumption Figures and Trends.].

[13] US-DHHS-CDCP-NCHS, Health, United States, 2008. Table 99 (Dietary supplement use among persons 20 years of age and over, by selected characteristics: United States, 1988-1994 and 2001-2004). 2008. p. 370.

[14] Bessems, J.G. and N.P. Vermeulen, Paracetamol (acetaminophen)-induced toxicity: molecular and biochemical mechanisms, analogues and protective approaches. *Crit. Rev. Toxicol*, 2001. 31(1): p. 55-138.

[15] Hinson, J.A., D.W. Roberts, and L.P. James, Mechanisms of acetaminophen-induced liver necrosis. *Handb. Exp. Pharmacol*, 2010(196): p. 369-405.

[16] Jaeschke, H., Role of inflammation in the mechanism of acetaminophen-induced hepatotoxicity. *Expert Opin. Drug Metab. Toxicol*, 2005. 1(3): p. 389-97.

[17] Hanawa, N., et al., Role of JNK translocation to mitochondria leading to inhibition of mitochondria bioenergetics in acetaminophen-induced liver injury. *J. Biol. Chem*, 2008. 283(20): p. 13565-77.

[18] Masubuchi, Y., C. Suda, and T. Horie, Involvement of mitochondrial permeability transition in acetaminophen-induced liver injury in mice. *J. Hepatol*, 2005. 42(1): p. 110-6.

[19] Burke, A.S., L.A. MacMillan-Crow, and J.A. Hinson, Reactive nitrogen species in acetaminophen-induced mitochondrial damage and toxicity in mouse hepatocytes. *Chem. Res. Toxicol*, 2010. 23(7): p. 1286-92.

[20] Roberts, D.W., et al., Immunohistochemical localization and quantification of the 3-(cystein-S-yl)-acetaminophen protein adduct in acetaminophen hepatotoxicity. *Am. J. Pathol*, 1991. 138(2): p. 359-71.

[21] Mahady, G.B., et al., United States Pharmacopeia review of the black cohosh case reports of hepatotoxicity. *Menopause*, 2008. 15(4 Pt 1): p. 628-38.

[22] Firenzuoli, F., L. Gori, and P.R. di Sarsina, Black Cohosh Hepatic Safety: Follow-Up of 107 Patients Consuming a Special Cimicifuga racemosa rhizome Herbal Extract and Review of Literature. *Evid Based Complement Alternat Med*, 2011. 2011: p. 821392.

[23] Teschke, R., et al., Black cohosh hepatotoxicity: quantitative causality evaluation in nine suspected cases. *Menopause*, 2009. 16(5): p. 956-65.

[24] Teschke, R., et al., Suspected black cohosh hepatotoxicity--challenges and pitfalls of causality assessment. *Maturitas*, 2009. 63(4): p. 302-14.

[25] Johnson, B.M. and R.B. van Breemen, In vitro formation of quinoid metabolites of the dietary supplement Cimicifuga racemosa (black cohosh). *Chem. Res. Toxicol,* 2003. 16(7): p. 838-46.

[26] Batchelor, W.B., J. Heathcote, and I.R. Wanless, Chaparral-induced hepatic injury. *Am. J. Gastroenterol*, 1995. 90(5): p. 831-3.

[27] Sheikh, N.M., R.M. Philen, and L.A. Love, Chaparral-associated hepatotoxicity. *Arch. Intern Med*, 1997. 157(8): p. 913-9.

[28] Alderman, S., et al., Cholestatic hepatitis after ingestion of chaparral leaf: confirmation by endoscopic retrograde cholangiopancreatography and liver biopsy. *J. Clin. Gastroenterol*, 1994. 19(3): p. 242-7.

[29] Stickel, F., G. Egerer, and H.K. Seitz, Hepatotoxicity of botanicals. *Public Health Nutr*, 2000. 3(2): p. 113-24.

[30] Katz, M. and F. Saibil, Herbal hepatitis: subacute hepatic necrosis secondary to chaparral leaf. *J. Clin. Gastroenterol*, 1990. 12(2): p. 203-6.

[31] Ye, Y.N., et al., Protective effect of polysaccharides-enriched fraction from Angelica sinensis on hepatic injury. *Life Sci*, 2001. 69(6): p. 637-46.

[32] Wang, E.J., et al., Protective effects of garlic and related organosulfur compounds on acetaminophen-induced hepatotoxicity in mice. *Toxicol. Appl. Pharmacol*, 1996. 136(1): p. 146-54.

[33] Kalantari, H. and M. Salehi, The protective effect of garlic oil on hepatotoxicity induced by acetaminophen in mice and comparison with N-acetylcysteine. *Saudi Med. J,* 2001. 22(12): p. 1080-4.

[34] Anoush, M., et al., The protective effects of garlic extract against acetaminophen-induced oxidative stress and glutathione depletion. *Pak. J. Biol. Sci*, 2009. 12(10): p. 765-71.

[35] Gwilt, P.R., et al., The effect of garlic extract on human metabolism of acetaminophen. *Cancer Epidemiol. Biomarkers Prev*, 1994. 3(2): p. 155-60.

[36] Zhao, C. and H. Shichi, Prevention of acetaminophen-induced cataract by a combination of diallyl disulfide and N-acetylcysteine. *J. Ocul. Pharmacol. Ther,* 1998. 14(4): p. 345-55.

[37] Salminen, W.F., Jr., R. Voellmy, and S.M. Roberts, Effect of N-acetylcysteine on heat shock protein induction by acetaminophen in mouse liver. *J. Pharmacol. Exp. Ther*, 1998. 286(1): p. 519-24.

[38] Lin, M.C., et al., Protective effect of diallyl sulfone against acetaminophen-induced hepatotoxicity in mice. *J. Biochem. Toxicol*, 1996. 11(1): p. 11-20.
[39] Hu, J.J., et al., Protective effects of diallyl sulfide on acetaminophen-induced toxicities. *Food Chem. Toxicol*, 1996. 34(10): p. 963-9.
[40] Hattori, A., et al., Protective effect of ajoene on acetaminophen-induced hepatic injury in mice. *Biosci. Biotechnol. Biochem*, 2001. 65(11): p. 2555-7.
[41] Sumioka, I., et al., Mechanisms of protection by S-allylmercaptocysteine against acetaminophen-induced liver injury in mice. *Jpn. J. Pharmacol*, 1998. 78(2): p. 199-207.
[42] Sumioka, I., T. Matsura, and K. Yamada, Therapeutic effect of S-allylmercaptocysteine on acetaminophen-induced liver injury in mice. *Eur. J. Pharmacol*, 2001. 433(2-3): p. 177-85.
[43] Sener, G., et al., Protective effects of ginkgo biloba against acetaminophen-induced toxicity in mice. *Mol. Cell Biochem*, 2006. 283(1-2): p. 39-45.
[44] Rajaraman, G., J. Chen, and T.K. Chang, Ginkgolide A contributes to the potentiation of acetaminophen toxicity by Ginkgo biloba extract in primary cultures of rat hepatocytes. *Toxicol. Appl. Pharmacol*, 2006. 217(2): p. 225-33.
[45] Liu, J., Y. Liu, and C.D. Klaassen, The effect of Chinese hepatoprotective medicines on experimental liver injury in mice. *J. Ethnopharmacol*, 1994. 42(3): p. 183-91.
[46] Sarma, D.N., et al., Safety of green tea extracts : a systematic review by the US Pharmacopeia. *Drug Saf*, 2008. 31(6): p. 469-84.
[47] Mazzanti, G., et al., Hepatotoxicity from green tea: a review of the literature and two unpublished cases. *Eur. J. Clin. Pharmacol*, 2009. 65(4): p. 331-41.
[48] Verhelst, X., et al., Acute hepatitis after treatment for hair loss with oral green tea extracts (Camellia Sinensis). *Acta Gastroenterol. Belg*, 2009. 72(2): p. 262-4.
[49] Chan, P.C., et al., Fourteen-week toxicity study of green tea extract in rats and mice. *Toxicol. Pathol*, 2010. 38(7): p. 1070-84.
[50] Lambert, J.D., et al., Hepatotoxicity of high oral dose (-)-epigallocatechin-3-gallate in mice. *Food Chem. Toxicol*, 2010. 48(1): p. 409-16.
[51] Roomi, M.W., et al., A nutrient mixture prevents acetaminophen hepatic and renal toxicity in ICR mice. *Hum. Exp. Toxicol*, 2008. 27(3): p. 223-30.
[52] Oz, H.S., et al., Diverse antioxidants protect against acetaminophen hepatotoxicity. *J. Biochem. Mol. Toxicol*, 2004. 18(6): p. 361-8.
[53] Oz, H.S. and T.S. Chen, Green-tea polyphenols downregulate cyclooxygenase and Bcl-2 activity in acetaminophen-induced hepatotoxicity. *Dig. Dis. Sci*, 2008. 53(11): p. 2980-8.
[54] Chitturi, S. and G.C. Farrell, Hepatotoxic slimming aids and other herbal hepatotoxins. *J. Gastroenterol. Hepatol*, 2008. 23(3): p. 366-73.
[55] Teschke, R., Kava hepatotoxicity--a clinical review. *Ann. Hepatol*, 2010. 9(3): p. 251-65.
[56] Wooltorton, E., Brief safety updates: acetaminophen, ASA and kava. *CMAJ*, 2002. 167(9): p. 1034.
[57] US-FDA. Consumer Advisory: Kava-Containing Dietary Supplements May be Associated With Severe Liver Injury. March 25, 2002 [cited 2011 08-11-2011]; Available from: http://www.fda.gov/Food/Resources ForYou/Consumers/ucm085482.htm.

[58] Yang, X. and W.F. Salminen, Kava extract, an herbal alternative for anxiety relief, potentiates acetaminophen-induced cytotoxicity in rat hepatic cells. *Phytomedicine*, 2011. 18(7): p. 592-600.

[59] Wan, X.Y., et al., Hepatoprotective and anti-hepatocarcinogenic effects of glycyrrhizin and matrine. *Chem. Biol. Interact*, 2009. 181(1): p. 15-9.

[60] Shen, C., et al., Acetaminophen-induced hepatotoxicity of gel entrapped rat hepatocytes in hollow fibers. *Chem. Biol. Interact*, 2006. 162(1): p. 53-61.

[61] Nakagiri, R., H. Oda, and T. Kamiya, Small scale rat hepatocyte primary culture with applications for screening hepatoprotective substances. *Biosci. Biotechnol. Biochem*, 2003. 67(8): p. 1629-35.

[62] Moon, A. and S.H. Kim, Effect of Glycyrrhiza glabra roots and glycyrrhizin on the glucuronidation in rats. *Planta Med*, 1997. 63(2): p. 115-9.

[63] McLean, A.E. and P.A. Day, The effect of diet on the toxicity of paracetamol and the safety of paracetamol-methionine mixtures. *Biochem. Pharmacol*, 1975. 24(1): p. 37-42.

[64] Stramentinoli, G., C. Pezzoli, and M. Galli-Kienle, Protective role of S-adenosyl-l-methionine against acetaminophen induced mortality and hepatotoxicity in mice. *Biochem. Pharmacol*, 1979. 28(24): p. 3567-71.

[65] Carrasco, R., et al., Effect of different doses of S-adenosyl-L-methionine on paracetamol hepatotoxicity in a mouse model. *Methods Find. Exp. Clin. Pharmacol*, 2000. 22(10): p. 737-40.

[66] Terneus, M.V., et al., Comparison of S-Adenosyl-L-methionine and N-acetylcysteine protective effects on acetaminophen hepatic toxicity. *J. Pharmacol. Exp. Ther*, 2007. 320(1): p. 99-107.

[67] Terneus, M.V., et al., Comparison of S-adenosyl-L-methionine (SAMe) and N-acetylcysteine (NAC) protective effects on hepatic damage when administered after acetaminophen overdose. *Toxicology*, 2008. 244(1): p. 25-34.

[68] Pratt, S. and C. Ioannides, Mechanism of the protective action of n-acetylcysteine and methionine against paracetamol toxicity in the hamster. *Arch. Toxicol*, 1985. 57(3): p. 173-7.

[69] Miners, J.O., R. Drew, and D.J. Birkett, Mechanism of action of paracetamol protective agents in mice in vivo. *Biochem. Pharmacol*, 1984. 33(19): p. 2995-3000.

[70] Song, Z., C.J. McClain, and T. Chen, S-Adenosylmethionine protects against acetaminophen-induced hepatotoxicity in mice. *Pharmacology*, 2004. 71(4): p. 199-208.

[71] Valentovic, M., et al., S-Adenosylmethionine (SAMe) attenuates acetaminophen hepatotoxicity in C57BL/6 mice. *Toxicol. Lett*, 2004. 154(3): p. 165-74.

[72] Hahn, R., A. Wendel, and L. Flohe, The fate of extracellular glutathione in the rat. *Biochim. Biophys. Acta*, 1978. 539(3): p. 324-37.

[73] Vina, J., et al., Effect of oral glutathione on hepatic glutathione levels in rats and mice. *Br. J. Nutr*, 1989. 62(3): p. 683-91.

[74] Stargrove, M.B., J.T. Treasure, and D.L. McKee, Vitamine B3 (Niacin), in Herb, Nutrient, and Drug Interactions, M.B. Stargrove, J.T. Treasure, and D.L. McKee, Editors. 2008, Mosby Elsevier: St. Louis. p. 281 - 305.

[75] Riley, T.R., 3rd and A.M. Bhatti, Preventive strategies in chronic liver disease: part I. Alcohol, vaccines, toxic medications and supplements, diet and exercise. *Am. Fam. Physician*, 2001. 64(9): p. 1555-60.

[76] Linnebur, S.A., O.C. Rapacchietta, and M. Vejar, Hepatotoxicity associated with chinese skullcap contained in Move Free Advanced dietary supplement: two case reports and review of the literature. *Pharmacotherapy*, 2010. 30(7): p. 750, 258e-262e.

[77] Sanchez, W., et al., Severe hepatotoxicity associated with use of a dietary supplement containing usnic acid. *Mayo Clin. Proc*, 2006. 81(4): p. 541-4.

[78] Yellapu, R.K., et al., Acute liver failure caused by 'fat burners' and dietary supplements: a case report and literature review. *Can. J. Gastroenterol*, 2011. 25(3): p. 157-60.

[79] Durazo, F.A., et al., Fulminant liver failure due to usnic acid for weight loss. *Am. J. Gastroenterol*, 2004. 99(5): p. 950-2.

[80] Stargrove, M.B., J.T. Treasure, and D.L. McKee, Vitamine A (Retinol), in Herb, Nutrient, and Drug Interactions, M.B. Stargrove, J.T. Treasure, and D.L. McKee, Editors. 2008, Mosby Elsevier: St. Louis. p. 235 - 252.

[81] Bray, B.J. and R.J. Rosengren, Retinol potentiates acetaminophen-induced hepatotoxicity in the mouse: mechanistic studies. *Toxicol. Appl. Pharmacol*, 2001. 173(3): p. 129-36.

[82] Bray, B.J., et al., The effect of retinol on hepatic and renal drug-metabolising enzymes. *Food Chem. Toxicol*, 2001. 39(1): p. 1-9.

[83] Rosengren, R.J., et al., The interactions between retinol and five different hepatotoxicants in the Swiss Webster mouse. *Fundam. Appl. Toxicol*, 1995. 25(2): p. 281-92.

[84] elSisi, A.E., et al., Characterization of vitamin A potentiation of carbon tetrachloride-induced liver injury. *Toxicol. Appl. Pharmacol*, 1993. 119(2): p. 280-8.

[85] Hargreaves, R.J., et al., Studies on the effects of L-ascorbic acid on acetaminophen-induced hepatotoxicity. II. An in vivo assessment in mice of the protection afforded by various dosage forms of ascorbate. *Toxicol. Appl. Pharmacol*, 1982. 64(3): p. 380-92.

[86] Jonker, D., et al., Comparison of the effects of ascorbyl palmitate and L-ascorbic acid on paracetamol-induced hepatotoxicity in the mouse. *Toxicology*, 1988. 52(3): p. 287-95.

[87] Madhu, C., Z. Gregus, and C.D. Klaassen, Biliary excretion of acetaminophen-glutathione as an index of toxic activation of acetaminophen: effect of chemicals that alter acetaminophen hepatotoxicity. *J. Pharmacol. Exp. Ther*, 1989. 248(3): p. 1069-77.

[88] Mitra, A., et al., Influence of ascorbic acid esters on acetaminophen-induced hepatotoxicity in mice. *Toxicol. Lett*, 1988. 44(1-2): p. 39-46.

[89] Mitra, A., et al., Effect of ascorbic acid esters on hepatic glutathione levels in mice treated with a hepatotoxic dose of acetaminophen. *J. Biochem. Toxicol*, 1991. 6(2): p. 93-100.

[90] Abdel-Zaher, A.O., et al., The potential protective role of alpha-lipoic acid against acetaminophen-induced hepatic and renal damage. *Toxicology*, 2008. 243(3): p. 261-70.

[91] Hill, A.S., et al., Effects of dietary antioxidant supplementation before and after oral acetaminophen challenge in cats. *Am. J. Vet. Res*, 2005. 66(2): p. 196-204.

[92] Amimoto, T., et al., Acetaminophen-induced hepatic injury in mice: the role of lipid peroxidation and effects of pretreatment with coenzyme Q10 and alpha-tocopherol. *Free Radic. Biol. Med*, 1995. 19(2): p. 169-76.

[93] Lewerenz, V., et al., Antioxidants protect primary rat hepatocyte cultures against acetaminophen-induced DNA strand breaks but not against acetaminophen-induced cytotoxicity. *Toxicology*, 2003. 191(2-3): p. 179-87.

[94] Mitra, S.K., et al., Protective effect of HD-03, a herbal formulation, against various hepatotoxic agents in rats. *J. Ethnopharmacol*, 1998. 63(3): p. 181-6.

[95] Girish, C., et al., Hepatoprotective activity of six polyherbal formulations in paracetamol induced liver toxicity in mice. *Indian J. Med. Res*, 2009. 129(5): p. 569-78.

[96] Olaleye, M.T., et al., Antioxidant activity and hepatoprotective property of leaf extracts of Boerhaavia diffusa Linn against acetaminophen-induced liver damage in rats. *Food Chem. Toxicol*, 2010. 48(8-9): p. 2200-5.

[97] Mukazayire, M.J., et al., Evaluation of the hepatotoxic and hepatoprotective effect of Rwandese herbal drugs on in vivo (guinea pigs barbiturate-induced sleeping time) and in vitro (rat precision-cut liver slices, PCLS) models. *Exp. Toxicol. Pathol*, 2010. 62(3): p. 289-99.

[98] Yan, S.L., et al., Protective effects from carnosine and histidine on acetaminophen-induced liver injury. *J. Food Sci*, 2009. 74(8): p. H259-65.

[99] Datta, S. and P. Bhattacharyya, Effect of a herbal protein CI-1, purified from Cajanus indicus on the ultrastructural study of hepatocytes, in models of liver failure in mice. *J. Ethnopharmacol*, 2001. 77(1): p. 11-8.

[100] Girish, C., et al., Hepatoprotective activity of picroliv, curcumin and ellagic acid compared to silymarin on paracetamol induced liver toxicity in mice. *Fundam. Clin. Pharmacol*, 2009. 23(6): p. 735-45.

[101] Yen, F.L., et al., Nanoparticles formulation of Cuscuta chinensis prevents acetaminophen-induced hepatotoxicity in rats. *Food Chem. Toxicol*, 2008. 46(5): p. 1771-7.

[102] Wang, A.Y., et al., Gentiana manshurica Kitagawa prevents acetaminophen-induced acute hepatic injury in mice via inhibiting JNK/ERK MAPK pathway. *World J. Gastroenterol*, 2010. 16(3): p. 384-91.

[103] Yamada, S., Y. Murawaki, and H. Kawasaki, Preventive effect of gomisin A, a lignan component of shizandra fruits, on acetaminophen-induced hepatotoxicity in rats. *Biochem. Pharmacol*, 1993. 46(6): p. 1081-5.

[104] Yapar, K., et al., Hepatoprotective effect of L-carnitine against acute acetaminophen toxicity in mice. *Exp. Toxicol. Pathol*, 2007. 59(2): p. 121-8.

[105] Sener, G., A.O. Sehirli, and G. Ayanoglu-Dulger, Protective effects of melatonin, vitamin E and N-acetylcysteine against acetaminophen toxicity in mice: a comparative study. *J. Pineal. Res*, 2003. 35(1): p. 61-8.

[106] Shon, Y.H. and K.S. Nam, Protective effect of Moutan Cortex extract on acetaminophen-induced hepatotoxicity in mice. *J. Ethnopharmacol*, 2004. 90(2-3): p. 415-9.

[107] Ray, S.D., et al., Pre-exposure to a novel nutritional mixture containing a series of phytochemicals prevents acetaminophen-induced programmed and unprogrammed cell deaths by enhancing BCL-XL expression and minimizing oxidative stress in the liver. *Mol. Cell Biochem*, 2006. 293(1-2): p. 119-36.

[108] Devi, K.P., et al., Assessment of the protective potential of Premna tomentosa (L. Verbenaceae) extract on lipid profile and lipid-metabolizing enzymes in acetaminophen-intoxicated rats. *J. Altern. Complement. Med*, 2004. 10(3): p. 540-6.

[109] Ray, S.D., M.A. Kumar, and D. Bagchi, A novel proanthocyanidin IH636 grape seed extract increases in vivo Bcl-XL expression and prevents acetaminophen-induced programmed and unprogrammed cell death in mouse liver. *Arch. Biochem. Biophys*, 1999. 369(1): p. 42-58.

[110] Sharma, S., R.L. Singh, and P. Kakkar, Modulation of Bax/Bcl-2 and caspases by probiotics during acetaminophen induced apoptosis in primary hepatocytes. *Food Chem. Toxicol*, 2011. 49(4): p. 770-9.

[111] Sharma, S., et al., Probiotic Enterococcus lactis IITRHR1 protects against acetaminophen-induced hepatotoxicity. *Nutrition*, 2011.

[112] Ramachandran, V. and B. Raja, Protective effects of syringic acid against acetaminophen-induced hepatic damage in albino rats. *J. Basic Clin. Physiol. Pharmacol*, 2010. 21(4): p. 369-85.

[113] Balaji Raghavendra Rao, H., A. Sathivel, and T. Devaki, Antihepatotoxic nature of Ulva reticulata (Chlorophyceae) on acetaminophen-induced hepatoxicity in experimental rats. *J. Med. Food*, 2004. 7(4): p. 495-7.

In: Acetaminophen: Properties, Clinical Uses
Editors: Atash Javaherian and Pasha Latifpour
ISBN: 978-1-61942-374-9

Chapter 7

SESAME OIL AND SESAMOL AS THERAPEUTIC AGENTS AGAINST ACETAMINOPHEN-INDUCED ACUTE LIVER INJURY

Victor Raj Mohan Chandrasekaran and Ming-Yie Liu*
Department of Environmental and Occupational Health, National Cheng Kung University, College of Medicine, 138 Sheng-Li Road, Tainan 70428, Taiwan

ABSTRACT

Acetaminophen is an analgesic and antipyretic. It is safe when taken as directed but can cause extreme harm and even death in amounts above recommended doses. N-acetylcysteine is the standard clinical antidote for treating overdoses of acetaminophen. However, the optimal dose, route, and duration of N-acetylcysteine therapy remain unknown despite more than 30 years of experience with this antidote. The search for a novel and effective antidote for acetaminophen overdose continues. Sesame oil has been widely used in Chinese and Indian herbal medicine. Sesame oil and its lignan sesamol have been proved effective for treating various drug-induced and chemically induced liver injuries. Sesame oil and sesamol not only maintain glutathione levels but also reduce mitochondrial oxidative stress by inhibiting the generation of reactive oxygen species during acetaminophen intoxication. Sesame oil and sesamol's multi-beneficial actions may be useful for treating acetaminophen-overdose-associated liver injuries.

DRUG-INDUCED LIVER INJURY

The liver is vital for the bodily disposition of drugs. Because of its strategic location as the delta of the portal blood stream, it is massively exposed to drugs and other foreign compounds absorbed through the intestine [1]. Drug-induced liver injury (DILI) is broadly classified into intrinsic and idiosyncratic types; intrinsic DILI is generally dose-dependent and predictable (e.g., acetaminophen toxicity), whereas idiosyncratic DILI is unpredictable

* myliu@mail.ncku.edu.tw

and does not depend directly on dose [2]. Patients with DILI have a wide variety of clinical presentations. Clinically, biochemically, and histologically, DILI can simulate almost all forms of acute and chronic liver injuries. Thus, patients with DILI can present with acute liver failure with severe encephalopathy, with acute hepatitis with or without jaundice, and with chronic hepatitis with both symptomatic and asymptomatic elevated liver tests [3]. Several different drugs have been associated with liver injury [4]. Antibiotics, different analgesics, and non-steroidal anti-inflammatory drugs are the most common type of drugs associated with DILI [5-8].

ACETAMINOPHEN

Acetaminophen (also called paracetamol (N-(4-hydroxyphenyl)-acetamide)) is a commonly used effective analgesic and antipyretic agent, which is available as an over-the-counter medication. Acetaminophen is considered safe at therapeutic doses, but higher doses may cause acute liver failure and even death, which is a major problem in countries such as the United States, the United Kingdom, Denmark, Australia, and Taiwan [9-13]. According to poison centers in the United States, acetaminophen poisoning was responsible for more than 70,000 visits to health care facilities and about 300 deaths in 2005 [14]. Acetaminophen poisoning can be caused by a single overdose (usually as an attempt at self-harm), or by repeated excessive doses or too-frequent standard doses, with therapeutic intent. Repeated supratherapeutic doses are increasingly recognized as a significant clinical problem [11, 15]. Regardless of whether acetaminophen poisoning occurs because of a single overdose or after repeated supratherapeutic ingestion, its progression can be categorized into four stages: preclinical toxic effects (a normal serum alanine aminotransferase concentration), hepatic injury (an elevated alanine aminotransferase concentration), hepatic failure (hepatic injury with hepatic encephalopathy), and recovery. This categorization is useful because each stage has a different prognosis and is managed differently. Transient liver injury may develop in patients who are treated during the preclinical stage, but they recover fully [11, 15-17]. Patients who are not treated until hepatic injury has developed have a variable prognosis, and patients who present with hepatic failure have a mortality rate of 20% to 40% [11, 15, 18].

ACETAMINOPHEN METABOLISM AND TOXICITY

When taken in therapeutic doses, acetaminophen is safely metabolized and excreted by glucuronidation and sulfation reactions [19]. However, when taken in toxic doses, acetaminophen is metabolized by the cytochrome P450 enzyme system into the highly electrophilic N-acetyl-p-benzoquinoneimine (NAPQI) [20]. NAPQI is extremely toxic to the liver, possibly because of its covalent binding to proteins and nucleic acids [21]. However, NAPQI is rapidly detoxified by interaction with glutathione to form cysteine and mercapturic acid conjugates [22]. As long as sufficient glutathione is present, the liver is protected from injury. Overdoses of acetaminophen (either a single large ingestion or repeated supratherapeutic ingestion) deplete hepatic glutathione stores and cause liver injury [23]. Metabolic activation of acetaminophen results in the generation of reactive oxygen species, which leads to oxidative stress and liver damage [24, 25]. Because acetaminophen toxicity depletes glutathione [26], the major peroxide detoxification system is predictably inhibited. Thus, an increase in the generation of superoxide, which is formed by several enzymatic reactions, including acetaminophen oxidation to NAPQI, may lead to an increase in hydrogen peroxide and to the initiation of oxidative stress via the Fenton mechanism. Excess hydrogen peroxide and ferrous ions react and form the hydroxyl radical, a potent oxidant that may oxidize lipids, which then causes lipid peroxidation [27-30]. It has been proposed [31] that mitochondria are the primary target of reactive metabolite. Oxidative stress and mitochondrial oxidative damage have been implicated in the etiology of numerous common diseases. The development of various mitochondrial dysfunctions has been observed with acetaminophen toxicity, including the inhibition of respiration, the downregulation of hepatic ATP levels and membrane potential, and the loss of mitochondrial calcium ions [32-35].

Acetaminophen and N-Acetylcysteine

In the late 1960s, physicians recognized that an acute acetaminophen overdose caused a dose-related liver injury and that, without treatment, many patients died [36]. Animal studies describing the metabolism of acetaminophen to NAPQI [22, 37] have shown that the prolonged presence of hepatic glutathione prevented cytotoxicity. Thereafter, reports [38, 39] showed that methionine and cysteamine prevent acetaminophen-induced hepatic injury. The use of these agents resulted in dramatic increases in survival, but their side effects led researchers to seek alternative treatments. N-Acetylcysteine was first suggested as an antidote for acetaminophen toxicity in 1974 [40]. Intravenous N-acetylcysteine was efficacious after a 20-hour regimen, but oral N-acetylcysteine was efficacious only after a 72-hour regimen. N-acetylcysteine has an unpleasant odor and taste, and vomiting is common with the oral form of the drug. The intravenous form also has some adverse effects. Hence, the duration of treatment and side effects spurred researchers to seek an alternative agent for acetaminophen-induced acute hepatic injury.

Sesame Oil

Description

Sesame oil is derived from the plant species *Sesamum indicum* L. and belong with Pedaliaceae family [41]. Sesame has been used for millennia in Chinese and Indian herbal medicine. Although often recommended as a laxative, sesame was used as early as the 4th century A.D. as a Chinese folk remedy for toothache and gum disease. In modern times, sesame has been embraced by Western herbalists for a variety of therapeutic purposes. The oil is also used in cooking and as an ingredient in margarine and salad dressings as well as in certain cosmetics and skin softening products. Native to Asia and Africa, sesame is primarily cultivated in India, China, Africa, and Latin America. Only the seeds and oil of the sesame plant are used for medicinal purposes. Sesame oil consists of olein, stearin, palmitin, myristin, linolein, sesamin, and sesamolin [42].

Beneficial effects of Sesame Oil

Sesame oil is effective against various diseases, including atherosclerosis, hypertension, and the effects of aging [43-45]. Along with sesaminol, which is the principle antioxidant component in sesame oil [46], the lignans in the oil contributes its antioxidant and anti-mutagenic properties [47, 48]. Sesame oil contains phenol, sesamin, sesamol, and sesamolin and a relatively small amount of tocopherol, which contributes to its superior oxidative stability [49]. Sesame oil is a better antioxidant than canola oil [50]. Compared with other dietary oils, such as those from ground nuts and sunflower seeds, sesame oil offers better protection against increased blood pressure, hyperlipidemia, and lipid peroxidation by increasing enzymatic and non-enzymatic antioxidants [51]. Sesame oil and its active ingredient sesamol are stronger antitumor agents than are resveratrol and sunflower seed oil [52]. Sesamol is one of the nonfat antioxidants in sesame oil [53]. It is effective against drug-induced and chemically induced organ injuries [54, 55]. Sesamol is anti-photo-oxidative because it scavenges singlet oxygen [56]. It inhibits lipid peroxidation, hydroxyl radical-induced deoxyribose degradation, and DNA cleavage [57]; it attenuates the production of nitric oxide and hydrogen peroxide; and it reduces monoamine oxidase activity in glial astrocytes [58].

Sesame Oil and Sesamol protect against Acetaminophen-induced Liver Injury

Sesame oil significantly attenuates acetaminophen-induced acute hepatic injury. It maintains the glutathione level and hepatic architecture and scavenges oxygen-free radicals in hepatic tissue injured by acetaminophen-induced oxidative stress [29]. Sesame oil does not alter the concentration of acetaminophen in serum, which shows that the huge oil load on the stomach in acetaminophen-overdosed rats does not affect the absorption of acetaminophen. Sesamol is water-soluble and has the same active constituents as natural sesame seed oil. It is a potent anti-inflammatory agent during lipopolysaccharide intoxication [59]. It is also active against various drugs and chemically induced organ injuries [59, 60]. It maintains glutathione levels and protects against acetaminophen-induced liver injury in rats [30]. It protects the liver by maintaining mitochondrial aconitase activity and inhibiting iron and hydrogen peroxide levels in the Haber-Weiss and Fenton reactions in acetaminophen-overdosed rats [30]. Acetaminophen-induced acute hepatic injury or failure that requires liver transplantation is a major concern in developing and developed countries [61, 62]. It is important to provide an alternative to reduce the incidence of liver transplantation after acetaminophen-induced acute hepatic injury or failure. Thus, sesame oil's and sesamol's protection against acetaminophen-induced liver damage [29, 30, 63, 64] suggests its high therapeutic value.

SUMMARY

In sesame's long history as a crop and oil, no harmful effects of sesame seed extracts have been reported. Sesame oil and sesamol show no observable adverse effects when treating acetaminophen intoxication in rats. Sesame oil's and sesamol's multi-actions may be important in treating acetaminophen-overdosed patients. However, their efficacies in humans are yet to be tested.

REFERENCES

[1] McLean, A. J.; Morgan, D. J. Clinical pharmacokinetics in patients with liver disease. *Clin. Pharmacokinet.* 1991, *21,* 42–69.

[2] Chalasani, N.; Björnsson, E. Risk factors for idiosyncratic drug-induced liver injury. *Gastroenterology* 2010, *138,* 2246–2259.

[3] Björnsson, E. Review article: drug-induced liver injury in clinical practice. *Aliment. Pharmacol. Ther.* 2010, *32,* 3–13.

[4] Zimmerman, H. *Hepatotoxicity: the adverse effects of drugs and other chemicals on the liver;* Lippincott, Williams & Wilkins: Philadelphia: 1999.

[5] Fontana, R. J.; Watkins, P. B.; Bonkovsky, H. L.; Chalasani, N.; Davern, T.; Serrano, J.; Rochon, J.; DILIN Study Group. Drug-Induced Liver Injury Network (DILIN) prospective study: rationale, design and conduct. *Drug Saf.* 2009, *32,* 55–68.

[6] Lammert, C.; Einarsson, S.; Saha, C.; Niklasson, A.; Björnsson, E.; Chalasani, N. Relationship between daily dose of oral medications and idiosyncratic drug-induced liver injury: search for signals. *Hepatology* 2008, *47,* 2003–2009.

[7] De Valle, M. B.; Av Klinteberg, V.; Alem, N.; Olsson, R.; Björnsson, E. Drug-induced liver injury in a Swedish University hospital out-patient hepatology clinic. *Aliment. Pharmacol. Ther.* 2006, *24,* 1187–1195.

[8] Larrey, D. Epidemiology and individual susceptibility to adverse drug reactions affecting the liver. *Semin. Liver Dis.* 2002, *22,* 145–155.

[9] Ott, P.; Dalhoff, K.; Hansen, P. B.; Loft, S.; Poulsen, H. E. Consumption, overdose and death from analgesics during a period of over-the-counter availability of paracetamol in Denmark. *J. Intern. Med.* 1990, *227,* 423–428.

[10] Hawton, K.; Fagg, J. Trends in deliberate self-poisoning and self-injury in Oxford, 1976–90. *Br. Med. J.* 1992, *304,* 1409–1411.

[11] Schiodt, F.V.; Rochling, F. A.; Casey, D. L.; Lee, W. M. Acetaminophen toxicity in an urban county hospital. *N. Engl. J. Med.* 1997, *337,* 1112–1117.

[12] Gow, P. J.; Smallwood, R. A.; Angus, P. W. Paracetamol overdose in a liver transplantation centre: An 8-year experience. *J. Gastroenterol. Hepatol.* 1999, *14,* 817–821.

[13] Tsai, C. L.; Chang, W. T.; Weng, T. I.; Fang, C. C.; Walson, P. D. A patient-tailored N-acetylcysteine protocol for acute acetaminophen intoxication. *Clin. Ther.* 2005, *27,* 336–341.

[14] Lai, M. W.; Klein-Schwartz, W.; Rodgers, G. C.; Abrams, J. Y.; Haber, D. A.; Bronstein, A. C.; Wruk, K. M. 2005 Annual report of the American Association of Poison Control Centers' national poisoning and exposure database. *Clin. Toxicol (Phila).* 2006, *44,* 803–932.

[15] Daly, F. F.; O'Malley, G. F.; Heard, K.; Bogdan, G. M.; Dart, R. C. Prospective evaluation of repeated supratherapeutic acetaminophen (paracetamol) ingestion. *Ann. Emerg. Med.* 2004, *4,* 393–398.
[16] Trey, C.; Davidson, C. S. In *Progress in Liver disease;* Popper, H., Schaffner, F., Eds.; The management of fulminant hepatic failure; Grune & Stratton: New York (NY), 1970, Vol. 3, pp 282–298.
[17] Smilkstein, M. J.; Knapp, G. L.; Kulig, K. W.; Rumack, B. H. Efficacy of oral N-acetylcysteine in the treatment of acetaminophen overdose: analysis of the national multicenter study (1976 to 1985). *N. Engl. J. Med.* 1988, *319,* 1557–1562.
[18] Makin, A. J.; Wendon, J.; Williams, R. A 7-year experience of severe acetaminophen-induced hepatotoxicity (1987-1993). *Gastroenterology* 1995, *109,* 1907–1916.
[19] Farrell, G. In *Drug-Induced Liver Diseases;* Farrell, G., Ed.; Paracetamol-induced hepatotoxicity; Churchill Livingstone: New York (NY), 1994, pp 205–224.
[20] Jollow, D. J.; Thorgeirsson, S. S.; Potter, W. Z.; Hashimoto, M.; Mitchell, J. R. Acetaminophen-induced hepatic necrosis. VI. Metabolic disposition of toxic and non-toxic doses of acetaminophen. *Pharmacology* 1974, *12,* 251–271.
[21] Jollow, D. J.; Mitchell, J. R.; Potter, W. Z.; Davis, D. C.; Gillette, J. R.; Brodie, B. B. Acetaminophen-induced hepatic necrosis. II. Role of covalent binding *in vivo. J. Pharmacol. Exp. Ther.* 1973, *187,* 195–202.
[22] Mitchell, J. R.; Jollow, D. J.; Potter, W. Z.; Gillette, J. R.; Brodie, B. B. Acetaminophen-induced hepatic necrosis. IV. Protective role of glutathione. *J. Pharmacol. Exp. Ther.* 1973, *187,* 211–217.
[23] Potter, W. Z.; Thorgeirsson, S. S.; Jollow, D. J.; Mitchell, J. R. Acetaminophen-induced hepatic necrosis. V. Correlation of hepatic necrosis, covalent binding and glutathione depletion in hamsters. *Pharmacology* 1974, *12,* 129–143.
[24] Adamson, G. M.; Harman, A. W. Oxidative stress in cultured hepatocytes exposed to acetaminophen. *Biochem. Pharmacol.* 1993, *45,* 2289–2294.
[25] Kamiyama, T.; Sato, C.; Liu, J.; Tajiri, K.; Miyakawa, H.; Marumo, F. Role of lipid peroxidation in acetaminophen-induced hepatotoxicity: comparison with carbon tetrachloride. *Toxicol. Lett.* 1993, *66,* 7–12.
[26] Roberts, D. W.; Bucci, T. J.; Benson, R. W.; Warbritton, A. R.; McRae, T. A.; Pumford, N. R.; Hinson, J. A. Immunohistochemical localization and quantification of the 3-(cystein-S-yl)-acetaminophen protein adduct in acetaminophen hepatotoxicity. *Am. J. Pathol.* 1991, *138,* 359–371.
[27] Samokyszyn, V. M.; Thomas, C. E.; Reif, D. W.; Saito, M.; Aust, S. D. Release of iron from ferritin and its role in oxygen radical toxicities. *Drug Metab. Rev.* 1988, *19,* 283–303.
[28] Dai, Y.; Cederbaum, A. I. Cytotoxicity of acetaminophen in human cytochrome P4502E1-transfected HepG2 cells. *J. Pharmacol. Exp. Ther.* 1995, *273,* 1497–1505.
[29] Chandrasekaran, V. R.; Wan, C. H.; Liu, L. L.; Hsu, D. Z.; Liu, M. Y. Effect of sesame oil against acetaminophen-induced oxidative hepatic damage in rats. *Shock* 2008, *30,* 217–221.
[30] Chandrasekaran, V. R.; Hsu, D. Z.; Liu, M. Y. The protective effect of sesamol against mitochondrial oxidative stress and hepatic injury in acetaminophen-overdosed rats. *Shock* 2009, *32,* 89–93.

[31] Masubuchi, Y.; Suda, C.; Horie, T. Involvement of mitochondrial permeability transition in acetaminophen-induced liver injury in mice. *J. Hepatol.* 2005, *42,* 110–116.

[32] Moore, M.; Thor, H.; Moore, G.; Nelson, S.; Moldeus, P.; Orrenius, S. The toxicity of acetaminophen and N-acetyl-p-benzoquinone imine in isolated hepatocytes is associated with thiol depletion and increased Cytosolic Ca^{2+}. *J. Biol. Chem.* 1985, *260,* 13035–13040.

[33] Burcham, P. C.; Harman, A. W. Acetaminophen toxicity results in site-specific mitochondrial damage in isolated mouse hepatocytes. *J. Biol. Chem.* 1991, *266,* 5049–5054.

[34] Harman, A. W.; Kyle, M. E.; Serroni, A.; Farber, J. L. The killing of cultured hepatocytes by N-acetyl-p-benzoquinone imine (NAPQI) as a model of the cytotoxicity of acetaminophen. *Biochem. Pharmacol.* 1991, *41,* 1111–1117.

[35] Nazareth, W. M.; Sethi, J. K.; McLean, A. E. Effect of paracetamol on mitochondrial membrane function in rat liver slices. *Biochem. Pharmacol.* 1991, *42,* 931–936.

[36] Davidson, D. G.; Eastham, W. N. Acute liver necrosis following overdose of paracetamol. *Br. Med. J.* 1966, *2,* 497–499.

[37] Mitchell, J. R.; Jollow, D. J.; Potter, W. Z.; Gillette, J. R.; Brodie, B. B. Acetaminophen-induced hepatic necrosis. IV. Protective role of glutathione. *J. Pharmacol. Exp. Ther.* 1973, *187,* 211–217.

[38] Prescott, L. F.; Newton, R. W.; Swainson, C. P.; Wright, N.; Forrest, A. R.; Matthew, H. Successful treatment of severe paracetamol overdosage with cysteamine. *Lancet* 1974, *1,* 588–592.

[39] Prescott, L. F.; Sutherland, G. R.; Park, J.; Smith, I. J.; Proudfoot, A. T. Cysteamine, methionine, and penicillamine in the treatment of paracetamol poisoning. *Lancet* 1976, *2,* 109–113.

[40] Heard, K. J. Acetylcysteine for acetaminophen poisoning. *N. Engl. J. Med.* 2008, *359,* 285–292.

[41] Sugano, M.; Akimoto, K. A. Multifunctional gift from nature. *J. Chin. Nutr. Soc.* 1993, *18,* 1–11.

[42] Simon, J. E.; Chadwick, A. F.; Craker, L. E. In *Herbs: An Indexed Bibliography, 1971-1980. The Scientific Literature on Selected Herbs, and Aromatic and Medicinal Plants of the Temperate Zone;* Archon Books: Hamden (CT), 1984. Available at: http://www.hort.purdue.edu/newcrop/med-aro/factsheets/SESAME.html. Accessed October 11, 2011.

[43] Fukuda, Y.; Osawa, T.; Namiki, M.; Ozaki, T. Studies on antioxidative substances in sesame seed. *Agric. Biol. Chem.* 1985, *49,* 301–306.

[44] Fukuda, Y.; Osawa, T.; Namiki, M. In *Food Phytochemicals for Cancer Prevention II: Teas, Spices and Herbs;* Ho, C. T., Osawa, T., Huang, M. T., Rosen, R. T., Eds.; A.C.S. Symposium Series: 1994, Vol. 547, pp 264–274.

[45] Namiki, M. The chemistry and physiological function of sesame. *Food Rev. Int.* 1995, *11,* 281–329.

[46] Osawa, T.; Kumon, H.; Namiki, M.; Kawakishi, S.; Fukuda, Y. Antimutagenic heat stable anti-oxidants. *Prog. Clin. Biol. Res.* 1990, *342,* 223–238.

[47] Kang, M. H.; Katsuzaki, H.; Osawa, T. Inhibition of 2,2′-azinobis(2,4-dimethylvaleronitrile)-induced lipid peroxidation by sesaminols. *Lipids* 1998, *33,* 1031–1036.

[48] Kang, M. H.; Naito, M.; Tsujiohara, N.; Osawa, T. Sesamolin inhibits lipid peroxidation in rat liver and kidney. *J. Nutr.* 1998, *S128,* 1018–1022.

[49] White, J. P. *Fatty acids in oil seeds. Fatty Acids in Foods and Their Health Applications;* Dekker M. Incorporated: New York (NY), 1992, pp 237–262.

[50] Baba, N. H.; Antoniades, K.; Habbal, Z. Effects of dietary canola, olive, and linolenic acid enriched olive oils on plasma lipids, lipid peroxidation and lipoprotein lipase activity in rats. *Nutr. Res.* 1998, *49,* 41–45.

[51] Sankar, D.; Sambandam, G.; Ramakrishna Rao, M.; Pugalendi, K. V. Modulation of blood pressure, lipid profiles and redox status in hypertensive patients taking different edible oils. *Clin. Chim. Acta* 2005, *355,* 97–104.

[52] Kapadia, G. J.; Azuine, M. A.; Tokuda, H.; Takasaki, M.; Mukainaka, T.; Konoshima, T.; Nishino, H. Chemopreventive effect of resveratrol, sesamol, sesame oil and sunflower oil in the Epstein–Barr virus early antigen activation assay and the mouse skin two-stage carcinogenesis. *Pharmacol. Res.* 2002, *45,* 499–504.

[53] Fukuda, Y. Food chemical studies on the antioxidants in sesame seed. *Nippon Shokuhin Kogyo Gakkaishi* 1990, *37,* 484–492.

[54] Hsu, D. Z.; Li, Y. H.; Chu, P. Y.; Chien, S. P.; Chuang, Y. C.; Liu, M. Y. Attenuation of endotoxin-induced oxidative stress and multiple organ injury by 3,4-Methylenedioxyphenol in rats. *Shock* 2006, *25,* 300–305.

[55] Hsu, D. Z.; Chien, S. P.; Chen, K. T.; Liu, M. Y. The effect of sesamol on systemic oxidative stress and hepatic dysfunction in acutely iron-intoxicated mice. *Shock* 2007, *28,* 596–601.

[56] Kim, J. Y.; Choi, D. S.; Jung, M. Y. Antiphoto-oxidative activity of sesamol in methyleneblue-and chlorophyll-sensitized photo-oxidation of oil. *J. Agric. Food Chem.* 2003, *51,* 3460–3465.

[57] Joshi, R.; Kumar, M. S.; Satyamoorthy, K.; Unnikrisnan, M. K.; Mukherjee, T. Free radical reactions and antioxidant activities of sesamol: pulse radiolytic and biochemical studies. *J. Agric. Food Chem.* 2005, *53,* 2696–2703.

[58] Mazzio, E. A.; Harris, N.; Soliman, K. F. Food constituents attenuate monoamine oxidase activity and peroxide levels in C6 astrocyte cells. *Planta Med.* 1998, *64,* 603–606.

[59] Hsu, D. Z.; Chu, P. Y.; Liu, M. Y. The non-peptide chemical 3,4-methylenedioxyphenol blocked lipopolysaccharide (LPS) from binding to LPS-binding protein and inhibited pro-inflammatory cytokines. *Innate Immun.* 2009, *15,* 380–385.

[60] Hsu, D. Z.; Wan, C. H.; Hsu, H. F.; Lin, Y. M.; Liu, M. Y. The prophylactic protective effect of sesamol against ferric-nitrilotriacetate-induced acute renal injury in mice. *Food Chem. Toxicol.* 2008, *46,* 2736–2741.

[61] Litovitz, T. L.; Klein-Schwartz, W.; White, S.; Cobaugh, D. J.; Youniss, J.; Drab, A.; Benson, B. E. 1999 annual report of the American Association of Poison Control Centers Toxic Exposure Surveillance System. *Am. J. Emerg. Med.* 2000, *18,* 517–574.

[62] Larson, A. M. Acetaminophen hepatotoxicity. *Clin. Liver Dis.* 2007, *11,* 525–548.

[63] Chandrasekaran, V. R.; Chien, S. P.; Hsu, D. Z.; Chang, Y. C.; Liu, M. Y. Effects of sesame oil against after the onset of acetaminophen-induced acute hepatic injury in rats. *J. Parenter. Enteral. Nutr.* 2010, *34,* 567–573.

[64] Chandrasekaran, V. R.; Chien, S. P.; Hsu, D. Z.; Liu, M. Y. Anti-hepatotoxic effects of 3,4-methylenedioxyphenol and *N*-acetylcysteine in acutely acetaminophen-overdosed mice. *Hum. Exp. Toxicol.* 2011, *30,* 1609–1615.

In: Acetaminophen: Properties, Clinical Uses
Editors: Atash Javaherian and Pasha Latifpour
ISBN: 978-1-61942-374-9

Chapter 8

PARACETAMOL USE IN THE ELDERLY

Gisèle Pickering*

Clinical Pharmacology Centre, University Hospital, Clermont-Ferrand, France and INSERM U766, Pharmacology Department, Faculty of Medicine, University Hospital, Clermont-Ferrand, France

ABSTRACT

Paracetamol is an effective agent for pain relief and is generally regarded as a safe medication at therapeutic doses. It is widely used in elderly patients with recommendations that are common to those for adults. Recent reports have however questioned the safety of recommended doses and suggest that the elderly patient might be at an increased risk of developing adverse events when on paracetamol treatment. Glutathione depletion, polymedication including CYP450 inducing drugs and anticoagulant therapy, increased incidence of organ insufficiency with age, malnutrition, dehydration, fragility are factors that may favour the development of serious adverse events. While the benefit/risk ratio of paracetamol is evident in clinical practise, clinicians should be aware of the potential and preventable adverse side-effects of this centenarian pain treatment favourite analgesic.

Keywords*:* Pain, aging, acetaminophen, France

INTRODUCTION

Paracetamol is one of the most widely prescribed and used drugs for the treatment of pain and fever and is generally regarded as a safe medication at therapeutic doses. Although it has been used for the past century, its mechanism of action is just starting to be more clearly defined, and paracetamol appears to produce analgesia through a central rather than a

---

* Correspondence: Gisèle Pickering, Clinical Pharmacology Centre, Bâtiment 3C, CHU, Hopital G Montpied, 63001 Clermont-Ferrand cedex, France. Tel: 33(0)4 73 17 84 10; Fax 33(0)4 73 17 84 12; Email :gisele.pickering@u-clermont1.fr

peripheral mechanism (1,2). In recommended doses (1g three to four times daily) its efficacy, safety, availability and low cost justify its worldwide use for pain treatment. Adverse effects are rare, with hepatotoxicity the principle safety concern. Paracetamol is widely used in the elderly, mainly because of the high prevalence of joint pathologies but elderly age per se is not considered to be a risk factor of developing hepatotoxicity. Recent reports have however questioned the safety of recommended doses (3,4) and of the chronic use of paracetamol: in the light of these studies, we look at how the elderly patient might be at risk of developing adverse events when on paracetamol treatment.

Efficacy and Prescribing of Paracetamol in the Elderly

Paracetamol is an effective agent for pain relief due to osteoarthritis as can be seen from a large meta-analysis focused on paracetamol use in osteoarthritis, by far the commonest chronic pain pathology of the elderly (5). Non-steroidal anti-inflammatory (NSAIDs) drugs display a higher efficacy score than paracetamol, especially as regards stiffness which is very disabling in the elderly population, but weighed against the good safety record of paracetamol, the latter is recommended as the first line oral analgesic in the management of osteoarthritis. Consumption and potential dangers of acetaminophen in elderly patients are however poorly documented in the literature and are shadowed by the prescription of NSAIDs and opiates because of their high risk of side-effects. There is a tendency in outpatient settings to use NSAIDs more frequently and opioids less so than younger patients, and a study on more than 7000 nursing home elderly patients showed that 28.8% and 17.3% use NSAIDs and opiates respectively, with only 3,7% using paracetamol (6). Addition of paracetamol to NSAIDs reduces opioid consumption and improves pain relief during the early post-surgery period (7), and intravenous acetaminophen, 1 g, administered over a 24-h period in patients with moderate to severe pain after orthopedic surgery, provides rapid and effective analgesia and is well tolerated (8). Paracetamol is commonly prescribed in elderly patients without risk factors at the recommended dose of 500-1000mg every 4-6 hours to a maximum of 4000 mg daily. There are, to our knowledge, no studies in very old patients or in fragile elderly patients, and most clinical studies refer to “young older” people around 65 years. Patients at risk of hepatotoxicity may be found in this group of old, very old and fragile patients, and there are no real guidelines for at risk patients when dose modifications of paracetamol have to be envisaged. Officially, an increased risk of hepatotoxicity concerns several patient groups: first, patients with depleted glutathione stores, associated usually with malnutrition or prolonged fasting or underweight. Secondly, patients with hepatic, renal or cardiac impairment, dehydration. Thirdly, patients taking CYP-450 enzymes inducing drugs. It is obvious that the elderly patient fits in well with these three risk factors as will be exposed below.

Pharmacology and Toxicity of Paracetamol

Liver is typically and by far the most involved organ in paracetamol metabolism and acute toxicity. Following absorption, 90% of paracetamol normally undergoes hepatic glucuronide (40–67%) and sulphate (20–46%) conjugation to form inactive, harmless metabolites, which are eliminated in urine. 5 to 15% of paracetamol is oxidized by the CYP-450 oxidase system (CYP2E1,CYP1A2, CYP3A4, and CYP2A6), resulting in the formation of N-acetyl-p-benzoquinoneimine (NAPQI). Glutathione combines with NAPQI and the resulting complex is converted to non-toxic cysteine or mercaptate conjugates, which are eliminated in urine. With appropriate paracetamol dosing, glutathione supply far exceeds that which is required to detoxify NAPQI. After paracetamol overdose glutathione stores are depleted below a critical value (about 30% of normal stores). NAPQI covalently binds cell proteins, inducing a series of events that may result in cell death with possible DNA fragmentation and mitochondrial injury. Fatal liver damage occurs unless sulphydryl replacement therapy is given, usually in the form of N-acetyl cysteine, but transplantation may be necessary in patients with a poor prognosis. Over the past 15 years especially in Europe and in the USA, paracetamol has become the most important cause of liver failure, and intentional overdoses (more than 10g a day in one administration) have been for a number of years the cause of paracetamol-related hepatotoxicity and liver failure, accounting for a high number of emergency room visits, hospital admissions and deaths. More recently however, unintentional overdoses have overridden intentional overdoses (with doses as low as 7g a day), and the safety of paracetamol has been under considerable debate by the US Food and Drug Administration (3), focusing on legal restriction in the availability of paracetamol. But a review concluded that no change was needed in how the drug was sold (9). There are however a number of issues about the safety of paracetamol at therapeutic doses.

Are Therapeutic Doses of Paracetamol Safe in the Elderly?

A number of studies have shown that therapeutic doses of paracetamol might be associated with increased concentrations of transaminases and with liver injury, especially in the context of a clinical onset of liver injury (viral hepatitis (10) or antitubercular drug (9). A recent study (11) showed that healthy volunteers with 4g paracetamol daily had concentrations of alanine aminotransferase that were more than three times over the normal upper limit while the placebo group had a normal hepatic profile ($p<0.001$). This questioning study should be repeated on a larger scale in healthy volunteers to be confirmed, and there are today no such studies in elderly persons.

At normal doses of paracetamol, only trace amounts of NAPQI are formed, which is bound and inactivated by glutathione. Excess doses are known to deplete glutathione stores and NAPQI binds covalently to hepatocyte proteins and leads to cell death. Depleted glutathione stores may however occur outside paracetamol overdoses, as in fasting (12), poor nutritional status or alcoholism (13). Animal studies have shown that a 24-h fasting period depletes hepatic glutathione stores (14) and that these begin to decline at therapeutic levels of paracetamol at doses of 0.5 to 3 g (15). A case of paracetamol-induced hepatotoxicity is described in a study (12) after intake of paracetamol at a recommended dosage in a severely malnourished woman. The absence of hepatotoxicity in the same patient after a re-challenge at a lower dose a few months later led the authors to conclude that this phenomenon may be dose-related rather than idiosyncratic. Other studies report hepatotoxicity with chronic paracetamol intake at therapeutic doses, and suggest that this could be due to an idiosyncratic (with hypersensitivity/allergy) or non idiosyncratic origin (associated with malnutrition and fasting). A clinical trial in healthy young volunteers showed a significant reduction in serum 'total' antioxidant capacity when paracetamol is taken in therapeutic doses (1 g four times a day) for 14 days, and the authors conclude that reduction in glutathione is probably associated with chronic ingestion of maximum therapeutic doses of paracetamol. (16). Several studies report changes of antioxidant status in ageing, with a diminution of glutathione stores with age and a correlation between age reduced/oxidised glutathione ratio (17). Also, comparing gene expression in young and older rats, glutathione transferase is lower in older rats, suggesting that detoxification is less with age (18).Concerning the elderly patient, drug intake is known to influence nutritional status, and inversely (19). This applies also to paracetamol, considered generally as one of the most secure drugs for pain treatment. This corpus of clinical reports suggests that paracetamol administration should be carefully implemented in fasting patients and that nutritional status should be fully assessed, especially in suspected underweight and malnourished elderly patients.

Cytochrome CYP3A13 plays a role in hepatotoxicity linked to paracetamol, and cytochrome CYP3A13 has been shown to be higher with age, suggesting that paracetamol metabolites production is also higher with age. Humans tend to show interindividual variations in P450-catalyzed reactions of drugs and chemicals, which have been associated with different susceptibilities of humans to toxicological and pharmacological products, and a number of genetic polymorphisms have been described for the human CYP2E1 gene (20). Use of cytochrome P450 enzyme-inducing drugs (isoniazide, carbamazepine…) increases the risk of hepatotoxicity when associated with a wide range of paracetamol doses including therapeutic doses. Drug consumption in the elderly is very high, with elderly patients being administered not infrequently with more than ten drugs a day, leading to an increased risk of side-effects (19).

Recommended doses for the elderly are similar to recommendations for adults, including caution in the use of paracetamol in the case of hepatic, renal, cardiac insufficiency and dehydration. These pathologies affect more often the elderly and the very elderly than the younger population. Available studies in patients with chronic liver disease are somewhat discordant: some have shown that even if the half-life of acetaminophen may be prolonged, cytochrome P-450 activity is not increased and glutathione stores are not depleted to critical levels in those taking recommended doses. Furthermore, acetaminophen has been studied in a variety of liver diseases without evidence of increased risk of hepatotoxicity at currently recommended doses (21). A study in patients with viral hepatitis has however shown that the risk of hepatotoxicity may be increased (10). Despite discordant studies, acetaminophen can be used safely in patients with liver disease and is a preferred analgesic/antipyretic because of the absence of platelet impairment, of gastrointestinal toxicity and of nephrotoxicity associated with NSAIDs (21).

Another reported adverse side-effect of paracetamol concerns its interaction with warfarin. The most plausible hypothesis to explain the in vivo interaction is that paracetamol (or its metabolites) interfere with enzymes involved in vitamin K-dependent coagulation factor synthesis (22). At the dosage of 4g daily, paracetamol potentiates the anticoagulant response produced by warfarin and increases the International Normalized Ratio (INR) by about one point, increasing the risk of warfarin-associated hemorrhage. Whether this interaction occurs when acetaminophen is taken in lower doses or is used sporadically requires further study. Warfarin is widely used for the prevention and treatment of venous and arterial thromboembolism, pathologies particularly associated with increased age. Clinicians should therefore be aware of this clinically significant and underestimated interaction especially in elderly patients (23), since both paracetamol and oral anticoagulants are increasingly used in clinical practice, especially in the post-operative period. As paracetamol is however still the safest analgesic to use in combination with oral anticoagulants, close monitoring of INR in patients receiving this drug combination must be recommended.

CONCLUSION

Tolerability of therapeutic doses of paracetamol is a major factor in the very wide use of the drug. The literature however reports a number of clinical cases or clinical trials where hepatotoxicity could occur with therapeutic doses of paracetamol. While the benefit/risk ratio of this drug remains very high compared to placebo or NSAIDs, clinicians should however be aware of 1- the potential risks of the diminished anti-oxydant capacity in the prescription of paracetamol in malnourished, underweight, dehydrated and ill elderly patients, 2- drug interactions with CYP450 inductors and warfarin, in order to avoid iatrogenic pathologies that are responsible for many hospital admissions in the geriatric population.

REFERENCES

[1] Bertolini A, Ferrari A, Ottani A, Guerzoni S, Tacchi R, Leone S. Paracetamol: new vistas of an old drug. CNS *Drug Rev* 2006;12(3-4):250-75.

[2] Pickering G, Loriot MA, Libert F, Eschalier A, Beaune P, Dubray C. Analgesic effect of acetaminophen in humans: first evidence of a central serotonergic mechanism. *Clin Pharmacol Ther* 2006;79(4):371-8.

[3] Ahmad SR. Safety of recommended doses of paracetamol. *Lancet* 2007;369(9560):462-3.

[4] Vitols S. Paracetamol hepatotoxicity at therapeutic doses. *J Intern Med* 2003;253(2):95-8.

[5] Zhang W, Jones A, Doherty M. Does paracetamol (acetaminophen) reduce the pain of osteoarthritis? A meta-analysis of randomised controlled trials. *Ann Rheum Dis* 2004;63(8):901-7.

[6] Federman AD, Litke A, Morrison RS. Association of age with analgesic use for back and joint disorders in outpatient settings. *Am J Geriatr Pharmacother* 2006;4(4):306-15.

[7] Legeby M, Sandelin K, Wickman M, Olofsson C. Analgesic efficacy of diclofenac in combination with morphine and paracetamol after mastectomy and immediate breast reconstruction. *Acta Anaesthesiol Scand* 2006;50(6):772.

[8] Sinatra RS, Jahr JS, Reynolds LW, Viscusi ER, Groudine SB, Payen-Champenois C. Efficacy and safety of single and repeated administration of 1 gram intravenous acetaminophen injection (paracetamol) for pain management after major orthopedic surgery. *Anesthesiology* 2005;102(4):822-31.

[9] Jalan R, Williams R, Bernuau J. Paracetamol: are therapeutic doses entirely safe? *Lancet* 2006;368(9554):2195-6.

[10] Yaghi C, Honein K, Boujaoude J, Slim R, Moucari R, Sayegh R. Influence of acetaminophen at therapeutic doses on surrogate markers of severity of acute viral hepatitis. *Gastroenterol Clin Biol* 2006;30(5):763-8.

[11] Watkins PB, Kaplowitz N, Slattery JT, Colonese CR, Colucci SV, Stewart PW, Harris SC. Aminotransferase elevations in healthy adults receiving 4 grams of acetaminophen daily: a randomized controlled trial. *JAMA* 2006;296(1):87-93.

[12] Kurtovic J, Riordan SM. Paracetamol-induced hepatotoxicity at recommended dosage. *J Intern Med* 2003;253(2):240-3.

[13] Zimmerman HJ, Maddrey WC. Acetaminophen (paracetamol) hepatotoxicity with regular intake of alcohol: analysis of instances of therapeutic misadventure. *Hepatology* 1995;22(3):767-73.

[14] Vogt BL, Richie JP. Fasting-induced depletion of glutathione in the aging mouse. *Biochem Pharmacol* 1993;46(2):257-63.

[15] Slattery JT, Wilson JM, Kalhorn TF, Nelson SD. Dose-dependent pharmacokinetics of acetaminophen: evidence of glutathione depletion in humans. *Clin Pharmacol Ther* 1987;41(4):413-8.

[16] Nuttall SL, Khan JN, Thorpe GH, Langford N, Kendall MJ. The impact of therapeutic doses of paracetamol on serum total antioxidant capacity. *J Clin Pharm Ther* 2003;28(4):289-94.

[17] Oztürk O, Gümüslü S. Changes in glucose-6-phosphate dehydrogenase, copper, zinc-superoxide dismutase and catalase activities, glutathione and its metabolizing enzymes, and lipid peroxidation in rat erythrocytes with age. *Exp Gerontol* 2004;39(2):211-6.

[18] Morishita K, Mizukawa Y, Kasahara T, Okuyama M, Takashima K, Toritsuka N, Miyagishima T, Nagao T, Urushidani T. Gene expression profile in liver of differing ages of rats after single oral administration of acetaminophen. *J Toxicol Sci* 2006;31(5):491-507.

[19] Pickering G. Frail elderly, nutritional status and drugs. *Arch Gerontol Geriatr* 2004;38(2):174-80.

[20] Cheung C, Yu AM, Ward JM, Krausz KW, Akiyama TE, Feigenbaum L, Gonzalez FJ. The cyp2e1-humanized transgenic mouse: role of cyp2e1 in acetaminophen hepatotoxicity. *Drug Metab Dispos* 2005;33(3):449-57.

[21] Benson GD, Koff RS, Tolman KG. The therapeutic use of acetaminophen in patients with liver disease. *Am J Ther* 2005;12(2):133-41.

[22] Parra D, Beckey NP, Stevens GR. The effect of acetaminophen on the international normalized ratio in patients stabilized on warfarin therapy. *Pharmacotherapy* 2007;27(5):675-83.

[23] Mahé I, Bertrand N, Drouet L, Bal Dit Sollier C, Simoneau G, Mazoyer E, Caulin C, Bergmann JF. Interaction between paracetamol and warfarin in patients: a double-blind, placebo-controlled, randomized study. *Haematologica* 2006;91(12):1621-7.

INDEX

B

C

D

E

H

L

M

N

O

P

Q

R

S

T

U

V

W

X

Y

Z